Key Clinical Topics in
Orthopaedic Trauma

Key Clinical Topics in Orthopaedic Trauma

Alex Trompeter BSc(Hons) MBBS FRCS(Tr&Orth)
Consultant Trauma and Orthopaedic Surgeon
St George's University Hospitals NHS Foundation Trust
London, UK

Piers Page MBBS MPhil MRCSEd
Orthopaedic Registrar
Royal Surrey County Hospital NHS Foundation Trust
Guildford, UK

Dominic Sprott MBBS MRCS FRCS(Tr&Orth)
Consultant Trauma and Orthopaedic Surgeon
Salford Royal NHS Foundation Trust
Salford, UK

Amir Qureshi MBBCh MRCS(Eng) FRCS(Tr&Orth)
Consultant Orthopaedic Surgeon
University Hospital Southampton NHS Foundation Trust
Southampton, UK

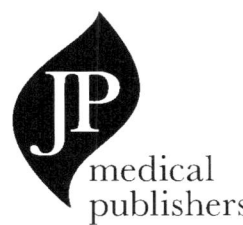

London • Panama City • New Delhi

© 2018 JP Medical Ltd.
Published by JP Medical Ltd,
83 Victoria Street, London, SW1H 0HW, UK
Tel: +44 (0)20 3170 8910   Fax: +44 (0)20 3008 6180
Email: info@jpmedpub.com   Web: www.jpmedpub.com

The rights of Alex Trompeter, Piers Page, Dominic Sprott and Amir Qureshi to be identified as the editors of this work have been asserted by them in accordance with the Copyright, Designs and Patents Act 1988.

All rights reserved. No part of this publication may be reproduced, stored or transmitted in any form or by any means, electronic, mechanical, photocopying, recording or otherwise, except as permitted by the UK Copyright, Designs and Patents Act 1988, without the prior permission in writing of the publishers. Permissions may be sought directly from JP Medical Ltd at the address printed above.

All brand names and product names used in this book are trade names, service marks, trademarks or registered trademarks of their respective owners. The publisher is not associated with any product or vendor mentioned in this book.

Medical knowledge and practice change constantly. This book is designed to provide accurate, authoritative information about the subject matter in question. However readers are advised to check the most current information available on procedures included and check information from the manufacturer of each product to be administered, to verify the recommended dose, formula, method and duration of administration, adverse effects and contraindications. It is the responsibility of the practitioner to take all appropriate safety precautions. Neither the publisher nor the editors assume any liability for any injury and/or damage to persons or property arising from or related to use of material in this book.

This book is sold on the understanding that the publisher is not engaged in providing professional medical services. If such advice or services are required, the services of a competent medical professional should be sought.

Every effort has been made where necessary to contact holders of copyright to obtain permission to reproduce copyright material. If any have been inadvertently overlooked, the publisher will be pleased to make the necessary arrangements at the first opportunity.

ISBN: 978-1-909836-43-3

British Library Cataloguing in Publication Data
A catalogue record for this book is available from the British Library

Library of Congress Cataloging in Publication Data
A catalog record for this book is available from the Library of Congress

Commissioning Editor:	Steffan Clements
Editorial Assistant:	Adam Rajah
Design:	Designers Collective Ltd

Preface

The day-to-day job of a junior doctor in orthopaedics and trauma can be daunting. During medical school, students rarely receive extensive teaching on trauma and orthopaedics; early placements in the orthopaedics department can therefore cause anxiety due to the range of conditions that may be encountered. Not knowing what will come in next when on call, the volume of cases in a busy fracture clinic and learning to perform procedures and operations all represent a significant challenge. Foundation and other doctors in their first years of practice may find their first surgical attachments are in orthopaedics, while surgical trainees in their later years should all expect to spend some time exposed to trauma. As they progress to their later years of specialist training, the questioning in the morning trauma meeting will inevitably fall to them with greater frequency.

Key Clinical Topics in Orthopaedic Trauma has been written to bridge the gap between qualification as a doctor and later years of orthopaedic specialty training. The 102 topics have been chosen on the basis of their clinical importance and the frequency with which they will be encountered in practice. By concentrating on the core knowledge required in these topics, the book provides a firm foundation and practical reference not just for junior doctors in the orthopaedic department and fracture clinic but also for trainee surgeons progressing through the middle years of their specialty training. Furthermore, the highly accessible writing style makes *Key Clinical Topics in Orthopaedic Trauma* ideal as a revision tool for the trauma element of the FRCS Tr&Orth (section 2) examination. Even though the book is written primarily for junior doctors and surgical trainees, we hope it will provide a helpful resource for those medical students and nurses seeking an overview of the principles of orthopaedic trauma in practice.

Imaging is necessarily a core tool in orthopaedic diagnosis, treatment and follow-up. Accordingly, numerous radiological images are included alongside clinical photographs to illustrate the appearance of topics discussed in the text. We also include diagrams to clarify anatomical structures and fracture classification systems. Finally, tables help to compare and summarise information while Further reading sections at the end of each topic point the reader towards useful sources of more detailed information.

We hope you will find *Key Clinical Topics in Orthopaedic Trauma* an invaluable guide to the subject, one which provides just the right amount of information on each condition or injury to enable readers to understand core principles and apply them in the everyday care of their patients.

Alex Trompeter
Piers Page
Dominic Sprott
Amir Qureshi
April 2018

Contents

		Page
Preface		v
Contributors		ix
Acknowledgements		xii
Dedication		xii
1	Amputations – mangled extremities and decision making	1
2	Amputations – prosthetics and rehabilitation	5
3	Ankle: Achilles tendon ruptures	8
4	Ankle: supination- and pronation-external rotation fractures	12
5	Ankle: supination-adduction and pronation-abduction fractures	17
6	Ankle: talar fractures	21
7	Bone grafts	25
8	Bone loss – options for reconstruction	29
9	Bone structure and physiology	32
10	Brachial plexus injury	38
11	Classification of fractures	42
12	Clavicle dislocations	46
13	Clavicle fractures	50
14	Compartment syndrome	53
15	Complex regional pain syndrome	57
16	Crush injuries and crush syndrome	61
17	Damage control orthopaedics and trauma physiology	64
18	Elbow – dislocations and associated fractures	67
19	Elbow – olecranon fractures	71
20	Elbow – radial head and neck fractures	74
21	Fat embolism and acute respiratory distress syndrome	77
22	Femoral fractures – distal	80
23	Femoral fractures – periprosthetic	83
24	Femoral fractures – shaft	88
25	Femoral fractures – subtrochanteric	92
26	Femoral neck fractures – extracapsular	96
27	Femoral neck fractures – intracapsular	100
28	Foot – calcaneal fractures	105
29	Foot – Lisfranc's fracture–dislocations	110
30	Foot – mid- and forefoot fractures	115

		Page
31	Foot – subtalar and Chopart's fracture–dislocations	120
32	Forearm – distal radial fractures	124
33	Forearm – Galeazzi's and Monteggia's fractures	128
34	Forearm – radius and ulna fractures	132
35	Fracture healing	136
36	Geriatric patients – perioperative management of hip fractures	138
37	Guidelines in trauma	142
38	Gunshot injuries	147
39	Hand and wrist – carpal dislocations	149
40	Hand and wrist – carpal fractures	153
41	Hand and wrist – metacarpal fractures	157
42	Hand and wrist – phalangeal fractures	163
43	Hand and wrist – scaphoid fractures	168
44	Hand and wrist – tendon ruptures	172
45	Head injury	177
46	Humeral fractures – distal	182
47	Humeral fractures – proximal	186
48	Imaging – description and interpretation	190
49	Imaging modalities	192
50	Implants – circular external fixators	195
51	Implants – monolateral external fixators	199
52	Implants – nails	202
53	Implants – plates	204
54	Implants – screws	206
55	Infection	209
56	Initial management of fractures	214
57	Knee – cruciate ligament injuries	217
58	Knee – extensor mechanism injury	221
59	Knee – meniscal injuries	225
60	Knee – patella fractures	228
61	Knee dislocations – multiligament injuries	232
62	Major trauma – Advanced Trauma and Life Support principles	235
63	Major trauma networks	239
64	Malunion and deformity correction	242
65	Multiple casualties	245
66	Nailbed injuries	250
67	Nonunion of fractures	254
68	Open fractures	258

		Page
69	Osteoporosis	261
70	Paediatric clavicle fractures	265
71	Paediatric distal tibial and ankle fractures	267
72	Paediatric femoral fractures	270
73	Paediatric forearm fractures	274
74	Paediatric fractures – nonaccidental injury	277
75	Paediatric humeral condylar fractures	280
76	Paediatric humeral fractures	284
77	Paediatric physeal fractures	286
78	Paediatric supracondylar humeral fractures	289
79	Paediatric tibial fractures	293
80	Pathological fractures	296
81	Pelvis – acetabular fractures	299
82	Pelvis – pelvic ring fractures	302
83	Peripheral nerve injury	305
84	Principles of nonoperative management of fractures	307
85	Principles of operative management of fractures	310
86	Resuscitation and massive transfusion	313
87	Septic arthritis – paediatric	316
88	Septic arthritis and crystal arthropathy – adult	319
89	Shoulder dislocations	321
90	Shoulder – scapula and glenoid fractures	324
91	Soft tissue coverage in trauma	326
92	Spine – atlas and axis cervical fractures and dislocations	329
93	Spine – cord injury	333
94	Spine – subaxial cervical fractures and dislocations	336
95	Spine – thoracic and lumbar fractures	339
96	Tibial pilon fractures	343
97	Tibial plateau fractures	347
98	Tibial shaft fractures	352
99	Trauma scoring systems	356
100	Trauma outcome scores: using patient-reported outcome measures	359
101	Triage	362
102	Whiplash	366
Index		369

Contributors

John Afolayan BSc(Hons) MBBS DPMSA MRCS
Topics 65, 66
Specialty Registrar, Surrey & Sussex Deanery, Kent, UK

Muhammad Ahsan MBBS MRCSEd
Topic 21
Clinical Fellow, Salford Royal Hospital Salford, UK

Gaurav S Batra MBBCh MRCS(Eng) PhD FRCS(Tr&Orth)
Topics 22, 23, 25
Consultant Orthopaedic Surgeon, Salford Royal Hospital, Salford, UK

Lucy Bailey BMBS MSc MRCS
Topics 26, 27, 37, 45
Specialty Trainee, North Hampshire Hospital Basingstoke, UK

Zine Beech MA(Cantab) MB BChir FRCS(Tr&Orth)
Topics 35, 38, 49
Specialty Trainee, Southampton General Hospital, Southampton, UK

Deepu Bhaskar MBBS MRCS DipSICOT MS(Ortho)
Topics 7, 8
Trauma and Orthopaedic Fellow, North Manchester General Hospital, Manchester, UK

Samer Bitar MD MRCSEd
Topics 1, 14
Senior Fellow, Trauma and Orthopaedic Surgery, Salford Royal Hospital, Salford, UK

Rob Boyd BM BSc MRCS FRCS
Topics 84, 85, 88
Post CCT Fellow, Royal Bournemouth General Hospital, Bournemouth, UK

John Dabis MBBS MRCS RCSEng FRCS(Tr&Orth)
Topics 70, 73, 74, 76
Knee Fellow, North Hampshire and Basingstoke NHS Trust, Basingstoke, UK

Edward JC Dawe BSc MBBS FRCS(Tr&Orth)
Topics 96, 98
Consultant Trauma and Orthopaedic Surgeon, St Richard's Hospital, Chichester, UK

Ankit Desai MBBS BSc MRCS
Topics 57, 58
Specialty Registrar, Ashford and St Peter's Hospital, Chertsey, UK

Ahmed Fadulelmola MBBS MSc MChOrtho MRCSEd
Topic 18
Specialty Training Registrar, Salford Royal Foundation Trust, Salford, UK

Sam Gallivan FRCS(Tr&Orth)
Topics 67, 68
Specialty Trainee, Kingston Hospital, Kingston upon Thames, UK

Kirsty Hutchinson MBBS BSc MRCP(UK)
Topics 36, 69
Consultant Physician and Ortho-geriatrician, Frimley Health NHS Foundation Trust, UK

Iliyasu Isah MBBS MSc
Topic 11
Specialty Trainee, Wrightington, Wigan and Leigh NHS Foundation Trust, UK

Muthu Jeyam MBBS FRCS MPhil FRCS(Tr&Orth)
Topics 13, 19
Consultant Shoulder and Upper Limb Surgeon, Salford Royal Hospital, Salford, UK

Rami Kallala BM MRCS
Topic 59
Specialty Registrar, Epsom and St Helier University Hospitals NHS Trust
UK

Andrew Keightley MBBs BSc FRCS (Tr&Orth)
Topics 51, 52, 53, 54
Upper Limb Fellow, Royal Surrey County Hospital, Guildford, UK

Al-Achraf Khoriati MBBS BSc MRCS
Topics 71, 72
Registrar, Department of Orthopaedics, Kingston Hospital, Kingston upon Thames, UK

Aiman Khunda MBChB PGCert PGDip(Health and Social Care) MRCSEd FRCSEd(Tr&Orth)
Topic 9
Knee Osteotomy Fellow, North Cumbria University Hospitals NHS Trust, UK

Will KM Kieffer MBBS BSc FRCS(Tr&Orth)
Topics 92, 93, 94, 95, 102
Spinal Fellow, Frimley Health Foundation Trust, UK

Jonny Lenihan MBBS(Hons) BSc(Hons) MRCS
Topics 56, 62
Specialty Registrar, West Suffolk Hospital, Bury St Edmunds, UK

Conrad Lee MBChB, MRCS, MSc
Topics 99, 100
Trainee Registrar, West Sussex NHS Trust, UK

Zoë Little MBBS BSc MRCS
Topics 60, 61, 97
Specialty Trainee St George's Hospital, London, UK

James S Logan MBBS BSc(Hons) PGdip(SEM) FRCS(Tr&Orth)
Topics 32, 33, 34, 42, 43
Senior Clinical Fellow in Hand Surgery, University Hospital Southampton, Southampton, UK

Ravi Kanth Mallina FRCS
Topic 80, 82
Specialty Registrar, St George's Hospital, London, UK

Dan Marsland MBChB MRCS MSc(SEM) FRCS(Tr&Orth)
Topics 28, 29, 30, 31
Specialty Registrar, University Hospital Southampton NHS Foundation Trust, UK

Josephine K McEwan BM MRCS
Topics 46, 47, 48, 50
Specialty Registrar, University Hospital Southampton, Southampton, UK

Majed Al Najjar MBBS, MRCS
Topics 12, 16
Clinical Fellow, Salford Royal NHS Foundation Trust, UK

Haris Naseem MBChB FRCS(Tr&Orth) MRes Dip Sports Med
Topic 17
Specialty Trainee, Salford Royal Hospital, Salford, UK

Paul D Nesbitt MbChB PgDip(Ortho) MRCS(Glasg)
Topic 15
Specialty Trainee, Salford Royal NHS Foundation Trust, UK

Greg Nicholls MBChB
Topic 2
Health Care Assessor, Centre for Health and Disability Assessments, Blackpool, UK

Alina Ortega-Briones MBBCh MD FEBOT
Topics 55, 63, 64
Consultant Trauma and Orthopaedic Surgeon, Rey Juan Carlos University Hospital, Madrid, Spain

Piers Page MBBS MPhil MRCSEd
Topic 81
Specialty Registrar, Royal Surrey County Hospital NHS Trust, UK

Stylianos Papalexandris MSc Med
Topics 3, 4, 5, 24
Hip and Knee Fellow, Wirral University Teaching Hospital NHS Foundation Trust, Upton, UK

Ali Phillips FRCS(Tr&Orth)
Topics 39, 40, 41, 44
Consultant Hand, Wrist and Elbow Surgeon, University Hospital Southampton, Southampton, UK

Asan Rafee MBBS FRCS(Orth)
Topic 10
Senior Orthopaedic and Reconstruction Surgeon, Salford Royal Hospital, Salford, UK

Shakeel M Rahman BA BMBS MRCS
Topic 83, 91
Specialty Registrar St George's Hospital, London, UK

Housameldin Raslan FRCS(Tr&Orth) PhD(Orth)
Topic 20
Major Trauma Fellow, Royal Preston Hospital, Preston, UK

Aisha Razik MBBS BSc MRCS
Topics 78, 79, 87
Specialty Registrar, Croydon University Hospital, London, UK

Ibrahim Roushdi BSc MBBS FRCS(Orth) DipHandSurg
Topics 89, 90
Consultant Orthopaedic Surgeon, Robert Jones and Agnes Hunt Orthopaedic Hospital, Oswestry, UK

Farid Saedi MBChB MRCS
Topic 10
Specialty Registrar, Salford Royal Hospital, Salford, UK

Brinda Somanchi MBBS MRCS MS(Orth) FRCS(Tr&Orth)
Topic 6
Locum Consultant Orthopaedic Surgeon, Royal Derby Hospital, Derby, UK

Avtar Singh Sur MBChB MRCS MSc
Topics 75, 77
Specialty Registrar, St George's Hospital, London, UK

Ben Taylor FRCA DipIMC MBChB(Hons) BSc
Topics 86, 101
Consultant Anaesthetist, Royal Stoke University Hospital, Stoke-on-Trent, UK

Acknowledgements

Figures 55.2, 57.1, 57.2 and 75.1 are reproduced from: Blucher N, Butler K, Platt S. Pocket Tutor Orthopaedics. London: JP Medical Publishers, 2017.

Dedications

I would like to thank my co-editors for their hard work in compiling this book. I also extend thanks to all the contributors who have worked hard to provide such excellent material. Finally, I thank my wife and children who always stand by me even when things are stressful and tough.

AT

For Caroline and William.

PP

I would like to acknowledge and thank the contributing authors who have given their time, energy and knowledge towards the preparation of this book. I would also like to thank my wife Lisa and children Ashley, Jade and Mateo, for their patience and understanding during this period. I am grateful to my parents for their never-ending support and encouragement.

DS

I would like to acknowledge and thank all the contributing authors who worked so hard for this book. For standing by me and always offering their support, I am grateful to my wife Javaria and children Isra, Yousuf, Haroon and Aalia. To my parents, I owe everything.

AQ

1 Amputations – mangled extremities and decision making

Key points

- The decision to salvage or amputate a severely injured extremity is one of the most difficult decisions that can face the orthopaedic surgeon
- The decision must be considered in the context of the severity of the injury, other associated injuries, patient's comorbidities and the social, economic and psychological background of the patient
- Multiple scoring systems have been designed to aid the decision process; however, many mangled extremities are borderline cases therefore scores should be used with caution and only as a guide to supplement the surgeon's clinical judgement

Introduction

A mangled extremity is an injury involving many or all components of a limb system, including soft tissue, bone, nerves and vessels. The management of these complex injuries, which is commonly associated with other life-threatening injuries, remains challenging.

The decision whether to salvage or amputate a mangled limb is a matter of debate. Amputation is without a doubt a devastating experience to both patient and surgeon, and with the current advancements in trauma life support and surgical techniques more mangled limbs are technically salvageable. However, the question remains as to whether the final functional outcome with salvage surgery outperforms the function following amputation with the currently available advanced prostheses. A nonfunctional limb that continues to be painful or insensate after prolonged attempts at reconstruction will certainly be inferior to amputation and a good prosthesis. On the other hand, lengthy unsuccessful attempts for reconstruction in a polytraumatised patient is associated with significant morbidity, high costs and even mortality. Furthermore when amputation is inevitable, performing early surgery can improve patient survival, reduce disability and pain, and decrease hospital stay.

Multiple factors affect the outcome in the management of mangled extremities and should be carefully considered when making the decision whether to salvage or amputate. These factors can be classified into:

- Local factors related to the severity of the injury
- Systemic factors like age, smoking and other associated injuries
- Factors related to the psychologic, social, and economic background of the patient like life-style, occupation, wishes and available resources

When considering the aforementioned factors, soft tissue injury was found to have the highest impact on amputation decision, other factors associated with poor outcome are irreparable vascular injury, warm ischaemia for >6 hours, infrapopliteal vascular injury involving all three vessels, loss of protective sensation in nerve injuries, age, smoking, pre-existing co-morbidities and the presence of concurrent injuries. If the need for amputation is not clear in the initial assessment, limb salvage should be attempted.

Mechanism of injury

Road traffic and industrial accidents are the leading causes for mangled upper and lower extremities, with other less common causes including fall from height, high-velocity gunshots, explosions and combat injuries.

Initial management

The management of mangled extremity begins in the emergency department with the standard trauma survey and resuscitation in accordance with the Advanced Trauma Life Support protocol. The examination of the extremity then starts with assessment of the degree of soft tissue damage and careful examination of the neurovascular status of the limb. If there is disruption to the arterial flow and reconstruction is considered, intraluminal shunt should be considered. Gross debris should be removed and any significant bleeding controlled by direct pressure. Photographs are useful tool to document the severity of the injury if amputation is considered and to monitor changes if reconstruction is planned. Appropriate dressing should then be used, gross deformities corrected and temporary splinting applied in order to improve pain, minimise further damage and reduce bleeding. Early prophylactic antibiotics and tetanus cover should be initiated and appropriate radiographs can then be planned.

Scoring systems

Different scoring systems have been designed in an attempt to help the decision-making process when dealing with mangled extremity. No single score has been found to be superior to the others and much controversy remains with regard to the ability of these systems to predict successful salvage of the mangled extremities or distinguish cases that are better managed with early amputation. The decision to amputate or salvage should be carefully assessed and should take into account the final functional outcome. A further limitation to scoring systems is that they are applied on the initial assessment of the injury and they do not provide guidance for the decision-making during the course of treatment.

The Mangled Extremity Severity Score (MESS) is the most commonly used and was originally described by Johansen et al. in 1990; a score of 7 or more was predictive of amputation in 100% of cases (**Table 1.1**). However, subsequent studies have been less convincing, reporting low sensitivity for predicting amputation. The limb salvage index (LSI) was proposed by Russell et al. in 1991. The LSI predicts the likelihood of salvage based on detailed intraoperative examination of the injury to six different tissues including artery, nerve, bone,

Table 1.1 Mangled Extremity Severity Score (MESS)

Skeletal/soft tissue injury (points 1–4)		
Low energy	e.g. stab, simple fracture, small calibre gunshot wound	1 point
Medium energy	e.g. open or multiple fractures, dislocation	2 points
High energy	e.g. high speed road traffic accidents	3 points
Very high energy	e.g. high speed trauma with gross contamination	4 points
Limb ischaemia (points 1–3)		
Mild	Pulse reduced or absent, perfusion normal	1 point*
Moderate	Pulse absent, paraesthesia, reduced capillary refill	2 points*
Severe	Pulse absent, cool, paralysed, insensate, no capillary refill	3 points*
Shock (points 0–2)		
Stable normotensive		0 points
Transient hypotension		1 point
Persistent hypotension		2 points
Age (points 0–2)		
<30 years		0 points
30–50 years		1 point
>50 years		2 points

*Score is doubled for ischaemia >6 hours

skin, muscle and deep veins. It takes into consideration limb ischaemia time. A score of 6 points or more predicts amputation (**Table 1.2**). Other scoring systems have been proposed like the mangled extremity syndrome index (MESI) developed in 1985 by Gregory et al., the predictive salvage index (PSI) by Howe et al. in 1987 and the NISSSA score (Nerve injury, Ischaemia, Soft-tissue injury, Skeletal injury, Shock, and Age) described by McNamara et al. in 1994.

It is important to note that the above mentioned scoring systems were specifically designed for the lower extremity. The currently available prostheses for the lower extremity support ambulation as the primary function of the lower extremity. However, prostheses for the upper extremity do not restore fine movements, and furthermore these movements are dependent on sensation, therefore a mangled upper extremity has a much larger effect on a patient's life than a mangled lower extremity and the decision-making process for salvage in these cases is quite different from those of the lower extremity. With better functional results following salvage and poorer functional prognosis after amputation, mangled upper extremity should be managed on a case-by-case basis.

Amputation

Amputations should be performed at the lowest possible level to preserve function and reduce metabolic demand. The level

Table 1.2 Limb salvage index (LSI)

Arterial trauma
- Contusion, intimal tear, partial laceration, palpable pulses — 0 points
- Occlusion of two or more shank vessels — 1 point
- Complete occlusion of femoral, popliteal or all three shank vessels — 2 points

Nerve trauma
- Contusion or stretch — 0 points
- Partial transection: sciatic, femoral, peroneal or tibial nerve. Complete transection: femoral, peroneal or tibial nerve — 1 point
- Complete transection: sciatic nerve or both peroneal and tibial nerves — 2 points

Bone trauma
- Closed or open fracture with minimum comminution — 0 points
- Closed fracture in at least three sites or open fracture with comminution or open joint with foreign body, or bone loss <3 cm — 1 point
- Bone loss >3 cm; type IIIB or IIIC — 2 points

Skin trauma
- Clean laceration, primary repair, 1st degree burn — 0 points
- Delayed closure due to contamination requiring skin grafts or flaps or 2nd and 3rd degree burns — 1 point

Muscle trauma
- One muscle or tendon avulsion or laceration — 0 points
- Two or more muscles or tendons laceration, or avulsion — 1 point
- Crush injury — 2 points

Deep vein trauma
- Contusion, partial laceration — 0 points
- Complete laceration, avulsion, or thrombosis — 1 point

Warm ischaemia time
- < 6 hours — 0 points
- 6–9 hours — 1 point
- 9–12 hours — 2 points
- 12–15 hours — 3 points
- 15 hours — 4 points

should allow prosthesis to be fitted securely and comfortably. Forequarter amputation (interscapulothoracic) and shoulder disarticulation are very rarely performed; forequarter is only indicated for traumatic avulsion. When shoulder disarticulation is considered, better appearance can be achieved by maintaining the humeral head. A prosthesis can be fitted if 2.5 cm of the proximal humerus is left. Other levels of amputations in the upper limb include transhumeral, transradial, wrist disarticulation and transcarpal. Wrist disarticulation has the advantage of improved pronation and supination and longer lever arm when compared with transradial amputation, however transradial is cosmetically more pleasing and easier for prosthetic application.

In the lower limb the ideal level for transfemoral, above-knee amputation is 12 cm above the knee joint to allow for prosthetic fitting. This level of amputation was found to be superior to through-the-knee amputation as the latter is associated with poorer functional, psychological and cosmetic outcomes. However, the main indication for amputation through the knee is in children, in order to preserve the lower femoral physis.

Transtibial, below-knee amputation, is ideally performed 12–15 cm below the joint. When possible preservation of the knee joint should be attempted as energy demand for below-knee amputation is only 10–30% more, as compared to 40–67% in transfemoral amputation. Excellent prostheses are currently available achieving satisfactory function and near normal gait. Prosthesis can be fitted with shorter stumps up to 5–6 cm.

Other levels of amputation include above-ankle Syme's amputation and partial foot amputations; Chopart amputation through the midtarsal joints; Lisfranc amputation through the tarsometatarsal joints; transmetatarsal amputation; and amputation through the metatarsophalangeal joints.

Further reading

Fodor L, Sobec R, Sita-Alb L, Fodor M, Ciuce C. Mangled lower extremity: can we trust the amputation scores? Int J Burn Trauma 2012; 2:51–58.

Ly TV, Travison TG, Castillo RC, et al. Ability of lower-extremity injury severity scores to predict functional outcome after limb salvage. J Bone Joint Surg Am 2008; 90:1738–1743.

MJ Bosse, MacKenzie EJ, Kellam JF, et al. An analysis of outcomes of reconstruction or amputation of leg-threatening injuries. N Engl J Med 2002; 347:1924–1931.

Related topics of interest

- *Topic 2* Amputations – prosthetics and rehabilitation
- *Topic 62* Major trauma – Advanced Trauma Life Support principles
- *Topic 68* Open fractures

2 Amputations – prosthetics and rehabilitation

Key points
- Amputation of a limb leads to a reduction in the level of function, sensation and appearance of the remaining limb. However, with a suitable prosthetic limb, appropriate wound care management and rehabilitation program, many reach a level of functionality that facilitates a return to work or participation in normal activities
- The most important decision regarding amputation is the anatomical level at which it should occur. The greater the skin, joint and muscle loss the greater the cost, loss of function and energy expenditure required to use a prosthetic limb. Soft tissue bleeding is a simple yet effective indicator of viable tissue
- Rehabilitation consists of expert advice from a variety of specialists enabling realistic goals to be set, and should provide knowledge of the different parts of the prosthetic limb, ongoing maintenance, complications and application. Awareness of alterations, reasons for pain or discomfort, and how to weight bear all help to reduce anxiety and worry

Prosthetic limb information

Prosthetic limbs can be used safely by the majority of people undergoing limb amputation. Exceptions for a prosthetic limb include poor muscle strength, short stumps, infected wounds or severe scarring.

Prosthetic upper and lower limbs have different roles to fulfil. However, a large part of their design principles is shared with a number of common parts. The following section will explore these in more detail.

Lower limb
Below-knee amputation
Socket
This area is in contact with the skin, therefore an ill-fitting socket will result in irritation pain and discomfort. The artificial limb should allow pressure to be placed on pressure-tolerant areas of the stump. Pressure tolerance occurs on areas where there is adequate muscle or soft tissue cover. The area with the greatest tolerance is over the patella tendon. Nonpressure tolerance occurs over areas of bone with poor tissue coverage.

An ill-fitting socket may be due to a poorly made prosthesis, change in the patient's habitus or composition including swelling, infection or shrinkage of the stump. Incorrect sock fitting can also lead to complications and will be discussed later.

A correct socket should be in tight contact with all of stump, restrict vertical movement but not be uncomfortable. It should not cause irritation, blisters or ulcers.

An insert may be needed to line the inside of the socket reducing the pressure on the stump and providing additional protection.

Suspension
This holds the prosthetic limb in place with straps or belts. A tight-fitting prosthesis is vital to minimise any irritation or discomfort.

Pylon and foot
The pylon connects the foot and the socket. A cover can be placed over the pylon for aesthetic design. The foot is designed to be the only part of the prosthetic limb that is in contact with ground. It is important to remember that different foot wear may cause

the limb to be misaligned applying pressure to nontolerant areas of the stump.

With above knee amputations, the loss of the knee joint makes ambulation more difficult and requires a higher energy usage compared to below-knee amputations.

Above-knee amputation

Socket
As with a below-knee amputation the socket remains in contact with the skin of the stump and must to be tight fitting to avoid complications. Two common socket designs are used in above-knee amputations:
1. Ischial ramal containment socket
2. Quadrilateral socket

Ischial ramal containment socket
This socket provides complete contact with the skin of the stump, with the ischium bone inside the socket encasing the medial aspect of the thigh. The gluteal fold should rest on the posterior wall of the socket without causing pain in the groin.

Quadrilateral socket
The quadrilateral socket is a subischial design that has four distinct walls fashioned to contain the thigh musculature with the ischium resting on the posteromedial aspect of the socket brim. The socket's primary functions are to provide for weight-bearing during the stance phase of gait.

Suspension
The prosthetic limb is held in place most commonly by a Silesian band fastening around the waist or alternatively a pelvic band with external hip joint if there is reduced muscle bulk. Suction suspension can be used providing an increased range of motion due to the lack of external fastening mechanisms.

A rigid knee provides the greatest level of safety but does impede on the level of mobility possible.

Upper limb

Prosthetic upper limbs are rarer than lower limbs but follow the same principles of design. The socket still needs to provide a firm continuous contact, but without the need to bear the body's weight.

The prosthetic limb is held in place via straps or a harness which can operate terminal mechanical devices or mobilise the elbow. Mechanical elbows are simple hinge joints allowing extension and flexion enabling objects to be brought to the mouth.

The distal end of the prosthesis can accommodate a variety of terminal devices, including hands or hooks assisting with day-to-day activities and improving aesthetic appearance.

A simple low-cost strap enables devices to be held in place on the distal aspect of the prosthesis, restoring a level of independence enabling simple tasks to be completed.

Prosthetic socks

Socks improve the fit of a prosthetic limb, but incorrect sizing and management of the sock causes irritation to the stump/skin, ulcers and an unstable fitting of the prosthesis.

As the stump heals, its dimensions will change with swelling or oedema, muscle and tissue loss and altered patient habitus resulting in a poorly fitting prosthesis.

The sock is placed over the stump between the socket and accommodates changes in the stump to maintain a correct fit.

Rehabilitation

After complete or partial loss of a limb the patient has to cope with both the physical and psychological loss as well as undergoing a challenging period of rehabilitation. Rehabilitation involves a co-ordinated multi-disciplinary team effort incorporating stump-care, pain management, physiotherapy and social support.

In the immediate postoperative period, management of the stump to allow wound healing, resolution of oedema and recovery is the primary concern and may take up to a month to occur. The stump should be attended to daily, reducing the risk of infection, promoting healing and preparing it for the prosthetic limb. Dressings are applied to provide a clean environment and compression to mould the stump to accommodate the socket.

Prosthetic rehabilitation is valuable to the majority of people following an amputation. Studies have shown quicker adaptation and better long-term outcomes are achieved if rehabilitation is combined with a strong support network of family and friends.

Prosthetic pain often originates from pressure on a nontolerant area or excessive movement on the stump. Altering the socket or using a sock can help to resolve the pain. If an ulcer develops the prosthetic limb should not be worn until the skin has healed.

Phantom limb pain is a common phenomenon in which the amputated limb still feels attached to the body, with the majority of sensations being painful. The symptoms may include tingling, itching, burning or aching. How to treat it remains a contentious issue.

Physical rehabilitation provides a highly individualised tailored programme with physiotherapists and occupational therapists working to set realistic outcome goals.

Exercises are initially simple in the immediate postoperative period, developing as the stump heals, maintaining strength and mobility in preparation for the prosthetic limb. It can take a number of months before both stump and user are ready for a prosthetic limb. This can be a long and frustrating period but ultimately reduces the time it takes to adjust to and be confident with the prosthesis.

Continuing and regular care is required. A prosthetic limb needs maintenance and adjustment to facilitate changes in the user's life. Modern prosthetic limbs allow for parts to be changed if necessary rather than the whole prosthesis.

If the outcome of rehabilitation is poor and the prosthetic limb limits use, limits function or is inconvenient to wear, the likelihood of the prosthesis being rejected increases. Prosthetic limbs should not be seen as a 'like-for-like' replacement of the amputated limb but as a means to provide a level of function that is appropriate for their circumstances.

Further reading

O'Keeffe B. Prosthetic rehabilitation of the upper limb amputee. Indian J Plast Surg 2011; 44:246–252.

World Health Organization. The rehabilitation of people with amputations. Philadelphia, PA: United States Department of Defense, MossRehab Amputee Rehabilitation Program, MossRehab Hospital; 2004.

Related topics of interest

- *Topic 1* Amputations – mangled extremities and decision making
- *Topic 62* Major trauma – Advanced Trauma Life Support principles

3 Ankle: Achilles tendon ruptures

Key points
- Imaging investigations are not always warranted for the diagnosis of a complete Achilles tendon rupture
- The long-term outcomes of nonoperative and operative treatment are comparable
- The most common complication of surgery is wound healing problems

Epidemiology

The annual incidence of Achilles tendon ruptures is 18 cases per 100,000 population (range 8–24). Most of them (68%) occur during athletic activities. Middle-aged men (average age 35–40 years) who exercise episodically are the typical sufferers of this injury. The male-to-female ratio is approximately 20:1. The diagnosis is missed in up to 25% of the cases, especially in patients older than 55 years with high body mass index (average 32.3 kg/m^2) who sustain the injury at work or during daily life activities. Rupture in one side increases the likelihood of a contralateral injury.

Pathophysiology

Mechanical, biological and biochemical factors have been associated with Achilles tendinopathy and ruptures. The hypovascular 'watershed area', 3–6 cm proximal to the Achilles tendon insertion, is susceptible to microscopic changes induced by hypoxia and cyclic mechanical loading. When there is extracellular matrix disruption this initiates an inflammatory response, mediated by cytokines like the hypoxia inducible factor-1 (HIF-1), the platelet-derived growth factor (PDGF) and the vascular endothelial growth factor (VEGF), resulting in neovascularisation and enhanced innervation. Metalloproteinases (MMPs) are overexpressed in order to degrade the disrupted matrix. The VEGF promotes angiogenesis, upregulates the expression of MMP and downregulates the tissue inhibitors of MMP.

The repair process fails when continuous traumatic impact exceeds the healing capacity of the tendon, which is rendered vulnerable to ruptures even with minor or moderate injury. In addition, an age-related decrease in collagen cross-linking alters the viscoelastic properties of the musculotendinous junction. Consequently, higher forcers are transmitted through the tendon as its tensile strength decreases.

Lower limb malalignment, cavus or varus deformity, hyperpronation of the foot, as well as overuse injuries, have been identified as risk factors for Achilles tendon ruptures. Inappropriate footwear may contribute by exacerbating the underlying biomechanical problems. Cigarette smoking, diabetes, preinjury steroid injection into or around the tendon and use of fluoroquinolones all predispose to Achilles tendon rupture. Fluoroquinolones exert a dose-independent cytotoxic effect on enzymes of the musculoskeletal tissue or directly affect type I collagen synthesis, promoting collagen degradation.

Clinical features

Achilles tendon ruptures can be partial or complete. Ruptures diagnosed within a month from the time of injury are classified as acute.

Patients usually describe a 'pop' or 'snap' at the back of the ankle as if they were hit or kicked from behind. There is sharp pain and difficulty or inability to walk. The ankle may be bruised or swollen. The Achilles tendon loses its normal contour and an indentation, corresponding to the rupture gap, might be visible and palpable. There is also tenderness on palpation of the rupture site. Resting ankle dorsiflexion in the prone position with the knee bent is increased whereas active plantarflexion is weak or impossible. Tibialis posterior and the toe flexors may mediate some active plantarflexion but there is typically inability to single leg tiptoe. In chronic ruptures, the calf muscles appear atrophied.

The Thompson's test, also known as Simmond's or calf squeeze test, is positive when squeezing the calf muscles does not produce ankle plantarflexion. It is positive only in complete tears of the Achilles tendon. The combination of a positive Thompson's test with a palpable Achilles tendon gap is reported to have 100% sensitivity in diagnosing an acute Achilles tendon rupture. Matle's, O'Brien's and Copeland's tests are rarely used.

Investigations

Radiographs are useful in ruling out other injuries, most commonly ankle fractures or avulsion of the Achilles tendon from the calcaneus. Pre-Achilles (Kager's) fat pad obliteration and soft tissue swelling are nonspecific signs of Achilles tendon rupture.

Ultrasound and MRI are requested when clinical examination is inconclusive. Ultrasound is reportedly 90–100% sensitive in the diagnosis of Achilles tendon ruptures but has significantly lower sensitivity for musculotendinous junction injuries. Partial tears appear as hypoechoic or anechoic intrasubstance areas usually with surrounding tendinosis. In complete tears there is a gap at the rupture site; the edges of the tendon are irregular, retracted with features of tendinosis, especially in chronic ruptures (**Figure 3.1**). Operative treatment is recommended if the gap between the tendon edges is >5 mm in full equinus. Achilles tendon ruptures are classified according to the degree of rupture and the retraction of the tendon edges (**Table 3.1**).

Interstitial or incomplete tears show a high signal on T2 sequence. The MRI findings of an acute Achilles tendon rupture (gap, irregularity and retraction of the tendon edges, oedema or hematoma) are similar to those seen on the ultrasound. Postoperative MRI may still show a gap at the rupture site which tends to disappear within 12 weeks.

Table 3.1 Classification of Achilles tendon ruptures	
Type	Description
I	Partial tears (<50%)
II	Complete rupture with <3 cm gap
III	Complete rupture with a gap >3 and <6 cm
IV	Complete rupture with >6 cm gap

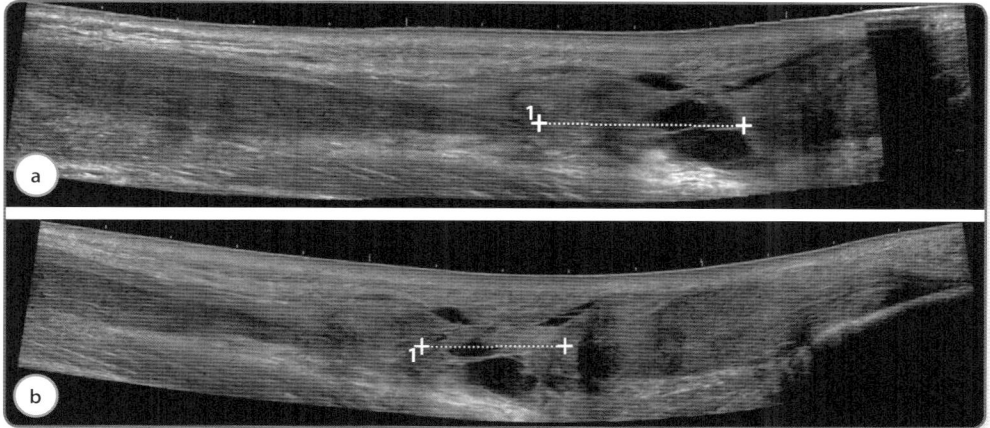

Figure 3.1 (a) Ultrasound scan of the left Achilles tendon showing re-rupture just distal to the musculotendinous junction. The initial rupture had been treated nonoperatively. (b) The gap at the rupture site does not reduce with plantarflexion. There is also moderate cystic and heterogeneous material consistent with haemorrhage and scar tissue.

Treatment

Nonoperative

Acute Achilles tendon ruptures can be treated nonoperatively depending on the type of rupture, the patient's expectations and the need to resume physical activity. Nonoperative treatment is usually preferred for those medically unfit to undergo surgery or low-demand, sedentary patients. It should also be considered for patients with decreased healing capacity (diabetes, peripheral neuropathy or vascular disease, smoking, immunocompromise, BMI > 30) who are prone to develop wound healing problems. The ankle is immobilised in the resting equinus position in a functional brace or cast. Ankle plantarflexion is gradually decreased to neutral within 8–12 weeks, usually at 2-week intervals. Once in a neutral position, functional rehabilitation is commenced which includes weight-bearing and a range of motion exercises.

Operative

Open end-to-end repair

A longitudinal incision slightly medial to the Achilles tendon is made and the paratenon is incised to expose the rupture site. The ragged tendon ends are debrided and the rupture is repaired with heavy nonabsorbable sutures, usually applied by the modified Kessler, Bunnell or Krackow technique. The repair tension should be equal or as close as possible to the contralateral side as excessive tension and shortening of the Achilles tendon will compromise function and the final outcome. The duration and type of postoperative ankle immobilisation and the rehabilitation regimen are dependent on the surgeon's preferences and the strength of the repair. It is recommended that the ankle is immobilized for 2 weeks in gravity equinus, to protect the repair and ease the soft tissue tension. As with conservative management the foot is brought to neutral over a period of 2–4 weeks with use of a protective device for mobilisation.

Percutaneous repair

Minimally invasive techniques aim to reduce the likelihood of wound healing problems or complications associated with open surgery. The Ma-Griffith technique and the use of dedicated devices through a transverse or longitudinal incision at the rupture level reduce the surgical impact to the soft tissues.

Reconstruction with gastrocnemius flaps or V-Y advancement

Achilles tendon ruptures with incomplete apposition but a rupture gap <3 cm can be reconstructed with gastrocnemius tendon and aponeurosis flaps or V-Y advancement. The flaps are 1–2 cm wide and 7–8 cm long. They are left attached 3 cm proximal to the rupture, reversed inferiorly and sutured onto the distal tendon stump. V-Y gastrocnemius advancement provides extra length to enable the approximation of the tendon edges.

Reconstruction with tendon transfer

Chronic ruptures may present with substantial (>3 cm) retraction of the tendon edges which cannot be approximated for a direct end-to-end repair. Flexor hallucis longus (FHL), flexor digitorum longus (FDL) and the peroneus brevis are most frequently transferred to facilitate the reconstruction. If the rupture gap is >6 cm long a gracilis autograft is indicated.

The main bulk of literature has shown higher re-rupture rate for nonoperatively treated patients. Recent evidence suggests comparable results if functional rehabilitation and early mobilisation are prescribed. Operative treatment has higher incidence of wound-related complications (wound breakdown and tethering of Achilles tendon to skin) and nerve (Sural) injury. Return to work and resumption of daily activities is quicker for operative treatment. Regaining the strength required for participation in athletic activities may take 6 months, although full strength may return after 1–2 years or may never return to the preinjury level.

Complications

- Re-rupture – several studies reported a rate of 10–30% for nonoperative treatment versus 2% for operative. However, recent research confirmed similar re-rupture rates for nonoperative and operative treatment

- Plantarflexion weakness – more common following nonoperative treatment and related to Achilles tendon slackness. The difference in range of motion and plantarflexion power between operative repair and treatment in a cast seems to disappear after 6 months
- Wound healing problems – the superficial wound infection rate is 5–10%. Deep infections are less common (approximately 1%) but may require surgical debridement and antibiotics for 6 weeks. Old age, corticosteroids, rupture during daily life activities and delay to treatment are risk factors for wound infection
- Sural nerve injury – more common with percutaneous repair techniques (0–10.5%)
- Reduced range of motion – repair under tension reduces ankle dorsiflexion
- Thromboembolic disease
- Skin necrosis

Further reading

American Academy of Orthopaedic Surgeons (AAOS). The diagnosis and treatment of acute Achilles tendon rupture guideline and evidence report. Rosemont: AAOS, 2009.

Erickson BJ, Mascarenhas R, Saltzman BM, et al. Is operative treatment of Achilles tendon ruptures superior to non-operative treatment? A systematic review of overlapping meta-analyses. Orthop J Sports Med 2015; 3.

Olsson N, Nilsson-Helander K, Karlsson J, et al. Major functional deficits persist 2 years after acute Achilles tendon rupture. Knee Surg Sports Traumatol Arthrosc 2011; 19:1385–1393.

Related topics of interest

- *Topic 4* Ankle: supination- and pronation–external rotation fractures
- *Topic 5* Ankle: supination–adduction and pronation–abduction fractures
- *Topic 28* Foot – calcaneal fractures

4 Ankle: supination– and pronation–external rotation fractures

Key points
- Anatomical structures around the ankle fail in a sequential, predictable pattern
- Assessment of fracture stability is crucial in determining optimal treatment
- Stable fractures can be treated nonoperatively in a boot, weight-bearing as tolerated

Epidemiology

Ankle fractures constitute 9% of all fractures, with an estimated annual incidence of approximately 100–200 fractures per 100,000 people. They have a bimodal distribution, most of them occurring in young men and elderly women. Age is related to the type of the fracture. The most common type is supination–external rotation (SER) which accounts for 40–70% of all ankle fractures. The incidence of open fractures is 2%. Smoking, alcohol, obesity and diabetes have been associated with increased likelihood of complications and worse outcomes.

Pathophysiology

Several classification systems have been implemented to describe ankle fractures according to their configuration on the radiographs. The Danis–Weber classification is based on the level of the lateral malleolus fracture. The AO/OTA classification provides a comprehensive description of the fracture location and pattern. The nomenclature of the Lauge-Hansen classification reflects its rationale. The first of the two terms used for each fracture refers to the position of the foot at the time of the injury and the second describes the direction of the deforming force. There are four main fracture types:
- supination–external rotation (SER)
- supination–adduction
- pronation–external rotation (PER)
- pronation–abduction (PAB)

The Lauge-Hansen classification, despite its limitations, facilitates a mental recreation of the injury circumstances which, in turn, is informative about the failed structures. Ligament ruptures and fractures occur in a sequential pattern, which is always the same for each given type of injury. Each main fracture type is subdivided into stages depending on the magnitude of the force exerted on the joint. Structures under tension are the first to fail and this is dictated by the position of the foot at the time of the injury. Ligament ruptures are equivalent to ipsilateral malleolar fractures. The age-related change in the ratio of bone and ligament strength determines whether the bone or the ligament will eventually fail.

The deforming force in both SER and PER fractures is torsional, although it has been suggested that SER injuries are not possible without an element of valgus force. The stages of SER injuries are presented in **Table 4.1**. The lateral malleolus fracture in SER II injuries is typically at the level of the syndesmosis but can be more proximal if an abduction moment was applied together

Table 4.1 Stages and injuries of supination external rotation ankle fractures

Stage	Injury
Stage I	Rupture of the AITFL or Chaput's fracture, or Wagstaffe's fracture
Stage II	Spiral fracture of the lateral malleolus at the level of the syndesmosis
Stage III	Rupture of the PITFL or posterior malleolus fracture
Stage IV	Rupture of the deltoid ligament or medial malleolus fracture

AITFL, anterior inferior tibiofibular ligament; PITFL, posterior inferior tibiofibular ligament

Ankle: supination- and pronation-external rotation fractures

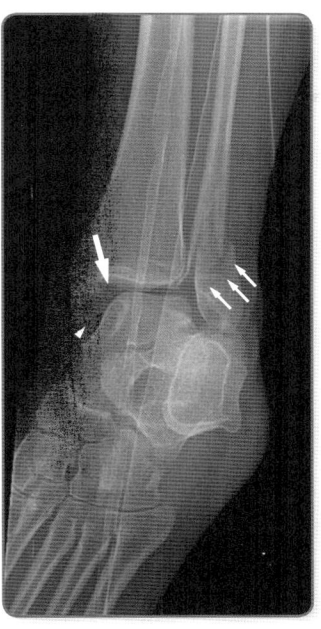

Figure 4.1 Supination–external rotation ankle fracture. The fracture of the lateral malleolus (smaller arrows) is at the level of the syndesmosis running from anterior–inferior to posterior–superior. The medial clear space (arrow head) is widened, and the talus is laterally shifted. The posterior malleolus fragment projects at the superomedial corner of the mortise (arrow).

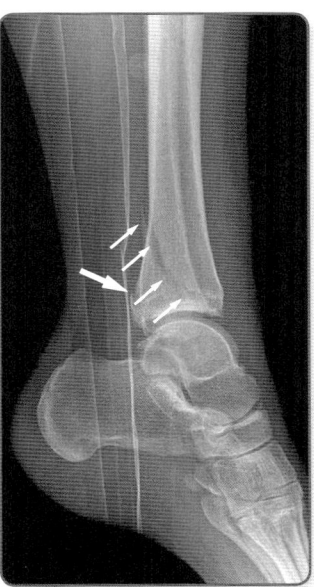

Figure 4.2 Lateral radiograph of the same patient as in Figure 3.1, depicting the direction of the lateral malleolus fracture (smaller arrows) and the size of the posterior malleolus fracture (larger arrow).

with the external rotation force (**Figure 4.1**). It has an anterior–inferior to posterior–superior direction (**Figure 4.2**). The medial malleolus fracture in SER IV injuries is mostly a transverse fracture but can also be oblique.

The sequence of injuries occurring in PER injuries is presented in **Table 4.2**. An isolated complete rupture of the deltoid ligament (PER I) is rather unlikely without disruption of the syndesmosis or a fibula fracture (**Figure 4.3**). The fibula fracture in PER III injuries is usually more than 6 cm proximal to the plafond and has reverse obliquity compared to the SER II fractures (**Figure 4.4**).

Clinical features

Serious, life or limb threatening injuries should be diagnosed and dealt with first, following the Advanced Trauma Life Support (ATLS) principles. In isolated ankle injuries, clinical examination should include the whole leg, the ankle and the foot.

Patients most commonly complain of pain and difficulty or inability to bear weight. Active and passive ankle movements may be reduced or even impossible. Swelling and ecchymosis over or distal to the malleoli are related to fractures or ligament ruptures. Fracture blisters may appear at a later stage.

Table 4.2 Stages and injuries of pronation–external rotation ankle fractures	
Stage	Injury
Stage I	Rupture of the deltoid ligament or medial malleolus fracture
Stage II	Rupture of the AITFL and the interosseous membrane
Stage III	Spiral or oblique fracture of the lateral malleolus above the syndesmosis
Stage IV	Rupture of the PITFL or posterior malleolus fracture

AITFL, anterior inferior tibiofibular ligament; PITFL, posterior inferior tibiofibular ligament

The entire length of the tibia and fibula, the base of the 5th metatarsal and the navicular should be palpated for tenderness. Concomitant injuries around the knee joint (e.g. Maisonneuve fracture) should not be missed. Collateral ligaments and syndesmosis should be examined for tenderness. Medial-sided tenderness, ecchymosis and swelling raise the suspicion but have poor positive predictive value for significant deltoid ligament injury.

The integrity of the syndesmosis should be assessed even though most clinical tests have questionable sensitivity. Positive dorsiflexion–external rotation (Kleiger's) and leg squeeze (Hopkin's) tests are indicative of syndesmotic disruption or a lateral malleolus fracture. Syndesmosis instability is better demonstrated on the sagittal rather than the coronal plane. The hook (Cotton's) test is performed intraoperatively to assess the tibiofibular clear space under fluoroscopy or even direct inspection. The anterior drawer and the talar tilt tests assess the anterior talofibular ligament and the calcaneofibular ligament, respectively. They are not advocated if a fracture is suspected. Their sensitivity and specificity are higher 4–7 days after the injury.

Clinical examination is also directed to elicit signs of Achilles or tibialis posterior tendon ruptures and subluxation or dislocation of the peroneal tendons.

The neurovascular status of the extremity should be assessed and documented at regular intervals, especially before and after reduction manoeuvres or application of plaster casts. The possibility of development of compartment syndrome should never be overlooked.

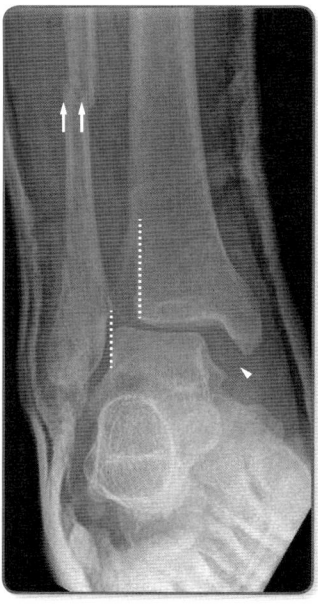

Figure 4.3 Pronation–external rotation fracture with significant widening of the medial clear space secondary to deltoid ligament rupture (arrow head), lateral talar displacement (dotted lines) and a high fibula fracture (arrows).

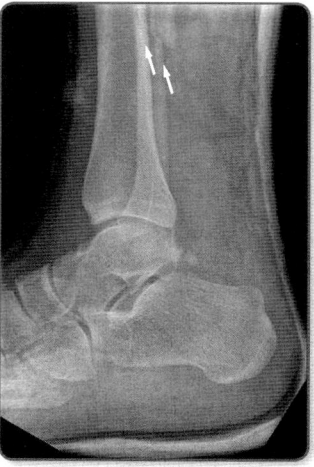

Figure 4.4 Lateral radiograph of the same patient as in Figure 4.3. The lateral malleolus fracture in PER injuries has reverse obliquity compared to SER fractures (posterior–inferior to anterior–superior).

Investigations

The Ottawa ankle rules (OAR) provide reliable guidance in identifying the skeletally mature patients who need radiographic investigation following an ankle injury. OAR applicability in children is debatable. Anteroposterior, lateral and mortise views are originally sufficient. Stress views can reveal ankle instability and distinguish between SER II and SER IV injuries. Gravity or manual external rotation stress views evaluate the stability of isolated lateral malleolus fractures when deltoid ligament rupture is suspected. These fractures are best assessed with weight-bearing views up to 1 week following the injury. Assessment of the medial and superior clear spaces should be undertaken with caution as these measurements are dependent on patient's age, gender and size, radiograph magnification, the position of the foot and rotation of the ankle.

Ultrasound, CT scan and MRI are not routine investigations. CT scans provide details about the size and configuration of a posterior malleolus fracture or the features of a pilon fracture. MRI is very useful for the evaluation of soft tissue injuries and occult fractures or chondral lesions of the talar dome or the tibial plafond.

Treatment

Treatment is guided by the fracture pattern and its stability with consideration to the patient's age, bone quality, comorbidities and previous mobility level. Stable SER I and II fractures can be treated nonoperatively. SER II fractures are immobilised in a below-knee cast or boot for 6–8 weeks or double the time in diabetic patients. Unstable SER II fractures require fixation of the lateral malleolus with one or more lag screws and a 1/3 tubular plate for neutralisation. Sturdier plates (DCP or locking) can be used for better rotational stability in larger patients or comminuted fractures but are associated with a higher rate of wound problems. The posterior malleolus fracture in SER III injuries is fixed with 4 mm partially threaded cancellous screws inserted preferably through a posteromedial or posterolateral approach. The medial malleolus fracture in SER IV injuries is also fixed with 4 mm partially threaded cancellous screws. If there is no medial maleolar fracture in SER IV then repair of the deltoid ligament is pursued to prevent subsequent instability.

Nondisplaced medial malleolus fractures in PER I injuries are treated in a below-knee cast or boot for 7–8 weeks with check radiographs obtained weekly for the first 2 weeks. Partial weight-bearing is usually allowed after 2–4 weeks. Displaced fractures are fixed with two 4 mm partially threaded cancellous screws. Tension band wire is applied when the fragment is small or comminuted and in osteoporotic bone. The lateral malleolus fracture in PER III injuries is fixed if it is within 7 cm from the plafond level with the same technique and hardware as the SER fractures. Fixation of a posterior malleolus fracture is important in maintaining the stability of the ankle. Antiglide screws or fixation with a plate should be considered.

The syndesmosis is fixed when the hook test is positive after fixation of the main fragments. One or two cortical screws, engaging the lateral malleolus and one or two tibial cortices are inserted from posterolaterally to anteromedially (**Figure 4.5**). They are maintained for at least 8–12 weeks.

Complications

Older age, vascular disease, diabetes and open fractures are predictors of early complications. The incidence of deep vein thrombosis (DVT) in operatively treated ankle fractures is 2–3%, even though subclinical peripheral DVT can be as high as 21–28%. Wound-healing problems occur in approximately 4–5% of patients with the infection rate being 1.5%. Injuries to the sural and the saphenous nerves are underestimated. Malunion is usually related to lateral malleolus rotational deformity. Post-traumatic arthritis manifested with persistent pain and stiffness may require ankle arthrodesis. Post-traumatic tibiofibular synostosis following syndesmosis injury can be up to 10%.

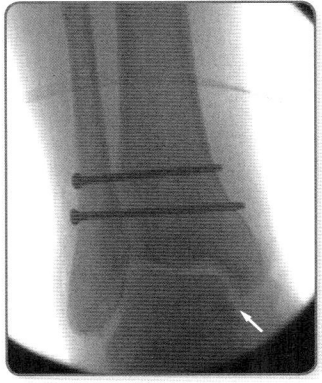

Figure 4.5 Intraoperative fluoroscopic image of the same patient as in Figures 4.3 and 4.4. The syndesmosis has been fixed with two cortical screws engaging four cortices. The deltoid ligament has been repaired with the use of an anchor-suture device (arrow).

Further reading

DeAngelis NA, Eskander MS, French BG. Does medial tenderness predict deep deltoid ligament incompetence in supination–external rotation type ankle fractures? J Orthop Trauma 2007; 21:244–247.

Koval KJ, Egol KA, Cheung Y, Goodwin DW, Spratt KF. Does a positive ankle stress test indicate the need for operative treatment after lateral malleolus fracture? A preliminary report. J Orthop Trauma 2007; 21:449–455.

Lambers KT, Van den Bekerom MP, Doornberg JN, et al. Long-term outcome of pronation-external rotation ankle fractures treated with syndesmotic screws only. J Bone Joint Surg Am 2013; 95:e1221–1227.

Related topics of interest

- *Topic 5* Ankle: supination–adduction and pronation–abduction fractures
- *Topic 62* Major trauma – Advanced Trauma and Life Support principles
- *Topic 68* Open fractures

5 Ankle: supination–adduction and pronation–abduction fractures

Key points

- Medial sided ecchymosis and swelling are not proof of significant deltoid ligament injury
- Stress radiographs may be necessary to illustrate ankle instability
- Supination–adduction and pronation–abduction fractures are often associated with osteochondral injuries of the tibial plafond and/or the talar dome

Epidemiology

Ankle fractures are common injuries caused by indirect trauma in 90% of the cases. The typical mechanism is either a twisting injury or a fall from a height. Supination–adduction (SAD) and pronation–abduction (PAB) fractures account for 10-20% and 2% of all ankle fractures, respectively. The incidence of ankle fractures stops increasing after the age of 60-70 years. Higher levels of physical activity in younger men and poor bone quality in older women make ankle fractures more common in these population groups. 13% of ankle fractures are associated with syndesmotic disruption.

Pathophysiology

The main advantage of the Lauge-Hansen classification is its ability to describe which structures have been injured, as they fail in a predictable sequence. However, it is compromised by its poor observer reliability and reproducibility. There are also specific fracture patterns that do not fit in any of the described types. The injuries occurring at each stage of the four main fracture types are shown in **Table 5.1**.

The deforming force in SAD and PAB fractures is predominantly translational. In SAD fractures the lateral structures are in tension, therefore they fail first when an adduction force acts on the ankle with the foot fixed in supination. The sequence of injuries sustained with this mechanism is shown in **Table 5.2**. The vast majority of the lateral malleolus fractures in SAD I injuries are transverse, located below the level of the syndesmosis. The tibial plafond may present impaction anteromedially (**Figures 5.1** and **5.2**).

The stages of a PAB fracture are shown in **Table 5.3**. The excessive abduction force drives the talus against the lateral edge of the tibial plafond and can potentially cause

Table 5.1 Sequence and type of injuries sustained in the four types of ankle fractures according to the Lauge-Hansen classification

	AITFL	Lateral malleolus	PITFL/posterior malleolus	Deltoid ligament/medial malleolus
SER	I	II	III	IV
PER	II	III	IV	I
SAD	–	I	–	II
PAB	II	III	–	I

AITFL, anterior inferior tibiofibular ligament; PAB, pronation–abduction; PER, pronation external rotation; PITFL, posterior inferior tibiofibular ligament; SAD, supination–adduction; SER, supination external rotation.

osteochondral injuries of the talar dome or impaction of the tibial plafond.

Clinical features

Before assessing an ankle injury, the attending doctor should ensure that life- or limb-threatening injuries have been addressed first, in accordance with the Advanced Trauma Life Support (ATLS) priorities.

Pain, difficulty or inability to bear weight, reduced ankle range of movement, swelling and ecchymosis are the most common manifestations of an ankle fracture. Ankle deformity depends on the type of the fracture and the degree of displacement. Nondisplaced fractures can be mistaken for ankle sprains, especially when the swelling is minimal.

Clinical examination of the whole leg is essential to rule out remote injuries (e.g. Maisonneuve fracture) or fractures of the foot. Ankle fractures can be associated with tibial, talar, calcaneal, midfoot or forefoot fractures, or dislocations. Ligament ruptures are considered as fracture equivalent injuries.

Table 5.2 Stages and injuries of supination–adduction ankle fractures

Stage I	Rupture of the ATFL and/or the CFL or transverse fracture of the lateral malleolus
Stage II	Vertical or oblique fracture of the medial malleolus

ATFL, anterior tibiofibular ligament; CFL, calcaneofibular ligament.

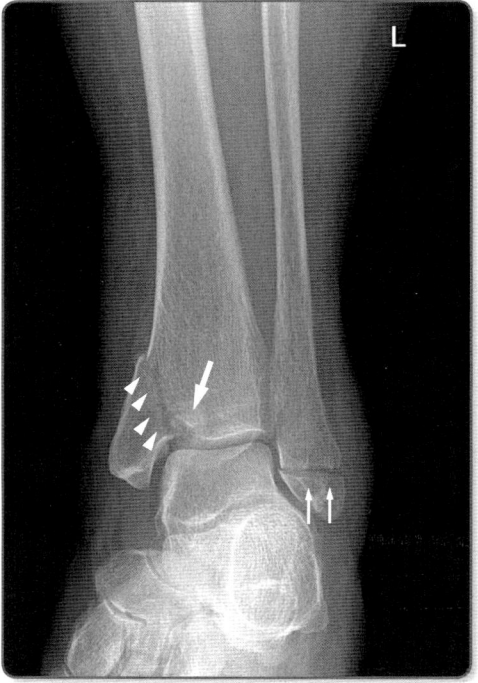

Figure 5.1 Anteroposterior radiograph of a supination–adduction ankle fracture with a typical horizontal lateral malleolus fracture distal to the syndesmosis level (small arrows) and a vertical medial malleolus fracture (arrowheads). Note the impaction of the anteromedial aspect of the tibial plafond (large arrow).

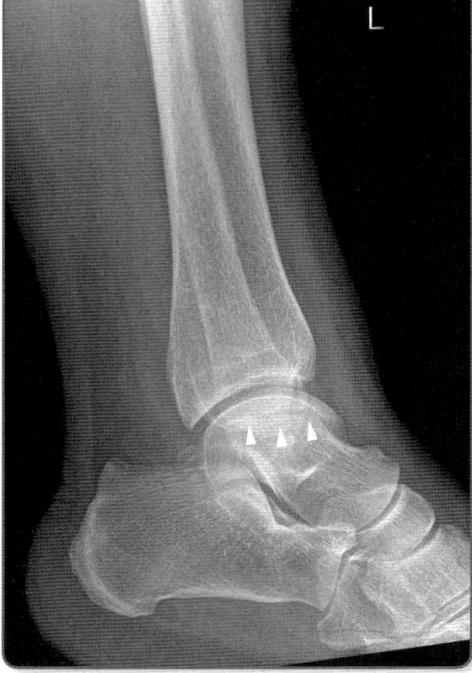

Figure 5.2 Lateral ankle radiograph of the same patient as in Figure 4.1 showing the low, horizontal lateral malleolus fracture (arrowheads).

Table 5.3 Stages and injuries of pronation–abduction PAB ankle fractures

Stage I	Rupture of the deltoid ligament or medial malleolus fracture
Stage II	Rupture of the AITFL the interosseous membrane and the PITFL
Stage III	Spiral or oblique fracture of the lateral malleolus above the syndesmosis

AITFL, anterior inferior tibiofibular ligament; PITFL, posterior inferior tibiofibular ligament; PAB, pronation–abduction; SAD, supination–adduction.

Deltoid ligament injuries cannot be excluded solely in the absence of medial-sided swelling and ecchymosis. The presence of these signs is only indicative and not evidence of significant ligamentous injury.

Disproportionate to the mechanism of injury anterolateral ankle pain, is the most specific symptom of syndesmotic disruption. The single leg hop test is the most sensitive but cannot be carried out in the acute phase. Equally, the dorsiflexion-external rotation (Kleiger's) and the squeeze (Hopkin's) test can be very painful or cause further displacement of the fracture. The intraoperatively performed hook (Cotton's) test is more useful in determining whether syndesmosis needs fixing or not. The lateral ligamentous complex is assessed with the anterior drawer and the talar tilt tests, which have increased sensitivity and specificity 4–7 days after the injury.

Tibialis posterior interposition may prevent anatomic reduction of the medial malleolus fracture. Tendon ruptures and ankle fractures may coexist or present with similar clinical picture. Examination of the neurovascular condition of the foot and the soft tissue envelope at regular intervals is essential, particularly if operative treatment is contemplated.

Investigations

The first-line investigations of an ankle injury are anteroposterior, mortise and lateral ankle radiographs. They are requested when the Ottawa ankle rules criteria are being met. Ambiguous history, inconclusive clinical examination, other distracting injuries and inability to communicate with the patient are also indications to obtain ankle radiographs. Persistent pain and swelling for more than 5–7 days warrant investigation.

PAB I and PER I injuries are indistinguishable on radiographs. The lateral malleolus fracture in PAB III injuries lies on the sagittal plane with an inferior-medial to superior-lateral direction. There may be lateral cortex comminution or a butterfly fragment. The medial malleolus fracture is usually transverse in PAB and vertical in SAD fractures.

When deltoid ligament injury is suspected, in the presence of a lateral malleolus fracture, gravity or stress views are indicated to assess ankle stability. The former is more reliable and better tolerated by the patients but tend to overestimate medial clear space widening and consequently ankle instability.

Posterior malleolus fractures, articular impaction and osteochondral fractures are better studied with CT scans than plain radiographs. MRI is valuable in evaluating soft tissue injuries.

Treatment

The fracture type and more specifically its stability dictate treatment. Displacement that is likely to cause functional restriction and inability of the joint to withstand routine forces without displacing mandate reduction and operative treatment. It is imperative that talotibial congruency is restored as soon as possible, in order to prevent further damage to the articular cartilage, the neurovascular structures and the soft tissue envelope.

Open fractures require meticulous wash out, surgical debridement and timely commencement of antibiotics. Definitive internal fixation is safe and effective practice if the joint is not heavily contaminated. An ankle spanning external fixator can be applied in open or unstable fractures when definitive treatment is contraindicated or expected to delay. Surgical incisions and clean or minimally contaminated wounds can be closed, whereas contaminated wounds are closed at a later stage or left to heal by secondary intention.

SAD I fractures can be treated with immobilisation in a cast or boot for 6–8 weeks with weight-bearing allowed after 1–2 weeks. Lateral malleolus fractures of considerable size can be fixed with screws, tension band or a plate. SAD II fractures with a displaced medial malleolus fragment render the ankle unstable, requiring reduction and fixation, which can be accomplished preferably with a buttress plate or screws. The screws are positioned perpendicular to the fracture line to provide adequate fixation. Washers distribute compression forces across a larger area; therefore they can be used in poor quality bone. Disimpaction, bone grafting and fixation of the anteromedial tibial plafond depression should aim at anatomic restoration of the articular surface.

Treatment of nondisplaced PAB I fractures is similar to this of PER I. Percutaneous or arthroscopically assisted reduction and fixation of the medial malleolus fracture may be negated by interposition of periosteum or the tibialis posterior tendon at the fracture site. Significant tibial plafond impaction in PAB III fractures is managed as in SAD II fractures.

Disruption of the syndesmosis requires reduction and fixation following the fixation of the main fragments. Regardless of whether screws or suture-button devices are used, syndesmosis needs to be properly reduced before it is fixed. There is no consensus about the optimum method of stabilisation, number and material of the screws, number of cortices engaged, weight-bearing restrictions, need for and timing of implant removal. Positional screws at the level of the syndesmosis are regarded as the gold standard. Overtightening of the syndesmosis screws may distort the distal fibula and result in widening of the lateral clear space.

Complications

Nonoperative treatment should aim at early mobilisation to prevent muscle atrophy, joint stiffness and reduced range of motion resulting from prolonged immobilisation until the fracture unites. Loss of anatomic reduction can lead to painful nonunion and mandate operative treatment. The risk of thromboembolic disease in patients with lower limb injuries treated in a plaster cast has been reported in the range of 1–20%.

Wound problems occur in 4–5% of operatively treated fractures. Deep infection complicates 1–2% of the cases with an up to ten-fold increase in diabetic patients. Diabetic peripheral neuropathy has been identified as an independent predictor for postoperative infection. Failure of implants may lead to revision of fixation. Post-traumatic arthritic changes may appear as early as 18 months after the injury, especially in nonanatomically reduced fractures. However, radiological changes do not always correlate with the functional level and the patient-reported outcome.

Further reading

Donken CC, Al-Khateeb H, Verhofstad MH, van Laarhoven CJ. Surgical versus conservative interventions for treating ankle fractures in adults. Cochrane Database Syst Rev 2012:CD008470.

Gardner MJ, Demetrakopoulos D, Briggs SM, Helfet DL, Lorich DG. The ability of the Lauge-Hansen classification to predict ligament injury and mechanism in ankle fractures: an MRI study. J Orthop Trauma 2006; 20:267–272.

Scolaro JA, Marecek G, Barei DP. Management of syndesmotic disruption in ankle fractures: A critical analysis review. JBJS Rev 2014; 2:e4.

Related topics of interest

- *Topic 3* Ankle – Achilles tendon ruptures
- *Topic 4* Ankle: supination– and pronation–external rotation fractures
- *Topic 6* Ankle – talar fractures

6 Ankle: talar fractures

Key points

- Talar fractures are relatively uncommon but are difficult to treat and potentially devastating to foot and ankle function
- Treating these fractures presents a significant challenge for orthopaedic surgeons
- Each fracture should be approached with a thorough understanding of the fracture pattern
- The prognosis is dependent on the affected area and the fracture displacement

Epidemiology

Talar fractures account for 3% of all foot and ankle fractures. The interest in talar fractures started during World War II when Aviator's astragalus was described by HG Anderson. Approximately 50% of these fractures are due to high-energy mechanical accidents such as car accidents. The average age of presentation is 30 years old, with a higher incidence in men than women. Talar fractures can occur in the head, neck, body and the lateral processes. Talar head fractures are very rare (10%), whereas talar neck (50%) and body fractures (40%) occur more frequently.

Pathophysiology

The talus is devoid of any muscular attachments and two thirds of its surface is covered with articular cartilage. The blood supply to the talar body is retrograde via the artery of the tarsal canal and medial calcaneal branches (from the posterior tibial artery), and from the anterior tibial artery via the artery of tarsal sinus, along with variable anastomotic contribution from the perforating peroneal artery. The blood supply to the body of the talus can be compromised following a displaced talar neck fracture leading to avascular necrosis with devastating consequences.

Talus fractures are often the result of high-energy injuries, such as falls from ladders and car accidents. Hyperdorsiflexion and axial loading of the foot against the tibia results in a talar neck fracture. The body of the talus is wider anteriorly than posteriorly, and therefore inversion and hyperplantar flexion of the foot can result in a fracture of the talar body.

Clinical assessment

A detailed history and a thorough clinical examination is essential. Patients present with high-energy injuries of foot and ankle. The patient's skin should be assessed for ischaemia and signs of an open fracture; and a neurovascular examination should be performed to rule out compartment syndrome.

Investigations

A radiographic assessment (**Figures 6.1** and **6.2**) is necessary to confirm the location, pattern and displacement of talar fractures. Plain anteroposterior (AP) radiographs of the ankle can identify the talar dome fractures and Hawkins' sign (a subchondral linear radiolucency on the Talar dome). Talar neck fractures are better analysed using the

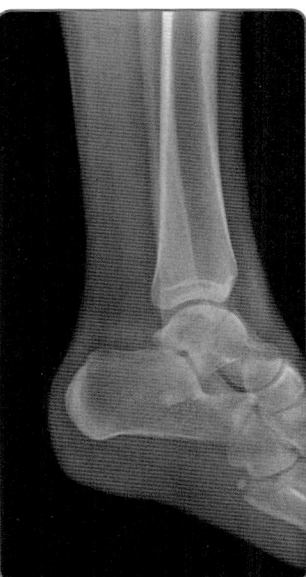

Figure 6.1 Preoperative lateral radiograph demonstrating a displaced talar body fracture.

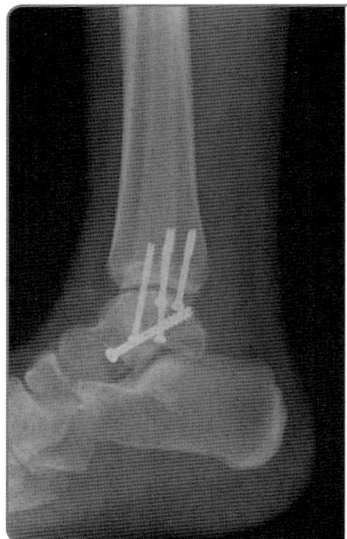 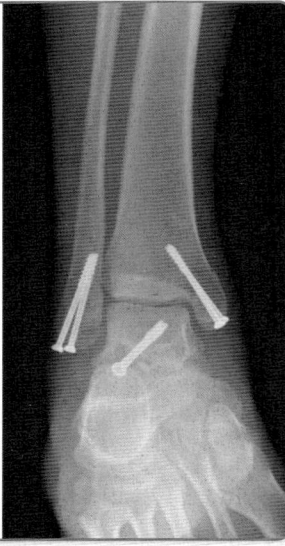

Figure 6.2 Postoperative AP and lateral radiographs demonstrating fixation of the talar body fracture with cannulated screw after medial malleolar osteotomy.

Canale view (described by Canale and Kelly) when the foot is in maximum plantar flexion position with a 15° internal rotation. The X-ray tube is tilted 75° cephalad from the surface of the table. This view enables identification of any displacement or malreduction of the neck of the talus.

CT scans are helpful to better understand the location, displacement and comminution of fractures of the talar body. An MRI is more appropriate for examining osteochondral fractures and for evaluation of avascular necrosis (AVN) in talar neck and body fractures as early as 3 weeks following injury.

Classification

Talar fractures are classified, according to the anatomical location: head, neck and body (**Table 6.1**).

Talar neck fractures were subdivided further by Hawkins (1970), and later modified by Canale and Kelly (1978) based on the displacement of the fracture and involvement of the tibiotalar, subtalar and talonavicular (TN) joints. Hawkins' classification for the neck of talus fractures takes into account the displacement of fracture and subluxation or dislocation of the joints around the talus. This classification is significantly prognostic (the risk of AVN of talus can be predicted using Hawkins' classification):
- Type 1 – undisplaced fractures
- Type 2 – displaced fractures with involvement of subtalar joint
- Type 3 – involve both subtalar and tibiotalar joints
- Type 4 – (added later by Kelly and Canale) includes type 3 fractures along with TN joint subluxation or dislocation, and carries the worst prognosis

Talar body fractures were divided into five types by Sneppen et al., on the basis of location and fracture pattern. These include:
- Osteochondral fractures
- Shear fractures
- Posterior tubercle fractures (more commonly posterolateral process)
- Lateral process fractures (also known as Snowboarder's ankle)
- Crush fractures

Treatment

Treatment of talar fractures varies according to the location, displacement and involvement of the articular surface.

Undisplaced talar head fractures without an articular step are treated in a below the knee nonweight-bearing cast for 8–12 weeks.

Table 6.1 Features of different types of talar fractures

Type	Incidence (%)	Classification	Incidence of AVN	Mechanism of injury	Treatment options	Site-specific complications
Head	10%	Nondisplaced Displaced fracture +/− TN subluxation	< 10% AVN of talar head	Axial compression on a plantar flexed foot	Nonweight-bearing cast for 6–12 weeks ORIF if there is articular step or TN joint instability	AVN of talar head (<10%) TN arthritis Midfoot instability
Neck	50%	Hawkins classification Type 1 Type 2 Type 3 Type 4	AVN of talar body < 10% 20–50% 85% 100%		Nonweight-bearing cast for 6–12 weeks for type 1 ORIF (for types 2, 3 and 4)	AVN of talar body Nonunion Malunion
Body	40%	Sneppen classification Osteochondral dome fracture Shear fracture Posterior process (Shepard's fracture) Lateral process (Snowboarder's ankle) Comminuted fracture	Body fracture without dislocation: 10% Body fracture with dislocation: 25%		Excision, drilling or curettage of the small osteochondral fractures ORIF Nonweight-bearing cast Transarticular external fixation or arthrodesis	Post-traumatic Osteoarthritis AVN of talar body

AVN, avascular necrosis; ORIF, open reduction and internal fixation; TN, talonavicular.

Displaced articular fractures with or without subluxation of the TN joint are treated by open reduction and internal fixation. For comminuted fractures, external fixation using ligamentotaxis can be advocated.

Treatment of talar neck fractures depends on the displacement of the fracture. Significantly displaced fractures with subluxation or dislocation of the talus resulting in skin ischaemia need to be treated as an emergency. There is no convincing evidence in the literature on the timing of surgery and incidence of avascular necrosis. It has been shown, however, that open fractures and comminuted fractures carry the least good prognosis.

Hawkins' type 1 talar neck fractures can be treated with a below the knee nonweight-bearing cast for 8–12 weeks with follow-up radiographs to ensure the fracture remains undisplaced. Displaced talar neck fractures (Hawkins' classification types 2, 3 and 4) are treated by anatomic reduction and internal fixation to reduce the risk of AVN and nonunion. Open reduction can be performed by anteromedial or anterolateral (or combined) approaches and internal fixation is by anterior to posterior, or posterior to anterior screw placement. Postoperatively, a nonweight-bearing cast is advocated until there is radiological evidence of healing. Follow-up radiographs are taken to look for Hawkins' sign (a subchondral linear radiolucency on the talar dome in the AP radiograph of ankle).

Osteochondral fractures of the talar dome are treated by excision, drilling or curettage of the small osteochondral fractures and fixation of the large fragments. Open reduction and internal fixation is performed for displaced shear fractures with an articular step of > 2 mm. A nonweight-bearing cast is advocated for 8–12 weeks for posterior and lateral process fractures, and excision of the fragment if symptomatic after nonoperative treatment. Comminuted talar body fractures are treated with either transarticular external fixation or arthrodesis (joint fusion).

Complications

The talus participates in various articulations and the risk of post-traumatic osteoarthritis is high following displaced fractures. There is also significant risk of AVN depending on the location and displacement of the fracture in the talus, especially in cases of talar neck fractures. Hawkins' classification of 'fracture neck of talus,' helps with predicting the risk of AVN and osteoarthritis. Other fracture complications include malunion, nonunion and arthrofibrosis.

Talar head fractures can result in AVN of the head in approximately 10% of cases. Midfoot osteoarthritis or instability can also result. Talar body fractures result in similar complications.

Further reading

Ahmad J1, Raikin SM. Current concepts review: talar fractures. Foot Ankle Int 2006; 27:475–482.

Higgins TF1, Baumgaertner MR. Diagnosis and treatment of fractures of the talus: a comprehensive review of the literature. Foot Ankle Int 1999; 20:595–605.

Related topics of interest

- *Topic 3* Ankle: Achilles tendon ruptures
- *Topic 4* Ankle: supination and pronation external rotation fractures
- *Topic 5* Ankle: supination–adduction and pronation–abduction fractures

7 Bone grafts

Key points

- Bone grafts have osteosynthetic, osteoconductive or osteogenic properties
- They are classified as autogenic, allogenic and synthetic substances
- Autografts are the gold standard but there is limited availability
- Graft substitutes are becoming more popular, especially injectable cement forms

Definition

A bone graft is a substance used to replace bone that has structural, osteoconductive (provides a scaffold for bone growth), osteogenic (introduces osteocytes and stem cells) or osteoinductive (contains growth factors that stimulate osteogenic cells already present) properties.

Bone grafts can be broadly classified into autogenic, allogenic and synthetic substances.

Autograft

This is the gold standard, however, they are in limited supply and are associated with donor site morbidity.

Cancellous grafts

These have optimum osteoconductive, inductive and genic properties, but they provide little initial structural strength. Examples include iliac crest, distal radius and proximal ulna grafts.

Impaction grafting using cancellous chips can be used to provide structural strength in revision surgery, e.g. revision hip replacement.

Cortical grafts

Although revascularisation takes longer with this type of graft, they provide initial stability. Being compact bone, this type of graft has less surface area for scaffold function and less inductive and genic material, therefore a cortico-cancellous graft, e.g. tricortical iliac crest grafts, is used more often than a pure cortical graft.

Vascularised grafts

These overcome some of the disadvantages of cortical grafts due to its quick incorporation and the ability to bring osteogenic and inductive material to the region. Examples include free fibular grafts.

Bone marrow aspirate

These are used to introduce osteogenic cells because an aspirate contains stem cells to the ratio of 1 osteoprogenitor cell to every 50,000 nucleated cells in the bone marrow.

Allograft

These are used when a large quantity of bone graft is required. Compared to autografts, allografts have lower osteogenic potential, a higher immunogenicity and may transmit disease, especially HIV and hepatitis C. When an allograft is obtained from a bone bank, it is processed in one of three ways: fresh, fresh frozen or freeze dried.

- Fresh grafts are highly immunogenic and carry risk of infection; therefore they are rarely used
- Fresh frozen grafts are most commonly used. They are tested for infection and also retain their structural strength
- Freeze dried grafts are the least immunogenic and can be stored at room temperature. However, they lose their strength over time, and therefore are not used as structural graft

Bone graft substitute

Calcium sulphate

This is the same substance as plaster of Paris. Due to its rapid resorption rates, it does not provide strength or structural support but it is useful as a carrier of antibiotics for treating bone infection. It is reabsorbed by a process of dissolution over a period of 5–7 weeks, but its properties can be altered by the addition of bone morphogenetic protein (BMP) or hydroxyapatite to increase its osteoinductive properties or prolong its reabsorption rate.

Calcium phosphate

Its use in cement form is growing in popularity. Similar to acrylic cement, it is a mixture of a powder containing monocalcium phosphate, tricalcium phosphate, calcium carbonate and liquid sodium phosphate. The paste sets in 10–15 minutes, and in 48 hours it has a compressive strength equal to that of cancellous bone. It is an almost nonexothermic reaction as no polymerisation happens. Its uses include bone defect filling where some structural support is required, i.e. in tibial plateau fractures, and to augment bone strength when using pedicle screws in spinal surgery.

Ceramics

These are formed when natural salts are subjected to a very high-temperature (sintering) to form highly crystalline material, e.g. tricalcium phosphate and hydroxyapatite.

Hydroxyapatite

This is produced from the exoskeleton of marine coral and has a porosity similar to that of cancellous bone and a very slow resorption rate.

In its natural marine form it is calcium carbonate. The carbonate is substituted in the manufactured form with phosphate to make coralline hydroxyapatite. It has high compressive strength but is brittle and has a low tensile strength.

Tricalcium phosphate

Its compressive strength is just less than that of cancellous bone, and it has the same uses as hydroxyapatite.

Demineralised bone matrix

This is prepared by removing the mineralised parts of cadaveric bone by acid extraction, leaving behind collagen, other proteins and a variable quantity of growth factors such as BMP. BMP availability is small and varies from batch to batch, and the sterilisation process also affects its availability. It acts mainly as an osteoconductor.

Collagen matrices (with incorporated graft substitutes)

Purified bovine Type I collagen into which substances such as hydroxyapatite is incorporated. Bone marrow can be added to provide osteogenic cells.

Bone morphogenic proteins

Also known as osteogenic proteins, BMP was originally obtained by extraction from cortical bone. It is now made from recombinant DNA technology and called 'recombinant human BMP' (rhBMP).

BMP2 and BMP7 are commercially available and produced by recombinant DNA technology. BMP reduces the risk of nonunion and promote faster bone healing.

A summary of the different types of bone grafts and their properties is shown in **Table 7.1**.

Method of incorporation of bone grafts

Following bone grafting, the process of incorporating the graft follows these steps, rather like the bone healing process:
- Haematoma formation around the graft
- Inflammation
- Vascular ingrowth
- Focal osteoclastic resorption
- Intramembranous and/or endochondral ossification on graft surface

Current concepts

There has been a huge surge in interest in osteogenic proteins since the discovery of BMPs. The current effort is to combine the different types of graft options to provide all the important properties of bone graft (osteoconductive, osteoinductive and osteogenic) along with initial stability and strength.

Bone grafts

Table 7.1 Bone grafts and their properties

Name	Type of graft	Osteoconductive	Osteoinductive	Osteogenic	Structural support	Other features
Cancellous graft	Autograft	Yes	Yes	Yes	No – except in impaction grafting	
Cortical graft	Autograft	Yes – but less than cancellous	Yes – but less than cancellous	Yes – but less than cancellous	Yes	
Vascularised graft	Autograft	Yes	Yes	Yes	Yes	
Bone marrow aspirate	Autograft	No	Yes	Yes	No	
Fresh allograft	Allograft	Yes	Yes	Yes	Yes	Highly immunogenic and risk of infection so rarely used
Fresh frozen	Allograft	Yes	Yes	Yes	Yes	Most commonly used. Tested for infections
Freeze dried	Allograft	Yes	No	No	No	Least immunogenic, stored at room temperature
Calcium sulphate	Substitute	Yes	No	No	No	Resorbed in 5–7 weeks. Antibiotics and osteoinductive material can be carried
Calcium phosphate	Substitute	Yes	No	No	Yes – similar to cancellous bone	Used as cement
Hydroxyapatite	Substitute	Yes	No	No	Yes – high compressive but brittle	Ceramic
Tricalcium phosphate	Substitute	Yes	No	No	Yes – less than cancellous bone	Ceramic
Demineralised bone matrix	Substitute	Yes	Yes – has variable small amounts of BMP	No	No	From acid extraction of mineralised parts
Recombinant human morphogenetic proteins	Substitute	No	Yes	Yes	No	Made from recombinant DNA technology

Abbreviations: BMP, bone morphogenetic protein

Further reading

Keating JF1, McQueen MM. Substitutes for autologous bone graft in orthopaedic trauma. J Bone Joint Surg Br 2001; 83:3–8.

Pape HC, Evans A, Kobbe P. Autologous bone graft: properties and techniques. Orthop Trauma 2010; 24:S36–40.

Related topics of interest

- Topic 8 Bone loss – options for reconstruction
- Topic 9 Bone structure and physiology
- Topic 35 Fracture healing

8 Bone loss – options for reconstruction

Key points

- Causes of bone loss include trauma, infection, tumour, natural development and iatrogenesis
- The initial management of traumatic bone loss follows Advanced Trauma Life Support (ATLS) principles
- Limb salvage versus amputation should be considered
- Options of management of bone loss includes acute shortening, autologous nonvascularised bone graft structural/nonstructural, membrane-induced techniques, vascularised free fibular bone graft, bone transport, structural allograft and endoprosthetic replacement

Causes of bone loss

Trauma is the leading cause of bone loss, but there are also a number of conditions where there can be loss of bone and the need for reconstruction. These include:

- Trauma – open fractures with bone loss; nonunions, especially those that are infected
- Infection – osteomyelitis, prosthetic and implant infection
- Tumour – postresection, limb salvage surgery
- Congenital/developmental – such as hip dysplasia, proximal focal femoral deficiency, pseudoarthrosis, e.g. tibia, clavicle
- Iatrogenic – osteolysis following joint arthroplasty

Classification

Robinson et al. classified severity of bone loss by modifying the Winquist and Hansen classification (**Table 8.1**). However, bone loss is often more usefully classified according to the condition causing the bone loss, e.g. Paprosky classification for bone loss around total hip replacement.

Initial management of traumatic bone loss

The initial management and stabilisation of a patient with traumatic bone loss is based on the ATLS principles, because they are mostly high-energy injuries.

The decision and timing on how to manage and treat long bone fracture(s) associated with major trauma has changed over the years from 'early total care', to 'damage control surgery' and currently to 'early appropriate care' (EAC). EAC is based on the adequacy of resuscitation of the patient and uses biochemical markers including lactate <4.0 mmol/L, pH ≥7.25 or a base excess ≥5.5 mmol/L. If these markers were maintained definitive treatment of fractures could proceed in one sitting if required.

Table 8.1 Classification of severity of bone loss (data from Robinson et al, 1995)

Grade	Maximal bone loss	Maximum length of bone loss (cm)
Trivial	Wedge <25%	
Minor	Wedge 25–50%	
	Wedge >50% but <100%	<2.5
Moderate	Wedge >50% but <100%	2.5–10
	Circumferential	<2.5
Severe	Wedge >50% but <100%	>10
	Circumferential	>2.5

Initial management of the bone loss depends on:
- General condition of the patient
- Extent of soft tissue injury
- Amount of bone loss
- Availability of expertise and resources
- Patient's wishes

In the more severe cases, the first question to ask is whether the limb can be salvaged or not. Scores such as mangled extremity severity score (MESS), the limb salvage index (LSI) and the predictive salvage index (PSI) help in making this decision, though recent studies have cast doubt on their usefulness.

Initial stabilisation ranges from external splintage to surgical splintage. External fixators, intramedullary nailing and plating can all the use in initial stabilisation.

Amputation versus limb salvage

Indications for amputation include major muscle loss, severe contamination and vascular injuries where revascularisation is not possible. Posterior tibial nerve injury and associated insensate foot used to be an indication as well which seems to have been refuted by literature.

Even where limb salvage is an option, sometimes the patient is better served by a surgery such as amputation and prosthetic limb fitting where the patient can return to rehab in a short time. It should be considered whether it is better to go through the process of reconstruction which may be more labour intensive and demands more patient motivation.

An amputation may not be acceptable to the patient and there may be other factors such as a lack of good prosthetic replacement, social stigma and that an amputation might alter the social and work style of the patient. Studies show that in the long run reconstruction is more cost effective than amputation.

Options for reconstruction in bone loss

Acute shortening

The acceptable shortening depends on the bone and surrounding soft tissues. Excessive shortening causes a kink in the blood vessels leading to vascular compromise, distal oedema and venous occlusion, e.g. up to 5 cm of acute shortening has been described in the tibia. Acute shortenings can be combined at the same time or later with bone transport to regain length.

Autologous nonvascularised bone graft – nonstructural/structural

This can be used for bone defects of up to 3 cm. This may be in the form of a cancellous bone graft in cases where there is continuity of bone or structural graft such as tricortical illiac crest graft or fibular strut graft. A special situation is the use of the proximal fibula to reconstruct the distal radius due to similarity in shape.

Masquelet technique of induced membrane

Antibiotic-impregnated cement beads or spacers are used for local antibiotics and maintaining a well-defined void to allow for later placement of graft, providing structural support, offloading the implant, and inducing the formation of a bio-membrane. This membrane prevents graft resorption and improves vascularity and corticalisation. It has been described that, after the initial placement of the antibiotic-impregnated spacer, an interval of 1 month but <2 is best for development and maturation of a biologically active membrane.

Bone transport distraction osteogenesis

Ilizarov discovered distraction osteogenesis by chance when a nonunion which was supposed to be treated by compression osteogenesis was in fact distracted. He developed his 'Law of tension stress' which showed that under the effect of slow and gradual distraction, bone and soft tissue including blood vessels, nerves, and skin would regenerate.

The principles are:
- Use of circular external fixator using tensioned wires – allows early weight bearing compared to monolateral fixators
- Low-energy corticotomy – such that endosteal and periosteal blood supply is maintained

- Distraction osteogenesis – used to treat shortness, deformity, bone loss, osteomyelitis
- Latency period – first 5–10 days where no distraction takes place
- Bone transport – Each segment is lengthened by 1 mm per day (0.25 mm × 4 mm) and up to 18 cm per segment can be achieved
- Consolidation phase – the patients continues walking in fixator that allows micromotion ossification of the regenerate
- Removal of fixator – 1 cm of lengthening takes about a month

Free vascularised fibula transfer

This is another option in bone defects >12 cm. It is important to leave enough bone at the distal end such that the ankle is stable, or conduct distal tibiofibular fusion. In cases where there is a soft tissue defect, this can be harvested along with a strip of skin overlying it called the free vascularised septocutaneous flap.

This surgery has fallen into disrepute due to significant donor site morbidity.

Bulk structural allograft

This option involves no donor site morbidity, however it is associated with a prolonged period of healing and fractures in the allograft.

Endoprosthetic replacement

Where the bone loss is next to or involving joints this is an option that can be considered to retain mobility, e.g. proximal or distal femoral replacements. Occasionally in segmental bone loss these may be used as an internal spacer device or definitive treatment, e.g. mid-shaft humeral bone loss.

Methods of initial stabilisation

Plating

In very small defects plating can be used especially in small wedge fractures.

Intramedullary fixation

This can be used to maintain the length in segmental bone loss, and depending on the extent of bone loss, can be combined later with bone graft or transport over a nail. It can also be used following acute shortening and where later transport over the nail is planned.

External fixation – ring fixators

In acute shortening, ring fixators carry the advantage that the bone transport can be carried out at a site distant to the injury that is more conducive to bone regeneration.

External ring fixators can be combined with a nail for transport over a nail. They can also be used to maintain length at the bone defect and bone transport carried out – typically in defects >5 cm where later the docking site may need to be opened and bone grafted.

Further reading

Keating JF, Simpson AH, Robinson CM. The management of fractures with bone loss. J Bone Joint Surg Br 2005; 87:142–150.

Masquelet AC, Fitoussi F, Begue T, Muller GP. Reconstruction of the long bones by the induced membrane and spongy autograft. Annales de Chirurgie Plastique et Esthetique 2000; 45:346–353.

Pipitone PS, Rehman S. Management of traumatic bone loss in the lower extremity. Orthop Clin North Am 2014; 45:469–482.

Robinson CM, McLauchlan G, Christie J, McQueen MM, Court-Brown CM. Tibial fractures with bone loss treated by primary reamed intramedullary nailing. J Bone Joint Surg Br 1995; 77:906-13.

Related topics of interest

- *Topic 7* Bone grafts
- *Topic 16* Crush injuries and crush syndrome
- *Topic 17* Damage control orthopaedics and trauma physiology

Bone structure and physiology

Key points

- Bone plays an important role in mineral homeostasis. Bone houses 99% of an individual's total body calcium
- The bone marrow located in the cancellous bone provides the haematopoietic elements, including erythrocytes, leukocytes and platelets
- Bone provides mechanical support, giving rise to body shape, protecting internal organs and facilitating movement by providing muscle attachments

Types of bone

Long bones form via endochondral ossification, the process by which bone forms in replacement of a cartilage model. Undifferentiated cells secrete a cartilage matrix and differentiate into chondrocytes. This is followed by mineralisation of the matrix and vascular invasion which brings about the osteoprogenitor cells. Osteoclasts reabsorb the calcified cartilage and osteoblasts produce bone. This form of bone formation applies not only to long bones but also to physeal growth and fracture callus.

Flat bones form via intramembranous ossification, the process by which bone forms without a cartilage model. Layers of undifferentiated mesenchymal cells differentiate into osteoblasts and start to produce organic matrix which undergo mineralisation. This form of bone formation applies to embryonic flat bones and distraction osteogenesis.

Anatomy

Long bones are made of three regions: the diaphysis, the metaphysis and the epiphysis.

The diaphysis is made of thick cortical bone surrounding a central intramedullary canal of trabecular bone. The inner aspect of the cortical bone is known as the endosteum and the outer surface as the periosteum. The periosteum has an outer layer of connective tissue and an inner layer of osteoprogenitor cells (**Figure 9.1**).

The metaphysis is made of trabecular bone surrounded by the thin layer of cortical bone.

The epiphysis is the specialised end of the bone that is involved in articulation. It is made of trabecular bone surrounded by a thin layer of cortical bone. The subchondral region underlines the articular cartilage.

Flat bones including the pelvis, scapula, skull and mandible are made purely of cortical bone with thin layers of trabecular bone in some regions.

Neurovascular supply

Bones receive blood supply from the nutrient arterial system, the metaphyseal–epiphyseal system and the periosteal system (**Figure 9.2**).

The nutrient artery enters the bone via a nutrient foramen. Once it reaches the medullary canal it divides into an ascending and a descending branch. The nutrient artery provides blood supply to the inner two thirds of the cortex. Branches from the nutrient artery run in the Volkmann's canals and Haversian systems. In a child these vessels do not cross the physis. Damage to this system results from intramedullary reaming.

The periarticular vascular supply penetrates the thin cortecis of the physis, metaphysis and epiphysis. Once the growth is complete, the metaphyseal vessels anastomose with the medullary and epiphyseal vessels.

The periosteum provides blood supply to the outer third of the cortex via capillaries at the site of major muscle attachments. Periosteal stripping as a result of fracture or plating damages this system.

In a normal bone the blood flow is centrifugal, from the high-pressure nutrient vessel system to the low-pressure periosteal system. The venous flow is therefore centripetal. In children and also in conditions

Bone structure and physiology

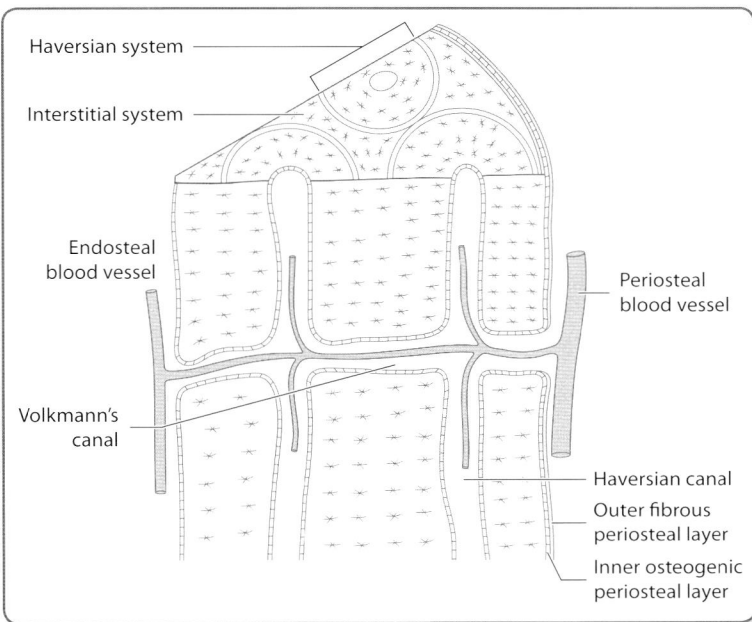

Figure 9.1 Bone structure, showing the periosteum, the endosteum, the Haversian and the interstitial systems.

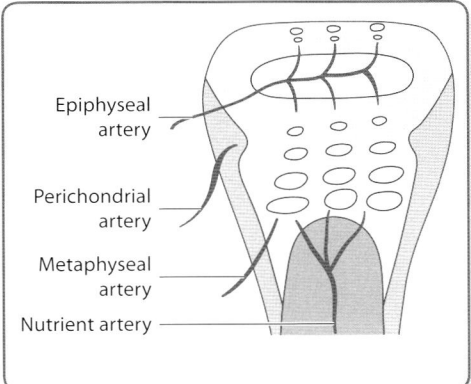

Figure 9.2 Vascular supply to the bone showing diaphyseal, metaphyseal and epiphyseal blood supply.

which result in disruption of the nutrient system the flow is reversed.

Nerves are found in the Haversians' systems and Volkmann's canals. Hilton's law states that the nerve supplying a muscle will also supply the bone to which the muscle is attached. Most of nervous supply is sympathetic and vasomotor and some is sensory which innervates the periosteum and articular ends of the bone.

Bone structure

Macroscopically, bone is either cortical, which is dense and compact, or trabecular, which is a loose network of struts.

Microscopically, bone is either woven, which is primary bone with random orientation of collagen matrix, or lamellar, which is secondary bone resulting from the remodelling of the primary bone. Woven bone therefore is weaker, more flexible and has isotropic characteristics. While lamellar bone is stress oriented, stronger and anisotropic.

The extracellular matrix is 40% organic and 60% mineral. The mineral matrix is made primarily from calcium and phosphate as hydroxyapatite and tricalcium phosphate. The tropocollagen helices give rise to the tensile strength of bone. They are organised in quarter-staggered arrangement with holes between the ends and pore between the fibrils. Mineral crystals form in the holes and pores, giving rise to the compressive strength of bone.

The organic matrix is made of collagen (90% type I), other proteins (osteocalcin, fibronectin, matricellular proteins and phosphoprotein), growth factors (bone morphogenic proteins, transforming growth factor-β, basic fibroblast growth factor, insulin growth factor and interleukins), proteoglycans and water.

Bone has unique cells that interact closely and respond to locally and systemically produced cytokines and hormones as well as physical and mechanical factors, bringing about the understanding of processes, such as remodelling, fracture healing, osteoporosis and pathological lesions.

Osteoblasts

Osteoblasts originate from mesenchymal stem cells, produce bone matrix and regulate osteoclasts. They can differentiate from periosteal membrane cells and marrow stromal cells. The mature osteoblast has a life span of 100 days before turning into a bone-lining cell or an osteocyte. It can also undergo apoptosis. Bone-lining cells are inactive cells that can undergo reactivation into functional osteoblasts.

Osteoblasts have several marker proteins including alkaline phosphotase, osteocalcin, osteonectin and osteopontin. Osteoblasts produce type I collagen and have parathyroid hormone receptors.

Osteocytes

When osteoblasts are embedded in the mineralised matrix they become osteocytes. They reside in lacunar spaces and have neumerus cell processes that lie within the canaliculi communicating with other osteocytes. Inter-osteocytes signalling occurs via complex proteins named gap junctions. There is increasing evidence of the important role of osteocytes in bone homeostasis.

Osteoclasts

Osteoclasts are haematopoietic cells, derived from the monocyte/macrophage lineage. They are multinucleated giants cells that reabsorb bone. They are made from the fusion of multiple mononuclear cells. A process stimulated by the receptor activator for nuclear factor-κ B ligand (RANKL) and macrophage colony-stimulating factors (M-CSF).

Osteoclasts have several marker proteins including tartarate-resistant acid phosphotase (TRAP), calcitonin receptors and cathespin-κ.

When osteoclasts are activated, they attach to bone surfaces and form a sealed enclosure at the bone–osteoclast interface. The plasma membrane within the enclosure forms a highly ruffled border and starts secreting ions and proteases dissolving bone.

Osteoclast activity is primarily governed by RANKL and osteoprotegerin (OPG). The latter is a decoy receptor that binds to and traps RANKL preventing it from differentiating and activating osteoclasts (**Figure 9.3**).

Bone homeostasis

Bone is a living dynamic tissue that is under constant remodelling through the action of its unique cells. The average turnover at adulthood is 5% of the bone mass per year.

In trabecular bone, osteoclasts activity leads to the development of a resorption pit called a Howship lacuna. Osteoblasts fill the defect with new bone matrix. The cement line is the region where resorption stopped and new bone formation begun.

In cortical bone, osteoclasts tunnel through bone with a cutting cone. Blood vessels grow in the defect giving rise to a Haversian system around which new bone is laid down by osteoblasts and is named the osteon (**Figure 9.4**).

Wolff's law states that bone remodels in line with the mechanical stress applied to it. This leads to bone gains where stress is applied. Bone also responds to piezoelectric charges. The compression side is electronegative stimulating osteoblasts while the tension side is electropositive stimulating osteoclasts. The Hueter-Volkmann law states that mechanical factors influence longitudinal growth, remodelling and fracture healing.

Osteoblast control of osteoclast function is well understood. Parathyroid hormone stimulation of osteoblast stimulates the

Bone structure and physiology

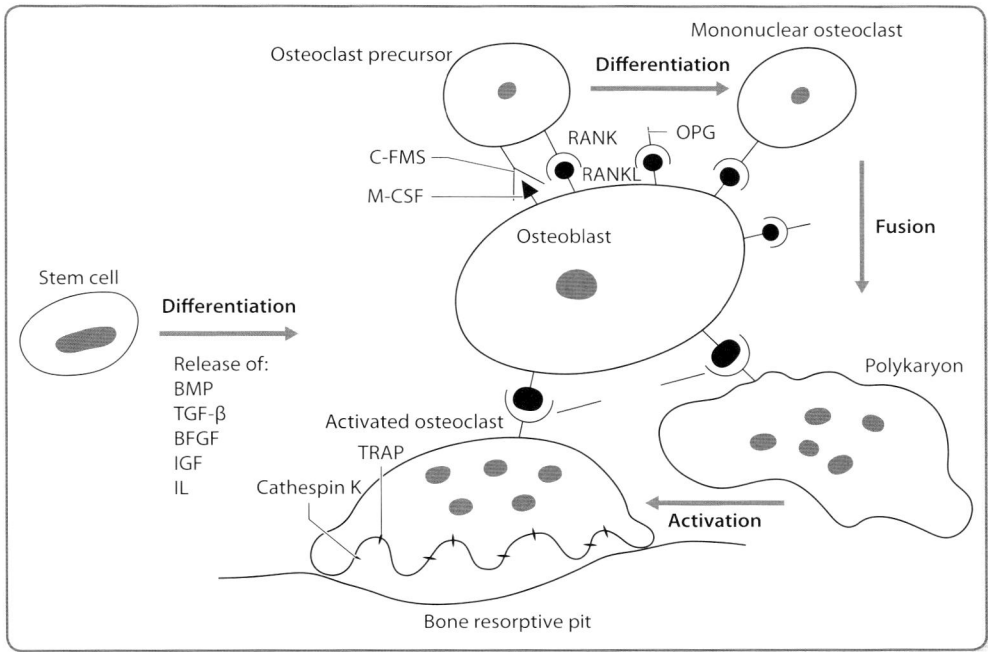

Figure 9.3 Schematic representation of osteoclast–osteoblast interaction. M-CSF, macrophage colony-stimulating factor; C-FMS, colony-stimulating factor 1 receptor; RANK, receptor activator for nuclear factor-κ B; RANKL, receptor activator for nuclear factor-κ B ligand; OPG, osteoprotegerin; TRAP, tartarate-resistant acid phosphatase; BMP, bone morphogenic protein; TGF-β, transforming growth factor-β; bFGF, basic fibroblast growth factor; IGF, insulin growth factor; IL, interleukins.

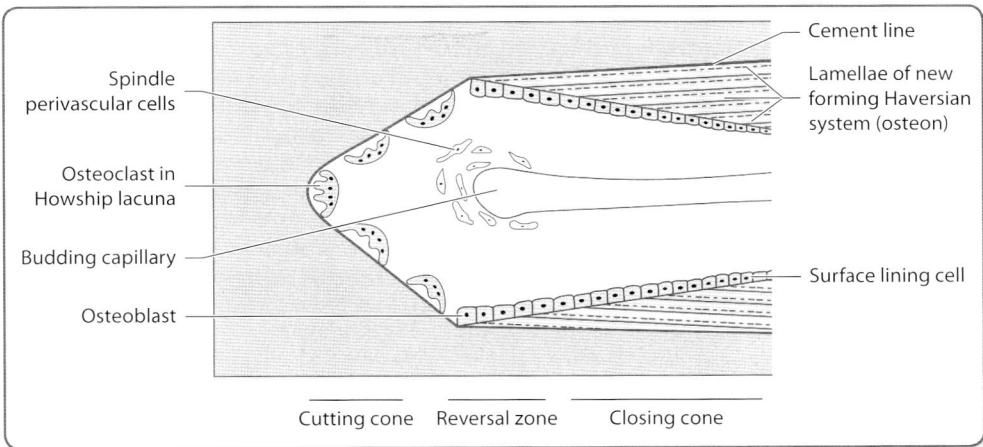

Figure 9.4 Bone remodelling. Osteoclasts are resorbing bone and forming a cutting cone while osteoblasts are building new Haversian systems in the defects created by osteoclasts.

synthesis of M-CSF and RANKL leading to the differentiation and activation of osteoclasts. Osteoblasts also produce OPG which sequesters RANKL. This means that osteoblasts can positively and negatively regulate osteoclasts. Osteoclasts are also affected by serum calcium levels and systemic hormones. Vitamin D and parathyroid hormone stimulate osteoclasts while calcitonin inhibits them.

Osteoclasts regulation of osteoblasts is via bone resorption which leads to the release of growth factors and cytokins that stimulate osteoblast differentiation.

A variety of cell types are able to produce RANKL, each comes into play at certain physiological or pathological condition. Chondrocytes produced RANKL is important in stimulating resorption of mineralised cartilage, a process essential in endochondral bone formation. Osteocytes derived RANKL plays a significant role in physiological bone remodelling. Bone homeostasis is also regulated by various hormones (**Table 9.1**).

Table 9.1 The regulatory effect of various hormones on bone

Hormone	Site of action	Effect
Thyroid hormone	- Physis - Mature bone	- Stimulates chondrocyte growth, type X collagen synthesis and alkaline phosphatise. - Increase resorption
Parathyroid hormone	- Osteoblasts: increase secretion of IL-1, IL-6, M-CSF and RANKL - Kidney: stimulates the conversion of vitamin D3 into its active form - Intestine: indirect action through increasing the production of the active form of vitamin D3	- Increase osteoclasts number and activity leading to bone resorption - Increases calcium resorption and phosphate excretion - Increase calcium absorption
Vitamin D3 (formed following exposure to UVB rays and undergoes hydroxylation in the liver and the kidney before the active form is produced)	- Kidney - Bone	- Increase reabsorption of calcium - Stimulates osteoclasts differentiation and promotes mineralisation of osteoid matrix by osteoblasts
Oestrogen	Hypertrophic zone of physis and the zone of calcification	- Prevents bone loss by decreasing the frequency of bone resorption and remodelling - Crucial in gaining peak bone mass
Growth hormone	- Intestine - Kidney	- Increase calcium absorption - Decrease calcium excretion
Steroids	- Intestine - Bone	- Decrease calcium absorption - Inhibit osteoblasts and decrease collagen synthesis
Calcitonin	Receptors on osteoclasts	Decrease osteoclasts count and activity

IL, interleukins; M-CSF, macrophage colony-stimulating factor; RANKL, receptor activator for nuclear factor-κ B ligand; UVB, ultraviolet B.

Further reading

Buckwalter JA, Glimcher MJ, Cooper RR, et al. Bone biology Part I: Formation, form, modelling and regulation of cell function. J Bone Joint Surg Am 1995; 77:1256–1275.

Buckwalter JA, Glimcher MJ, Cooper RR, et al. Bone biology Part II: Formation, form, modelling and regulation of cell function. J Bone Joint Surg Am 1995; 77:1276–1289.

Miller JD, McCreadie BR, Alford AI, Hankenson KD, Goldstein SA. Form and function of bone. In: Einhorn TA, O'Keefe RJ, Buckwalter JA (Eds). Orthopaedic Basic Science: Foundations of Clinical Practice, 3rd edn. Rosemont, IL: American Academy of Orthopaedic Surgeons 2007:129–159.

Weitzmann MN. The role of inflammatory cytokines, the RANKL/OPG Axis, and the immunoskeletal interface in physiological bone turnover and osteoporosis. Scientifica 2013; 2013:125705.

Related topics of interest

- *Topic 7* Bone grafts
- *Topic 8* Bone loss – options for reconstruction
- *Topic 35* Fracture healing

10 Brachial plexus injury

Key points

- The brachial plexus is formed by the anterior rami of the lower four cervical and first thoracic nerves (C5–C8, T1). These chains of nerves carry signals from the brain to the shoulder, arm and hand
- It has sensory, motor and autonomic out flow function, and provides sensation and facilitates movement of the upper limb [apart from the trapezius muscle which is innervated by the spinal accessory nerve (CN XI)]
- Sympathetic fibers from the first thoracic nerve (T1) provide autonomic function of the upper limb, head and neck, so injury at this level can be associated with Horner's syndrome
- Brachial plexus lesions can lead to severe functional impairment

Epidemiology

Brachial plexus injuries (BPIs) occur unpredictably and vary in presentation and severity. The BPIs can be broadly divided into two groups: obstetric injuries and nonobstetric injuries.

The incident of obstetric-associated injuries is approximately 2:1000 term births in the western world. The risk factors include: shoulder dystonia, gestational diabetes, forceps delivery, vacuum extraction, breech delivery, macrosomia and multiparity. Most infants (75%) present with upper root cervical injury (Erb-Duchenne palsy); 4–5% are bilateral.

The nonobstetric BPIs are much more common than obstetric injuries. The majority of these patients (<90%) are young adults who have been involved in a car or motorcycle accident. Other nonobstetric causes of BPI include: nerve entrapment (as a result of thoracic outlet obstruction), infections (viral plexopathy), radiation (fibrosis, malignant degeneration after radiation), tumors (schwannoma, pulmonary apices) and iatrogenic causes such as axillary or scalene anaesthesia, surgical biopsy, median sternotomy, and intraoperative positioning.

Pathophysiology

The degree of nerve damage varies from partial to complete involvement of the brachial plexus. It varies from a mild stretching of the plexus to a complete nerve transection. The injury may result in a transient weakness to complete paralysis of the limb. In minor BPIs, known as neuropraxia, the plexus is stretched and there is a transient conducting block; however, the axons and nerve sheaths are intact and Wallerian degeneration does not take place distal to the zone of injury. As soon as the block is resolved, nerve function to the target organ will return to normal. These patients usually recover fully with no surgical intervention. The moderate BPIs result from compression and/or traction of the plexus. These result in axon damage (axonotmesis) with or without nerve sheath disruption. Wallerian degeneration will occur distal to the injury, but regeneration in the surviving proximal stump is still possible and should regenerate by 1–4 mm per day. The recovery in these patients is variable from partial to full and may require surgical intervention. In severe types of BPIs (neurotmesis), there is an axonal and nerve sheath disruption. This happens as a result of rupture or avulsion of the nerve root from the spinal cord. These patients almost certainly require surgical intervention, although a successful outcome is not guaranteed.

Clinical assessment

Interpretation of clinical findings of BPI depends on knowledge of peripheral nervous system (PNS) structures and physiology. Multiple spinal nerves innervate extremity muscle groups and their corresponding peripheral nerves. Brachial plexus is a bundle of nerves originating from the lower cervical and upper thoracic spinal cord. It forms a network of the nerves in the posterior triangle, the posterior to the clavicle, and axilla and upper arm. The terminal branches of the brachial plexus are peripheral nerves which supply motor, sensory and autonomic out flow of the upper limb. The BP originates from C5–T1 nerve roots from the spinal cord, but occasionally can have contributions from C4–T2. (**Figure 10.1**).

In obstetric associated BPIs, although an early diagnosis and treatment is imperative for improved long-term outcome, clinical examination of a neonate following a difficult delivery should commence after the first 48 hours in order for the assessment to be reliable. Two main types of BPIs in neonates are Erb's palsy and Klumpke's palsy.

In Erb's palsy [an injury of the upper brachial plexus (C5, C6 nerve root involvement)], the arm is characteristically held in an adducted and internally rotated position with a forearm pronated and hand and wrist flexed (waiter's tip position). The infant is unable to move the arm and the shoulder. In Klumpke's palsy [an injury of the lower brachial plexus (C8, T1)], the intrinsic muscles of the hand are affected as well as the flexor of the wrist and fingers. The classic presentation of Klumpke's palsy is the 'claw hand' where the forearm is supinated and the wrist and fingers are flexed. Patients with Klumpke's palsy might also have constriction of a pupil (miosis) as well as a weak, droopy eyelid (ptosis), both of which are present in Horner's syndrome. These patients may have a decreased sweating tendency (anhidrosis).

BPI should be suspected when examining a patient following a major upper trunk and upper limb injury. A detailed examination of the brachial plexus and its terminal branches can be performed in the emergency department in a few minutes on a co-operative conscious patient. The median, ulnar and radial nerves can be examined by assessing the finger and wrist sensation and motions. The sensory modality of the brachial plexus in the hand can be examined by assessing the sensation of:
- The radial aspect of the palm for the median nerve
- The ulnar aspect of the palm for the ulnar nerve
- The dorsal aspect of the 1st web space for the radial nerve.
- Thumb sensation is supplied by C6, the middle finger by C7 and the little finger by C8

To assess the motor modality of the brachial plexus, we can assess the following ranges of motion to assess the integrity of the relevant nerve root of the brachial plexus:
- C5: shoulder movement in all directions, flexion of elbow (to some degree)
- C6: flexion of elbow, rotation of forearm, flexion of wrist (to some degree)
- C7: mainly a sensory trunk (produces a general loss of movement in the arm, without total paralysis in any given muscle group. Always supplies the latissimus dorsi
- C8: extension and flexion of fingers, flexion of wrist, hand movement
- T1: intrinsic muscles of the hand, e.g. adduction or abduction of fingers

Investigations

A plain radiograph can be useful to diagnose a hemidiaphragm (paralysis due to phrenic nerve involvement), or to rule out a fracture of the clavicle or humerus which can be associated with nerve injuries. Other investigations, such as a high-resolution MRI, can provide a detailed view of the brachial plexus. It is noninvasive and contains no radiation compared with CT myelography. Electromyography and nerve conduction studies are also useful tools, which are cheaper and more accessible. These tests can provide a rapid result and can also assess the nerve conduction modality.

Classification

The brachial plexus can be classified based on different criteria including: anatomical location, age of the patient and type of pathology. The Leffert classification combines the above criteria and categorises BPIs into four types which all have different management approaches and outcomes.

The Leffert classification has the following types (**Table 10.1**):
- Type I injuries are open injuries which require emergency surgical repair; they can be a pure nerve injury or as a result of major trauma associated with vascular injuries, fractures and chest or head injuries. The majority of these injuries are type 4 and 5 injuries based

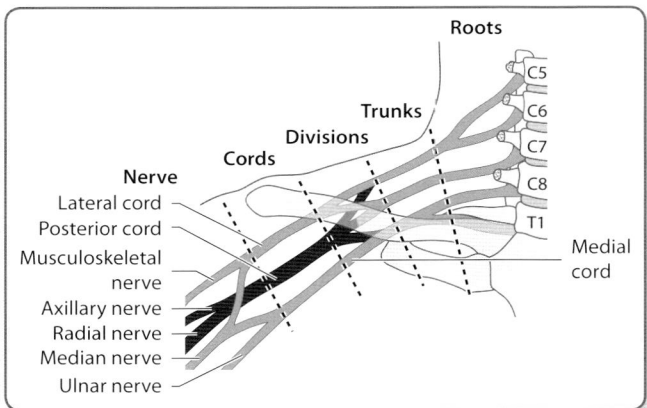

Figure 10.1 Anatomy of the brachial plexus.

Table 10.1 Leffert classification

Type	Description	Subtype
I	Open injuries	
II	Closed injuries	IIa – supraclavicular IIb – infraclavicular IIc – combined
III	Radiation induced	
IV	Obstetric	IVa – Erb's (upper root) IVb – Klumpke (lower root) IVc – mixed

on the Sunderland classification system and may also include segmental loss with multiple nerve roots or a trunk injury, making their management more complicated
- Type II injuries are divided into supraclavicular (IIA), infraclavicular (IIB) or combined (IIC) injuries. These injuries are usually traction type injuries. Type IIa injuries can be also occur pre- or postganglionic injuries, which can have a different presentation and management
- Type III injuries are radiation-induced injuries following head and neck tumor management. These are fibrosis types of injuries
- Type IV injuries are obstetric injuries which can be either an upper trunk injury (Erb's palsy, IVa), lower trunk injury (Klumpke's, IVb) or a mixed injury (IVc).

- Alternatively, the Seddon and Sunderland classifications can be used to assess a peripheral nerve injury (**Table 10.2**):

The Seddon classification categorises the injuries from mild (neuropraxia), moderate (axonotmesis) to severe (neurotmesis). Sunderland classifies nerve injuries as: 1st degree (essentially the same as neuropraxia), 2nd degree (axonotmesis), 3rd degree (axonotmesis plus endoneurium disruptions), 4th degree (axonotmesis plus endo- and perineurium disruption) and 5th degree (neurotmesis or complete transection of the nerve).

Treatment

The single most important factor in achieving a successful outcome is the preservation or restoration of the function of the muscle group which has been lost or compromised due to nerve damage. The type of treatment depends on the mechanism and the type of nerve injury, the duration since the injury occurred, the degree of functional loss and the age of the patients. Broadly speaking, the management can be divided into nonoperative or operative. If the injury of the nerve is due to traction with some conduction loss and minimal functional disability, physiotherapy would be an option. The use of a limb brace can also prevent contractures. In neonates, spontaneous recovery usually occurs and can start within days, but can take

Table 10.2 Seddon and Sunderland classifications

Seddon	Sunderland	Description
Neurapraxia (mild injury)	I	Complete motor paralysis
Axonotmesis (moderate injury)	II	Loss of axonal continuity
Neurotmesis (severe injury)	III	Type II and endoneurium
	IV	Type III and perineurium
	V	Complete transection of an entire trunk

months. Prevention of obstetric injuries is not always possible, as a significant proportion of injuries may occur in utero. Other nonsurgical treatments include a botulinum toxin injection and electrical stimulation to relieve the block and promote axonal firing. Neuromuscular electrical stimulation (NMES) is a treatment used in older children where muscles are stimulated by pulsating, alternating currents. It is usually titrated with guidance from the child to allow muscle contraction without causing pain. Surgery is recommended as an early intervention as the outcomes are best if the repair is undertaken within 3 months of injury. Surgery must be carried out in a specialist surgical unit by a specialist nerve surgeon. The options of surgery include: nerve transfer, nerve grafting, muscle transfer and neurolysis of the scar around the brachial plexus.

Complications

If an intervention is carried out as early as possible and allowed sufficient time to recover, many BPIs in both adults and children recover with no lasting damage. However, some injuries can cause temporary or permanent problems depending on the age of the patient, and the type, location and severity of the injury. BPIs can result in muscle atrophy or paralysis of the muscle group involved. This can lead to stiff joints and reduced function, causing progressive contractures which in turn can cause chronic pain. Bony deformities such as scoliosis or recurrent dislocation of a shoulder can leave the patients with a permanent postural disability.

Further reading

Foster MR. Traumatic brachial plexus injuries. Medscape; 2011.
National Institute for Health and Care Excellence (NICE). Phrenic nerve transfer in brachial plexus injury. Interventional procedures guidance [IPG468]. London: NICE, 2013.
Orebaugh SL, Williams BA. Brachial plexus anatomy: normal and variant. The Scientific World Journal 2009; 9:300–312.

Related topics of interest

- Topic 83 Peripheral nerve injury
- Topic 92 Spine – atlas and axis cervical fractures and dislocations
- Topic 93 Spine – cord injury

11 Classification of fractures

Key points

- Most modern fracture classification systems are based on the location, displacement and number of fracture lines seen on the radiograph
- Some systems require the classification of soft tissue injury associated with fractures which require direct viewing as well as systems that require use of CT, i.e. the Sanders classification of calcaneal fractures
- To classify a fracture, the location of the bone and its morphological characteristics are essential

Types of fracture classification

There are three broad categories of fracture classification systems:
1. Fracture-specific; these classify a given fracture in a single location in the body.
2. Based on the degree of soft tissue injury.
3. The generic fracture classification systems that use a unified methodology to the classification of fractures in all parts of the human body.

The generic or universal classification systems

This is also known as Arbeitsgemeinschaft für Osteosynthesefragen (AO)/Orthopaedic Trauma Association (OTA) classification systems (**Figure 11.1**). The AO/OTA classification was developed through a consensus panel of orthopaedic traumatologists based on the initial classification systems designed and proposed by Müller AO/Association for the study of internal fixation (ASIF) group in Europe and is essentially the only classification in wide use currently.

This classification system uses an alpha-numeric code that allows consistent in detail description of a fracture in a defined terminology that can be applied to most bones within the body. There are five basic steps to follow in order to classify a given fracture using this system, these steps allow localisation and morphological characterisation of every fracture. The first two steps are for localisation of the fracture in the body and the last three steps for the morphological characterisation:

i. **The bone in the body that is fractured.**
Major bones in the body are numbered as follows:

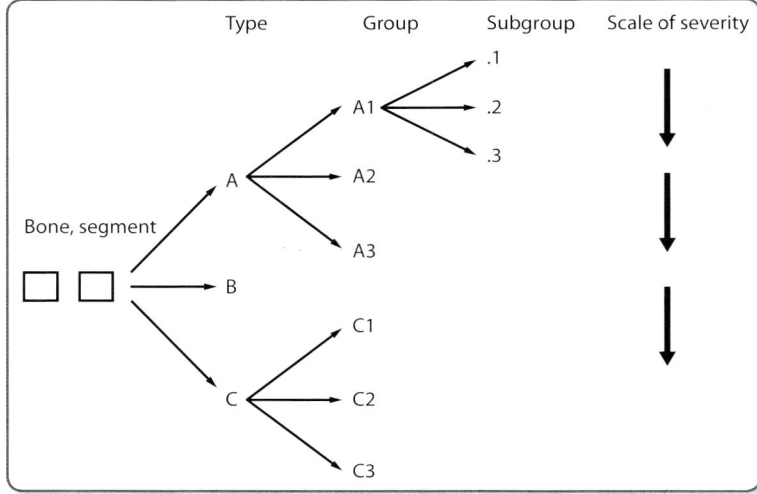

Figure 11.1 AO/OTA classification. As in Group A1, the classifications continue to the subgroup for each of the fracture types and group.

Classification of fractures

1. Humerus
2. Forearm bones (radius and ulna)
3. Femur
4. Tibia and fibular
5. Spine
6. Pelvis
7. Hand
8. Foot
9. All other bone

ii. The location of the fracture in the bone. This identifies a specific segment within the bone. Most long bones are divided into three segments: the proximal segment number 1; the shaft or the diaphyseal segment number 2; and the distal segment number 3. The dividing line between the shaft and the proximal and distal segments is the metaphysis. The tibia and fibular are given the 4th segment called the malleolar segment. For instance, the fracture involving the malleolar segment in either tibia or fibular is given the numeric number 44 (4 for tibia/fibula, 4 for malleolar segment). In the spine, the three segments are the cervical-51, thoracic-52 and the lumbar-53.

iii. The fracture type. Next, each fracture is given a letter (A, B or C) to either describe the joint involvement in a fracture at either end of the bone or to describe the complex nature in a fracture involving the other part.

In the case of the fracture of the proximal and distal segments, type A – is extra-articular; type B – partial articular with some continuity between the shaft and a portion of the articular cartilage and type C – is complete articular with disruption of the articular surface from the shaft. The exceptions to this step include:
- Proximal humerus (11): Type A – extra-articular, unifocal; Type B – extra-articular, bifocal; Type C – articular
- Proximal femur (31): Type A – extra-articular, trochanteric; Type B – extra-articular, neck; Type C – articular, head
- Malleoli (44): Type A – infrasyndesmotic; Type B – transyndesmotic; Type C – suprasyndesmotic

On the other hand, in the diaphyseal segment type A – is simple fracture with two fragments. Type B – is a wedge fracture with three or more fragments and the main fragments have contact after reduction. Type C is a complex fracture with three or more fragments and the main fragments have no contact after reduction. For the fracture involving both diaphyseal and end segments, if the articular component is displaced it is considered articular fracture, however if it is an undisplaced fissure then it is classified as diaphyseal fracture.

iv. The fracture group. Each fracture type is further divided into three groups with more specific descriptions. In the diaphyseal segment, type A is grouped into A1 (simple spiral), A2 (simple oblique) and A3 (transverse) fractures. The type B (wedge fracture) is divided into B1 (spiral wedge), B2 (bending wedge) and B3 (fragmented wedge) fractures. Lastly the type C (complex fracture) is divided into C1 (complex fracture, spiral), C2 (complex fracture, segmental) and C3 (complex fracture, irregular).

The grouping of the fracture of the proximal and distal segments follows a similar pattern. The type-A (extra-articular fracture) is further divided into A1 (simple), A2 (wedge) and A3 (complex) fractures. For the partial-articular type B; B1 = spilt, B2 = depression and B3 = split-depression while the complete articular type C is divided into C1 (simple articular, simple metaphyseal), C2 (simple articular, complex metaphyseal) and C3 (complex articular, complex metaphyseal) fractures.

v. The subgroup. This also differs from bone to bone and utilises specific features for any given bone in its classifications. Subgroups describe the fractures in terms of displacement, angulation, shortening and rotation. In-depth description of the subgroup is not normally needed for everyday clinical application and communication.

Classification of fractures based on associated soft tissue injury

The degree of soft tissue damage may reflect the energy level involved in a fracture. High energy level often leads to a multi-fragmented or comminuted fracture. The exception is in osteoporotic bone where a low energy level can result in comminuted fractures. Soft tissue damage can occur in an open fracture where there is a breech in the skin or the epithelial surfaces or in closed fracture. There are two widely used classification systems in soft tissue injury associated fracture; Gustilo open fracture classification system (**Table 11.1**) and Oestern and Tscherne classification of closed fracture (**Table 11.2**). The Gustilo classification can only be applied fully after the surgical debridement of open fracture. The Gustilo classification uses the amount of energy, the extent of soft-tissue injury and the extent of contamination for determination of fracture severity and the management.

Fracture-specific classification system

These classification systems are either based on the mechanism of injury as is the case of Lauge-Hansen classification of malleolar fractures or descriptive. The examples of the descriptive types are the Neer classification of proximal humeral fracture, the Schatzker classification of the proximal tibia fractures and the Garden classification of the femoral neck fractures and so on. Details of these can be found in Topics 27, 47 and 97.

Uses of fracture classifications

- Enhances communication between colleagues
- Serves as educational tool, it helps to understand various mechanism of injury that causes fracture and also provide an avenue to compare clinical research
- As a guide to the management of fractures
- Predict risk of infection and outcome after fracture care

Table 11.1 Gustilo–Anderson classification of open fractures

Classification	Wound (cm in length)	Level of contamination	Soft tissue injury
I	<1	Clean	Minimal
II	>1, <10	Moderate	Moderate, some soft tissue damage
III A	>10	High	Severe crushing injury, adequate periosteal coverage of the fracture
III B	>10	High	Severe loss of coverage with periosteal stripping and bone damage, usually require soft tissue coverage
III C	–	High	Associated with an arterial injury requiring repair, irrespective of degree of soft-tissue injury

Table 11.2 Oestern and Tscherne classification of closed fractures

Grade	Soft tissue injury	Bony injury
0	Minimal soft tissue damage	Pattern of fracture – simple
1	Superficial abrasion/contusion	Pattern of fracture – mild
2	Deep abrasion with skin or muscle contusion	Pattern of fracture – severe
3	Extensive skin contusion or severe damage to underlying muscle, subcutaneous avulsion	Pattern of fracture – severe

Further reading

Court-Brown CM, Heckman JD, Bucholz RW, et al. Rockwood and Green's Fractures in Adults, 6th edn. Philadelphia, PA: Lippincott Williams and Wilkins; 2006.

Fracture and dislocation compendium. Orthopaedic Trauma Association Committee for Coding and Classification. J Orthop Trauma 1996; 10:1–154.

Müller ME, Nazarian S, Kack P. CCF – Comprehensive Classification of Fractures. Bern: Murice E. Muller Foundation; 1996.

Related topics of interest

- *Topic 9* Bone structure and physiology
- *Topic 11* Classification of fractures
- *Topic 85* Principles of operative management of fractures

12 Clavicle dislocations

Key points
- The clavicle is an S-shaped bone that acts as a lever arm connecting the scapula and upper limb to the torso
- It connects the arm to the torso via the sternoclavicular (SC) joint, coracoclavicular (CC) ligaments, acromioclavicular (AC) joint and several muscles attachments
- Clavicle dislocations can be SC or AC

Sternoclavicular joint dislocation

Anatomy
The medial end of the clavicle is the first bone to ossify and the last physis to close (by the age of 25 years). It forms a shallow saddle diarthrodial synovial joint with the manubrium and part of the first costal cartilage.

The joint stability is provided by:
- Capsular ligament: formed by anterosuperior and posterior capsule thickening. It provides anteroposterior (AP) stability. Damage to this ligament may also cause superior translation
- Anterior SC ligament: resists superior dislocation
- Interclavicular ligment: prevents superior displacement of the clavicle
- Costoclavicular ligament, also known as rhomboid ligament: provides rotational, medial and lateral stability
- Intra-articular disc ligament
- Subclavius muscle, which can play a role in stabilising the joint even after the disruption of the joint ligaments

Shoulder movements through the SC joint allow the clavicle to move around 35° in the anterior and posterior plane, 30–35° in elevation, and 45–50° of rotation around its axis.

Aetiology and epidemiology
The SC dislocations account for 1% of all joint dislocation and 3% of upper limb dislocations. They can be classified by aetiology to traumatic and atraumatic, or by direction to anterior and posterior dislocations depending on the position of the displaced medial end of the clavicle. Anterior dislocations are more common than posterior dislocation.

Traumatic injuries can be categorised to mild sprain, moderate sprain or subluxation and acute dislocation. Traumatic dislocations generally occur from high-energy injuries, i.e. road traffic accidents, fall from height and athletic injuries. The dislocating force can be direct or indirect, with the indirect dislocations more common for posterior dislocations. Anterior dislocations are almost always indirect. A compression and internal rotation force on the shoulder causes posterior dislocation of the ipsilateral SC joint, whereas a compression and external rotation force on the shoulder causes anterior dislocation of the ipsilateral SC joint.

Atraumatic subluxation or dislocation of the SC joint often affects adolescents, and it is usually related to generalised ligamentous laxity. It occurs in overhead arm elevation.

Clinical features
Patients with anterior dislocation can present with pain and tender swelling at the SC join, as well as painful shoulder movements. In posterior SC joint dislocations patients also present with pain, less prominent SC joint, they can also present with respiratory symptoms (dry cough and hoarseness, shortness of breath, chocking and difficulty breathing), dysphagie, vascular symptoms (venous congestion in the neck or ipsilateral upper limb, and decreased circulation in the ipsilateral upper limb), or neurological ipsilateral upper limb symptoms due to brachial plexus injury.

Physical examination includes palpation of the joint and other components of the ipsilateral shoulder girdle, assessment of the range of movement and the neurovascular status of the upper limb, and chest auscultation.

Imaging

Visualising the SC joint in the plain radiographic AP view is normally difficult. Serendipity view is frequently used; the beam in this view is at 40° cephalic tilt, it is interpreted as anterior dislocation if the affected medial half of the clavicle projected above the normal contralateral clavicle, and posterior dislocation if projected below.

A CT scan is the method of choice for SC joint evaluation. The contralateral SC joint should be included in the CT scan study for comparison. MRI can be helpful in assessment of the joint ligaments and articular disc injuries.

Management

Most SC joint injuries are effectively treated nonoperatively. Chronic anterior dislocations and chronic subluxations are often treated with local symptomatic treatment with ice, rest, poly sling and nonsteroidal anti-inflammatories.

Manipulation and closed reduction is usually performed for acute anterior and posterior dislocations, this procedure is carried out under local or general anaesthetic.

For anterior dislocations, the patient is positioned supine on the table with a thick pad or a sand bag between the patient's shoulders. The clavicle may reduce with direct pressure while a downward traction is applied to the abducted arm. A figure-of-eight sling is then applied for 4–6 weeks. Abduction traction and adduction traction techniques were described for reducing posterior SC joint dislocations, in both methods the patient is supine with a thick pad between the shoulders. In the first method, lateral traction is applied to the abducted arm, the medial side of the clavicle is sometimes grasped with the surgeon's hand or a clamp for anterior traction. In the second method, traction is applied to the adducted arm with simultaneous anterior to posterior pressure on the shoulder. Post reduction a figure-of-eight sling is applied for 4–6 weeks.

Operative treatment in the means of open reduction and ligaments reconstruction with thoracic surgery support is indicated for posterior dislocation with respiratory compromise, dysphagia or neurovascular symptoms.

Acromioclavicular joint dislocation

A common injury that accounts for around 9% of all shoulder girdle injuries. It is more common in men.

Anatomy

The AC joint is a synovial diarthrodial joint between the lateral end of the clavicle and the medial surface of the acromion process of the scapula. It contains a fibrocartilaginous disc that is variable in shape and size.

The joint acquires its stability through the AC ligaments, CC ligaments, capsule and muscular attachments. The joint is surrounded by a thin capsule that is strengthened by the superior, inferior, anterior and posterior AC ligaments; they provide horizontal stability to the joint. The deltoid and trapezius muscles attachment on the superior aspect of the clavicle and acromion reinforces the stability of the joint.

The CC ligaments are strong ligaments that run between the coracoid process and the inferior surface of the clavicle, they consist of conoid (medial) and trapezoid (lateral) ligaments. They provide vertical stability to the AC joint.

Mechanism of injury

The most common mechanism is a direct fall on the lateral aspect of the adducted shoulder. The injury can happen indirectly resulting from a fall on the outstretched hand with the force transmitting through the humeral head into the AC joint.

Clinical assessment

Clinical examination is performed while the patient is standing or sitting. Abnormal outline of the shoulder girdle can be observed. The distal clavicle may displace superiorly resulting in skin tenting, or displace inferiorly giving a flat appearance of the shoulder with a prominent acromion. AC joint palpation is normally tender. A standard shoulder examination with neurovascular assessment of the ipsilateral upper limb should be conducted.

Imaging assessment

Anteroposterior view of both AC joints in one image should be obtained for comparison. Shoulder plain radiography (AP, scapular 'Y' and axillary views) are adequate. Zanca views are useful for projecting subtle distal clavicle fractures as they can be missed in the conventional AP images. These are taken with the beam in 10–15° cephalic tilt.

Stress views in which a ~7 kg weight is applied to the affected upper limb, can be helpful with the diagnosis of CC ligaments injury by assessing the CC space and comparing it the healthy contralateral side. They are no longer used as they are not clinically applicable in the acute injuries.

Classification

The Rockwood classification describes AC joint injuries depending on clavicle displacement degree and direction (**Table 12.1**).

Figure 12.1 The Rockwood classification of acromioclavicular joint injuries

Type	Illustration	Features
I	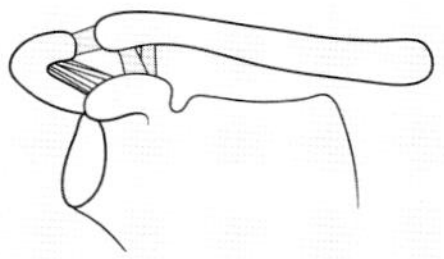	AC ligaments: sprained CC ligaments: intact Radiological appearance: normal
II	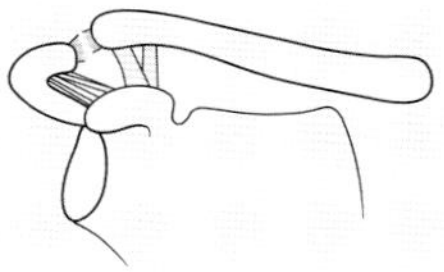	AC ligaments: torn CC ligaments: sprained Radiological appearance: superior distal clavicle subluxation
III	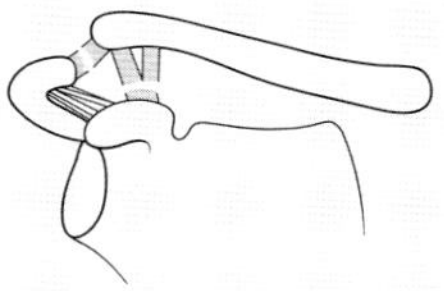	AC ligaments: torn CC ligaments: torn Radiological appearance: superior dislocation of the distal clavicle with the CC distance 25–100% > the contralateral normal side
IV	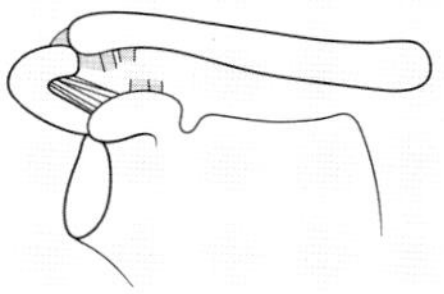	AC ligaments: torn CC ligaments: torn Radiological appearance: posterior distal clavicle dislocation through trapezius
V	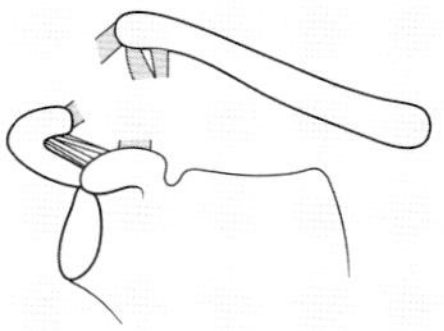	AC ligaments: torn CC ligaments: torn Radiological appearance: superior distal clavicle dislocation with CC distance >100% the contralateral normal side
VI	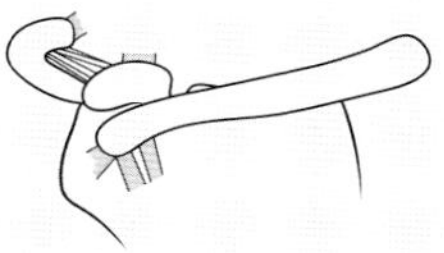	AC ligaments: torn CC ligaments: torn Radiological appearance: inferior displacement of the distal clavicle (sub-acromion or sub-coracoid)

AC, acromioclavicular; CC, coracoclavicular

Treatment

Nonoperative treatment with ice, rest, sling and early rehabilitation is indicted for types I, II, and type III injuries in older and low demand patients.

Type III injuries in active, athletes and high demand patients as well as types IV, V and VI are managed surgically with open reduction and ligaments repair or reconstruction.

Complications

The AC joint arthritis is the main long-term complication. Coracoclavicular ossification may develop.

Further reading

Bucholz RW, Heckman JD, Court-Brown C, et al. Rockwood and Green's Fractures in Adults, 6th edn. Philadelphia, PA: Lippincott Williams and Wilkins, 2005.

Pope TL Jr, Harris JH Jr. Harris and Harris. The Radiology of Emergency Medicine, 5th edn. Philadelphia, PA: Lippincott Williams and Wilkins, 2013.

Robinson CM, Jenkins PJ, Markham PE, Beggs I. Disorders of the sternoclavicular joint. J Bone Joint Surg Br 2008; 90:685–696.

Related topics of interest

- *Topic 10* Brachial plexus injury
- *Topic 13* Clavicle fractures

13 Clavicle fractures

Key points
- The severity of clavicle fractures depends on the mechanism of the injury
- Most fractures heal with conservative management, with little or no consequence
- Surgery is reserved for high-energy injuries, fractures with considerable shortening or displacement and fractures associated with ligamentous injuries. (recent evidence supports surgical management of these fractures to avoid the complications of symptomatic non-union and malunion.)
- The surgical aim is to bring the clavicle out to length and to correct the deformity

Epidemiology
The incidence of clavicle fractures is around 5–10% of all fractures. These fractures are common in three age groups:
- Toddlers and young children, due to falls. It is one of the common fractures to occur in childhood
- Young adults, due to sports injuries and high-energy injuries
- Elderly patients with low energy injuries

Fractures to the clavicle occur commonly in men. The male to female ratio is 2.6:1.

The high-energy injuries are associated with more complex fracture patterns and soft tissue disruption.

Pathophysiology
Clavicular fractures are mostly due to a direct injury to the point of the shoulder or a fall on an out-stretched hand. Low-energy injuries are common around the middle third of the clavicle. High-energy injuries are associated with comminution at the fracture site and soft tissue disruption. Disruption of the ligamentous structures that stabilise the clavicle, especially the coracoclavicular ligament, leads to displacement and instability of the lateral end of the clavicle. As the severity of these injuries increase there is also disruption of the deltotrapezial fascia.

Clinical assessment
There is swelling around the clavicle. There may be deformity that is clearly visible (**Figure 13.1**). The clavicle is tender to touch. Movements of the shoulder are painful especially above the level of the shoulder.

Careful assessment of the neurovascular status is mandatory. Clavicle fractures, particularly in relation to high-energy injuries are associated with brachial plexus injury and obstetric injuries during child birth. This is due to the close proximity of the plexus to the clavicle. The incidence of brachial plexus injury is low, around 1%, with the medial and posterior cords of the plexus commonly involved.

Investigations
A plain radiograph in two different views is usually sufficient to identify these fractures. A plain anteroposterior (AP) radiograph and AP radiograph with 30° cephalic tilt gives good information regarding the fracture pattern and displacement.

There are special radiographic views for medial and lateral end fractures. For medial end fractures, particularly involving the sternoclavicular joint, a serendipity view is useful. For the lateral end fractures a Zanca view gives sufficient information about the fracture characteristics.

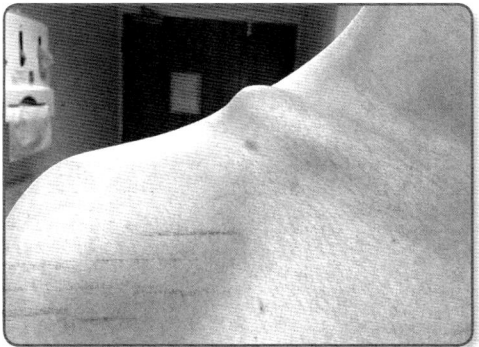

Figure 13.1 Deformity of clavicle visible with tenting of the skin.

In addition, other investigations such as a CT-scan with 3D reconstruction is useful in comminuted fractures or when dealing with nonunion or malunion.

Classification

There are different classifications for clavicle fractures.

Allman classification

The most common classification is the Allman classification. The fractures are classified according to the anatomic region in the descending order of frequency.

Type I: Middle third of clavicle
Type II: Lateral third of clavicle
Type III: Medial third of clavicle

Neer classification

Neer classified the lateral end of clavicle fractures into:

Type I: Fracture lateral to coracoclavicular ligaments. Conoid and/or trapezoid ligament remain intact. Minimal displacement - stable
Treatment: Nonoperative.

Type IIa: Fracture occurs medial to coracoclavicular ligaments. Conoid and trapezoid ligment remain intact. Significant medial clavicle displacement - unstable. Up to 56% nonunion rate with nonoperative management
Treatment: Operative recommended.

Type IIb: Two fracture patterns: (1) Fracture occurs either between the coracoclavicular ligaments. Conoid ligament torn. Trapezoid ligament intact. (2) Fracture occurs lateral to coracoclavicular ligaments. Conoid and trapezoid ligament torn. Signficant medial clavicle displacement - unstable. Up to 30–45% nonunion rate with nonoperative management.
Treatment: operative recommended.

Type III: Intra-articular fracture extending into AC joint. Conoid and trapezoid ligaments remain intact. Minimal displacement - stable injury. Patients may develop post-traumatic AC arthritis.
Treatment: Nonoperative.

Type IV: Physeal fracture that occurs in skeletally immature. Conoid and trapezoid ligaments remain intact. Displacement of lateral clavicle occurs superiorly through a tear in the thick periosteum. Clavicle pulls out of periosteal sleeve – stable.
Treatment: nonoperative.

Type V: Comminuted fracture pattern Conoid and trapezoid ligaments remain intact. Significant medial clavicle displacement – usually unstable
Treatment: operative.

Robinson classification

A more detailed descriptive classification by Robinson classifies the clavicle fractures as follows:

Table 13.1 Management of fractures of the medial third of the clavicle

Nonoperative	Operative
Majority of fractures	Open fractures
Polysling for 2–3 weeks	Severe displacement
Mobilise as pain dictates	Where there is risk to mediastinal structures
	'Floating shoulder'
	Open reduction and internal fixation using plate osteosynthesis

Table 13.2 Management of fractures of the middle third of the clavicle

Nonoperative	Operative
Majority of fractures, especially undisplaced or minimally displaced	Displaced fractures, open fractures, high-energy fractures with severe comminution and soft tissue injury, shortening of >1 cm, 'floating shoulder'
Polysling for 2–3 weeks	
Mobilise as pain dictates	Open reduction and internal fixation using plate osteosynthesis
	Intramedullary nail/pins

Table 13.3 Management of fractures of the lateral third of the clavicle

Nonoperative	Operative
Undisplaced or minimally displaced fractures where the coracoclavicular ligament is intact	Displaced fractures where the coracoclavicular ligament is disrupted leading to vertical instability, open fractures, 'floating shoulder'
Polysling for 2–3 weeks	
Mobilise as pain or discomfort allows	Open reduction and internal fixation using plate osteosynthesis with lateral clavicular plates
	Bone suture or graft sling techniques

Type I: Medial third fractures
Type II: Middle third fractures
Type III: Lateral third fractures

Each of these types are subdivided into type A, where the fractures are displaced < 100%, and type B, where the fractures are displaced more that 100%.

Type I medial fractures and type III lateral fractures are further subdivided into subgroup 1 with no articular involvement and subgroup 2 with involvement of the joint.

Type II middle third fractures are subdivided according to the degree of comminution. Subgroup 1 are simple and wedge type fractures. Subgroup 2 are comminuted and segmental fractures.

Treatment

Treatment is tailored to each patient. However, as a guide for management, the operative and nonoperative treatments for clavicular fractures are presented in **Tables 13.1, 13.2** and **13.3**.

The timing of operative intervention is important to achieve the best outcome, particularly for lateral end fractures and some middle third fractures.

Complications

Resulting from the fracture

Early: neurovascular injuries, especially injury to the brachial plexus.
Late: malunion with shortening and decreased shoulder function and painful nonunion.

The nonunion rates are around 8.3% for medial end fractures, 4.5% for middle third fractures and 11.5% for lateral end fractures.

The predictors of nonunion are advancing age, female gender, displacement of the fracture and comminution at the fracture site.

Arising due to surgery

There are a number of complications related to surgery such as infection, neurovascular injury, hardware failure, hypertrophic scarring, complex regional pain syndrome, nonunion, especially with the use of rigid locking plates and re-fracture after implant removal. The most common ones are related directly to the hardware.

Further reading

Allman FL Jr. Fractures and ligamentous injuries of the clavicle and its articulation. J Bone Joint Surg Am 1967; 49:774–784.
Neer CS II. Fractures of the distal third of the clavicle. Clin Orthop 1968; 58:43–50.
Robinson CM. Fractures of the clavicle in the adult. Epidemiology and classification. J Bone Joint Surg Br 1998; 80:476–484.
Robinson CM, Court-Brown CM, McQueen MM, Wakefield AE. Estimating the risk of no-union following non-operative treatment of clavicular fractures. J Bone Joint Surg Am 2004; 86:1359–1365.

Related topics of interest

- *Topic 10* Brachial plexus injury
- *Topic 11* Classification of fractures
- *Topic 12* Clavicle dislocations

14 Compartment syndrome

Key points
- Acute compartment syndrome (ACS) is one of the few true orthopaedic emergencies
- ACS is a condition where osteofascial intracompartmental pressure (ICP) increases to levels that critically compromises tissue perfusion hence creating tissue ischaemia
- A high index of suspicion for early diagnosis and prompt surgical intervention are of utmost importance to avoid the potential serious consequences to limb and even life

Epidemiology

The average annual incidence for compartment syndrome is 3.1 per 100,000 people (7.3 per 100,000 men and 0.7 per 100,000 women). Road traffic accidents and sport injuries are among the most common modes of injury, but ACS can occur after any injury regardless of the aetiology, velocity or degree of fracture comminution. It mostly affects young men, and it is thought that young individuals are more likely to have strong tight fascia with more muscle volume and are more likely to sustain a high-energy trauma. On the other hand, older people may have high blood pressure which may compensate for the increase in tissue pressure.

There is an associated fracture in approximately two thirds of cases, tibial diaphysial accounting for almost half. Distal radial and diaphyseal fractures of radius and ulna are the second most common fracture followed by femoral, hand, foot, ankle, elbow, pelvis and humeral fractures. ACS is equally likely following closed and open fractures. The incidence of ACS following tibial fractures varies from 2.7% to 11%. Other causes of ACS without fractures are injuries with soft tissue damage, i.e. in blunt trauma, crush injuries and burns. ACS can also result without trauma in medical conditions like nephrotic syndrome, viral myositis, bleeding disorders, diabetes mellitus and malignancies and following treatment with anticoagulants. It can also affect patients undergoing prolonged surgical interventions in lithotomy position or poorly positioned surgical patients.

Pathophysiology

ACS can be caused by restriction of compartment volume, like tight casts and bandages, or increase in the contents of compartment as in bleeding and oedema. As the pressure increases, venous capillary pressure also rises. This will lead to decreased arteriovenous pressure gradient and subsequently decreased tissue perfusion. The compromised venous drainage and continuing blood flow into the compartment in early stages lead to further swelling and oedema and hence further ICP increase. This vicious circle of compromised microcirculation results in critical reduction in perfusion and oxygenation which leads to myoneural ischaemia and necrosis.

Clinical features

The symptoms and signs are of a progressive nature, therefore it is essential that clinical examination is done repeatedly and preferably by the same clinician. Patients with ACS typically present with progressive pain out of proportion to the stimulus that usually does not respond to painkillers. Other features include altered sensation (distal to affected area of limb), tense firm swelling, pain on passive stretch of the affected muscle group, and late symptoms include paralysis and pulselessness as mentioned in the 5 'P's in literature: pain, paraesthesia, pallor, paralysis and pulselessness.

Pain with passive stretch is the most sensitive finding before the onset of ischaemia, whereas the presence of paraesthesia, and later on hypoesthesia, is indicative of nerve ischaemia. Although pain is the leading feature, it may not always be easy to assess in patients such as children and polytraumatised patients. Pain may be also absent in regionally anaesthetised patients and in sedated patients in ITU, therefore, a high index of suspicion and a low threshold for measuring intracompartmental pressure is essential to identify high-risk patients.

Paralysis and pulselessness are late findings, with full recovery being rare in the former and very unlikely in the latter. Pulselessness is therefore not a diagnostic criteria because peripheral pulses are usually present also with high ICP and it is more likely to be a sign of direct arterial injury.

Investigations

ICP measurement can aid early diagnosis especially in equivocal cases. Different techniques and devices can be used for measuring ICP, like Whitesides infusion technique, wick-and-slit catheters, Stryker ICP monitor system and regular needle with arterial line manometer. Whitesides infusion technique utilises a handheld needle mercury manometer to obtain a single pressure reading. This technique is simple, but it requires the injection of saline which could aggravate an impending compartment syndrome. The wick-and-slit catheters, on the other hand, provide continuous pressure recording over 24-hour period. The reading should be obtained within 5 cm of the fracture as this is usually the area of highest pressure. Noninvasive techniques have also been proposed. Near-infrared spectroscopy (NIRS) is a noninvasive tool that can play a role in continuous monitoring; it measures ischaemia by transmitting light at wavelengths that react with haemoglobin to obtain tissue oxygen saturation.

Diagnosis

The diagnosis is based on careful clinical examination. Unequivocally positive clinical findings warrant immediate surgical intervention without the need for ICP measurements. However, ICP measurement is indicated in polytraumatised patients and patients with altered level of consciousness or when clinical examination is inconclusive.

Normal resting ICP is 0–8 mmHg. Clinical symptoms of ischaemia first appear at an ICP of between 20–30 mmHg. Accepted thresholds for fasciotomy are an ICP of 30–45 mmHg or ICP within 30 mmHg of the patient's diastolic blood pressure ($\Delta P \leq 30$) at a single point in time. Continuous monitoring is also an effective way of assessing patients who are at risk.

Treatment

The objectives of treatment are to relieve increased ICP in order to normalise tissue perfusion and maintain function, and to debride any nonviable tissues. All constrictive plaster and bandages should be removed. High elevation is not recommended as it can lead to further reduction in perfusion. Fasciotomy should be performed urgently and incisions should be large enough to release the affected compartments. The viability of muscles should be assessed based on colour and presence of contraction on stimulus. If diagnosis is delayed more than 24 hours, fasciotomy is associated with high risk of infection and amputation; therefore, treatment should consist of observation and delayed reconstructive surgery as required.

Leg fasciotomy

- The two-incision technique is most commonly used. Use an anterolateral incision to approach anterior and lateral compartments. This is midway between tibial crest and fibular axis, starting 5 cm distal to fibular head and extending up to 5 cm proximal to lateral malleolus. The superficial peroneal nerve is at risk distally. The other incision is posteromedial, 2 cm posterior to medial border of the tibia. It is used to decompress superficial and deep posterior compartments. Soleus insertion should be released to adequately decompress the deep posterior compartment. Care must be taken to avoid injury to saphenous nerve and vein
- Single incision with or without fibulectomy are less popular techniques. They utilise an incision along the fibula axis to decompress all compartments

Forearm fasciotomy

The forearm compartments are interrelated and do not need to be individually addressed. Volar fasciotomy can significantly lower pressure in the dorsal compartment. Different incisions may be used, e.g. the 'lazy S' shaped or curved incisions. The incision should avoid exposing the median nerve distally but it should extend to the proximal palm to decompress the carpal tunnel. The dorsal compartment can be decompressed through a longitudinal incision which extends from 2 cm lateral and 2 cm distal to lateral epicondyle toward the middle of the wrist.

Hand, foot and arm fasciotomies (Table 14.1)

There are 10 compartments in the hand which comprise: hypothenar; thenar; adductor pollicis; four dorsal interosseous; three volar (palmar) interosseous.

ACS of the hand is typically released by a 5-incision technique: two dorsal incisions over the 2nd and 4th metacarpals; three palmer incisions, one each to the thenar and hypothenar region and a central carpal tunnel decompression incision.

Fasciotomy wound management

Wounds should be reviewed in theatre at 48–72 hours and debridement of any further nonviable tissues should be performed. If there is no residual necrotic tissue, skin can be loosely approximated. If tension free closure cannot be achieved, assisted closure methods can be utilised like negative pressure wound therapy (NPWT) or dynamic wound closure using vascular loop or shoelace technique. Split thickness skin grafting is a popular technique if closure cannot be achieved.

Table 14.1 Different compartments and their common surgical approaches

Region	Compartments	Surgical incisions
Leg	Anterior, lateral, superficial and deep posterior	Two-incision technique, lateral and medial One incision technique, lateral with or without fibulectomy
Forearm	Volar, dorsal, mobile wad, pronator quadratus	Volar, 'lazy S' shape including carpal tunnel Dorsal, distal to lateral epicondyle towards the middle of the wrist
Hand	Adductor pollicis Four dorsal interosseus Three palmar interosseus	Dorsum: Two incisions along 2nd and 4th metacarpals
	Central palmar Thenar Hypothenar	Palmar: Radial side along 1st metacarpal Ulnar side along 5th metacarpal
	Carpal tunnel	Carpal tunnel decompression
Thigh	Anterior and posterior	Lateral incision
Foot	Medial Lateral Four interosseus Three central (superficial, central and deep)	Two incisions along 2nd and 4th metatarsals

Complications

Volkmann's ischaemic contracture can result from delayed diagnosis or delayed, or incomplete fasciotomy which lead to irreversible ischaemia, necrosis and scarring.

Further reading

Elliott KG, Johnstone AJ. Diagnosing acute compartment syndrome. J Bone Joint Surg Br 2003; 85:625–632.

McQueen MM, Gaston P, Court-Brown CM. Acute compartment syndrome. Who is at risk? J Bone Joint Surg Br 2000; 82B:200–203.

Rorabeck CH. The treatment for compartment syndromes of the leg. J Bone Joint Surg Br 1984; 66:93–97.

Shadgan B, Menon M, Sanders D, et al. Current thinking about acute compartment syndrome of the lower extremity. Can J Surg 2010; 53:329–334.

Related topics of interest

- *Topic 34* Forearm – radius and ulna fractures
- *Topic 84* Principles of nonoperative management of fractures
- *Topic 85* Principles of operative management of fractures
- *Topic 98* Tibial shaft fractures

15 Complex regional pain syndrome

Key points
- Complex regional pain syndrome (CRPS) has wide ranging and variable symptoms accompanied by intractable pain that is out of proportion with the original insult or injury
- The Budapest criteria are used to diagnose CRPS and should be used as a guide for orthopaedic surgeons in the early recognition of CRPS and direction of investigations
- Once CRPS is suspected expedient referral to an appropriate MDT is vital to allow effective therapy before the onset of chronic signs and symptoms that lead to a worse prognosis

Epidemiology

CRPS is a group of painful and disabling conditions that occur after an insult or injury to the peripheral limbs. Seen most commonly within the upper limb (60% of cases) after fracture (45%), sprains (18%) and elective surgery (12%) with wide ranging symptoms and signs it is difficult to classify and definitively diagnose. CRPS is three times more common in females than males and classically presents in the fifth and sixth decades of life. Due to the inherent variability in presentation of CRPS, prevalence and incidence figures vary widely and interobserver reliability is poor. Epidemiological studies performed in the United States and the Netherlands place incidence at between 5.5 and 26 per 100,000 person years and prevalence of 21 per 100,000. Recovery from CRPS is also poorly defined with between 30% and 70% of sufferers seeing improvement at 6 years.

Pathophysiology

Pathological mechanisms explaining the occurrences in CRPS are numerous, wide-ranging and poorly understood. In particular the interaction between the pathways of inflammation the autonomic nervous system (ANS) and central nervous system (CNS) are of interest. It is thought that during the 'warm' phase of CRPS the inflammatory pathways play a pre-dominant role in causing symptoms. An overproduction of vasoconstrictors causes ischaemia and subsequent ANS damage. This in turn causes vasodilation and the painful 'warm' phase of CRPS. In response to reduced blood flow, up-regulation of receptors within the ANS occurs. As the inflammatory processes then recedes, ANS function returns to previous levels causing vasoconstriction and the 'cold' phase of CRPS. During the months that follow, persistent pain causes structural and functional changes in the CNS with sensitisation of nociceptive pathways and alteration in emotional and behavioural responses to pain.

Diagnosis

CRPS is a diagnosis of exclusion and a thorough history, investigation and examination is critical to rule out another cause. The Orlando criteria is endorsed by the International Association for the Study of Pain and has been used since 1994 to diagnose CRPS. More recently, a modified version known as the Budapest criteria with a higher specificity and inclusion of the motor symptoms of CRPS has been validated. In use since 2004, this appears to be the new standard in diagnosis of CRPS (**Table 15.1**). In orthopaedics, this should be used as a guide to aid the recognition of developing CRPS and direct investigations accordingly.

Investigations

CRPS remains a clinical diagnosis of exclusion with no specific tests. However investigations help in ruling out other possible causes and supporting referral to specialist services.

Table 15.1 Budapest criteria for diagnosis of CRPS

Budapest criteria for CRPS

All of the following criteria must be met to have a positive diagnosis of CRPS:
- Continuing pain disproportionate to the inciting event
- Patient must have 1 sign in 2 or more of the categories below
- Patient must have 1 symptom in 3 or more of the categories below
- No other diagnosis better explains the symptoms

Number	Category	Sign/symptom
1	Sensory	Allodynia (pain to light touch and/or temperature sensation and/or deep somatic pressure and/or joint movement and/or hyperalgesia (to pin prick)
2	Vasomotor	Temperature asymmetry and/or skin colour changes and/or skin colour asymmetry
3	Sudomotor/oedema	Oedema and/or sweating asymmetry
4	Motor/trophic	Decreased range of motion and/or motor dysfunction (weakness, tremor, dystonia) and/or trophic changes (hair, nail, skin)

MRI is widely available within a reasonable time frame and is useful in both assessing bone structure and ruling out nerve entrapment or injury. The discovery of bone oedema within the affected limb may also strengthen suspicion of CRPS, especially if away from the site of original insult.

Electromyography and nerve conduction studies are useful in excluding a generalised or focal neuropathy. However, they do not test small A and C delta fibres commonly affected in CRPS. Punch skin biopsies do allow analysis of the small axonal fibres but there are a plethora of conditions that cause pathological changes and specificity is very low.

Studies of skeletal bone density in CRPS reveal osteoporosis in chronic disuse from CRPS. Earlier detection via scintigraphy and/or densitometry is useful in strengthening a diagnosis but other causes must be ruled out. Bone densitometry may also be useful in monitoring the progress of treatment and has been shown to be useful in plotting recovery over time.

Thermography can also be used to monitor temperature differences between limbs. This form of investigation, often coupled with sensory testing, is currently in infancy but may be useful in quantifying temperature differences used to measure response to treatment.

Classification

CRPS is divided into:
- Type 1, where no nerve lesion can be identified
- Type 2, where there is a demonstrable peripheral nerve lesion

Type 1 is relevant in orthopaedics due to its inherent presentation in the limbs and in those with trauma. Type 2 CRPS is often referred onto specialist services dealing with the management and treatment of nerve injuries. Type 1 CRPS is then further classified into 'warm' or 'cold'. Although it is commonly observed that 'warm' CRPS progresses to 'cold' CRPS in the chronic stage of disease, 'cold' CRPS has been observed as the acute primary complaint.

Clinical features

The clinical features of CRPS are wide-ranging and highly variable amongst sufferers. As well as sensory dysfunction causing pain, symptoms also arise from dysfunction of the cardiovascular and integumentary systems.

Beginning after a noxious event (e.g. wrist fracture) CRPS develops over a period of months. Disproportionate pain in the affected limb and cardiovascular dysfunction are characteristic of early CRPS. Increase in blood flow causes swelling, erythema and increase in temperature (**Figure 15.1**). Described

Complex regional pain syndrome

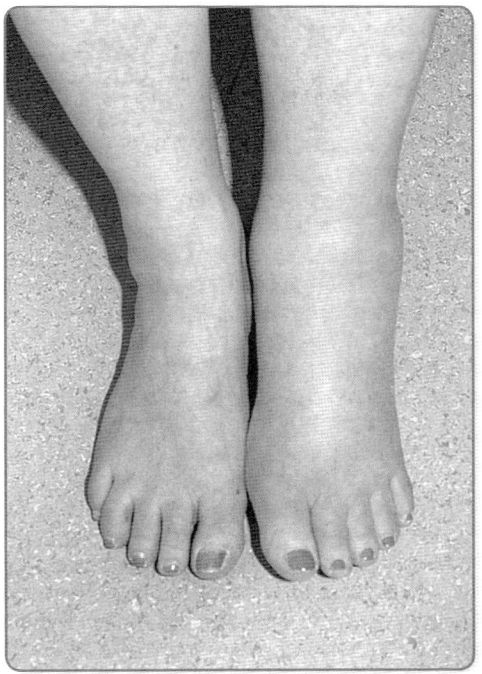

Figure 15.1 Warm type CRPS with acute swelling and shiny skin associated with early onset of CRPS.

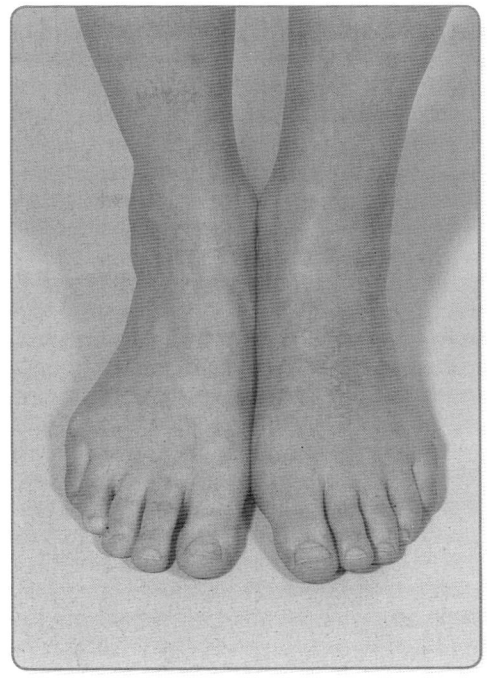

Figure 15.2 Trophic changes in CRPS include right sided discolouration, dry skin and loss of hair on the dorsum of the foot.

as the 'warm' phase of CRPS, symptoms follow no specific peripheral nerve or nerve root distribution. Over the following weeks, integumentary dysfunction effecting nail and hair growth (**Figure 15.2**) and disuse atrophy occurs. Further sensory dysfunction in the form of allodynia and hyperalgesia can also develop.

Months after development, pain persists and has often spread throughout the effected limb. Motor dysfunction is common with loss of voluntary control and dystonia, myoclonus and tremor. Cardiovascular dysfunction continues but blood flow is now reduced rendering the limb cold and discoloured (**Figure 15.3**). The 'cold' phase of CRPS begins and negative sensory dysfunction with hypoalgesia, hypoaesthesia and hypothermaesthesia compound debilitation and further reduce function.

Treatment

Due to its variable nature and wide ranging clinical manifestations CRPS is difficult to treat. In orthopaedics emphasis is placed on early recognition and appropriate investigation to allow expedient referral to a specialised multidisciplinary team (MDT). The MDT is often lead by anaesthetics and includes physiotherapy, occupational therapy, neurology and neurophysiology.

First line treatment often comes in the form of a combination of pharmacotherapy and physiotherapy. In the acute period the administration of ascorbic acid and glucocorticoids has shown some benefit. Other successful treatments include sympathetic nerve blockade or ablation, vasodilator therapy, bisphosphonates and immunoglobulin administration. Physiotherapy focuses on the restoration of

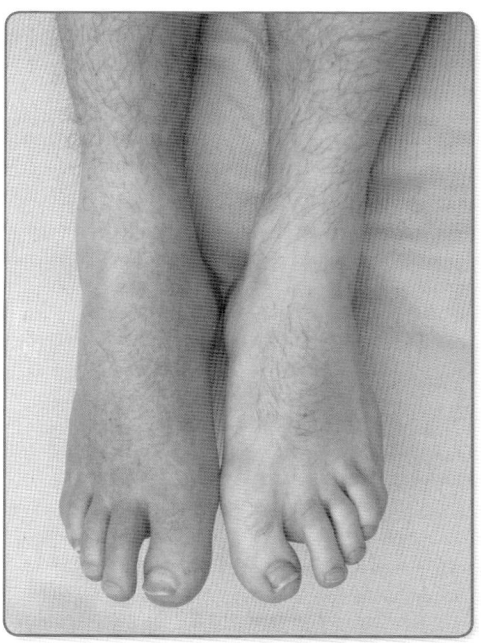

Figure 15.3 Cold type CRPS with severe discolouration, trophic changes including the nails and atrophy.

function and desensitisation. Transcutaneous electrical nerve stimulation with progressive weight bearing and tactile desensitisation are common therapies. Other interesting prospects include mirror box therapy, graded motor imagery and tactile discrimination testing.

If disablement and pain continue over many years without improvement amputation is often considered. Assessment from a psychologist and prosthetics team is essential in planning for the procedure and patient education is vital. This should take place in a specialist unit with an experienced team of anaesthetists and physiotherapists used to dealing with chronic pain.

Further reading

Gatti D, Rossini M, Adami S. Management of patients with complex regional pain syndrome type I. Osteoporos Int 2016; 27:2423–2431.

Kortekaas M, Niehof S, Stolker R, Huygen F. Pathophysiological mechanisms involved in vasomotor disturbances in complex regional pain syndrome and implications for therapy: A review. Pain Pract 2015; 16:905–914.

Marinus J, Moseley G, Birklein F, et al. Clinical features and pathophysiology of complex regional pain syndrome. Lancet Neurol 2011; 10:637–648.

Related topics of interest

- *Topic 1* Amputations – mangled extremities and decision making
- *Topic 2* Amputations – prosthetics and rehabilitation
- *Topic 37* Guidelines in trauma
- *Topic 83* Peripheral nerve injury

16 Crush injuries and crush syndrome

Key points
- Crush injuries are the result of a prolonged compression over the human body; this can lead to a systemic response, organ failure and death.
- Crush injuries and crush syndrome are common in areas of war and natural disasters. They also occur after road traffic accidents and crashes at industrial sites. Sometimes they result from body-weight-induced compression rather than trauma
- Crush syndrome manifestations include: rhabdomyolysis and the triad of reduced muscle power, myalgia and dark urine

Definition
Crush syndrome is the systemic manifestation of the mechanical muscle crush. It is produced by continuous, prolonged pressure over the human body. The duration and the scale of the force applied on the body, as well as the muscular mass that is affected, determine the severity of the injury.

Pathology and pathophysiology
Mechanical muscle damage results from an intense crush force that destroys the muscle cells, or from a combination of mechanical force and ischaemia to the muscle bulk due to the continuous compression force. The latter can be seen in patients who are not able to move for several hours, i.e. unconscious fallen patient with body-weight-induced compression.

The clinical presentation of crush syndrome is due to the traumatic rhabdomyolysis, thus the release of the myocytes components into the serum or urine. This mechanical muscle injury instigates local tissue and muscle damage, ischaemia of the affected region, and leads to the subsequent multiorgan failure and metabolic abnormalities.

Due to crush, the volume regulators of the myocytes are damaged, hence the impermeability of the sarcolemma and the cations balance of these myocytes are distorted. Since the myocytes' cytoplasm is negatively charged and hyperosmotic, this damage to their membrane shifts the extracellular fluid and cations (calcium and sodium) into the myocytes leading to swelling of these cells, and eventually fluid retention in the damaged extremities instigating hypovolaemia (due to loss of extracellular volume), shock and renal failure. Moreover, the excessive swelling and oedema in the muscle compartment may lead to local compartment syndrome, which is itself a high risk in hypovolaemic hypotensive patients, due to the decreased arteriolar-perfusion pressure.

The influx and efflux of the ions and myocytes constituents through the damaged membrane is disrupted. Along with the extracellular fluid, calcium and sodium are shifted into the damaged cell. The increased cytosolic calcium activates the cytotoxic protease and muscle necrosis. On the other hand, the decreased serum calcium levels may lead to hypocalcaemia. Conversely, the damaged myocytes release the following factors into the extracellular fluid and serum:

- Potassium: leading to hyperkalaemia and cardiac arrhythmias
- Phosphate: this may set off hyperphosphataemia that exacerbates hypocalcaemia and causes phosphate calculi, and renal failure
- Lactic acid and the resultant metabolic acidosis
- Creatine kinase
- Thromboplastin which may cause disseminated intravascular coagulation
- Myoglobin: the elevated concentrations of myoglobin are nephrotoxic, they eventually cause acute renal failure with the combination of renal vasoconstriction due to hypovolaemia and hypotension, metabolic acidosis, and high concentrates of phosphate and urate

Clinical presentation

The clinical picture of crush injuries is broad. Patients may present initially with no physical complaint or pain, or on the other hand, present with extensive body injuries, mangled extremities and compartment syndrome features.

In patients with closed compression injuries to the limbs, the affected skin is usually bruised. It can form blisters in the later course of the injury. Oedema and swelling of the limb is the most dominant clinical feature. It grows rapidly, however it usually takes few hours to fully develop.

Neurological deficiency is observed as patients may present with sensory loss or even with flaccid paralytic limb. These neurological features do not usually correspond to the limb nerve distribution, and the presence of normal anal sphincter and bladder function can be helpful with ruling out spinal injury. Pulses are usually weak but present, and the absence of pulses should raise concerns to other injuries.

Crushed patients can present with shock that can be caused by the mechanical muscle damage explained above, or by concomitant injuries in the head, chest, abdomen, pelvis, and fractures of pelvis, spine and long bones.

Treatment

Crush injury treatment should be initiated as soon as possible for the purpose of preventing this injury from developing into crush syndrome.

Crush injuries are common in warfare and natural disasters, hence the pre-hospital assessment and treatment is crucial in these situations.

In cases of multiple casualties a triage system should be applied upon arrival to prioritise patients' treatments.

After ensuring medical staffing safety, the following treatment should be instigated:
- Assessment of the airways, breathing and circulation is the first step of treatment
- Administration of high flow oxygen and external haemorrhage control
- Obtaining intravenous access and administering intravenous fluid therapy at a rate of 1 L per hour. The central venous pressure (CVP) and urinary output should be monitored as soon as possible.
- Patients should be freed from compression as soon as possible, with awareness of the possibility of spinal injuries and sustaining spinal precautions
- Assessment of the neurovascular status of the injured limb, and limb splinting if necessary. Care should be taken to avoid hypothermia
- Patients should be transported to a trauma centre that has intensive care unit and renal support

Hospital treatment

Upon arrival to the emergency department:
- Patient should be assessed as per Advanced Trauma Life Support algorithm and guidelines
- Blood tests to assess blood, bone and liver profile, creatine kinase, clotting and for blood transfusion if required
- Continuation of intravenous fluid therapy with hourly 500 mL of crystalloids
- Urinary catheterisation and hourly urine output assessment
- Central venous catheterisation and CVP monitoring should be considered in early stages of hospital treatment
- Imaging and other means of investigations should the patient be suspected to have any concomitant injury

Michaelson and Reis et al., both gave similar recommendations for treatment of crush injury and crush syndrome explaining their experience in managing this condition, and reviewing other articles in the management of these injuries following natural disasters.

They emphasised that the treatment should be planned to prevent acute renal failure. They explained that the treatment is dependent on two factors. First, is keeping the urine PH above 6.5 which will prevent tubular casts formation, hence protecting the kidneys from the toxic effect of the myoglobin. The second factor is the increase in the urine output of at least 300 mm/h (or 8 L/day); this diuresis plays a protective role on the kidneys and helps controlling the cations imbalance and acidemia. These factors are achieved with administration of large volumes of intravenous fluids, alkalinisation with sodium bicarbonate, and mannitol usage to produce osmotic diuresis.

Fasciotomy and amputation

The Mangled Extremity Severity Score can be helpful in distinguishing non-retrievable mangled limbs, and can be useful in the amputation decision making. However, few literature reviews have reported full recovery of terribly crushed limbs that have been managed conservatively. Additionally, there is no evidence that prophylactic amputation of the injured limb can prevent crush syndrome and acute kidney injury from occurring.

Compartment syndrome is classically managed with fasciotomy of the affected muscle compartment. Nevertheless, Michaelson (1992), Reis et al. (1992) and several other literature reports have advised against fasciotomy in closed muscle crush compartment syndrome, due to the high rate of subsequent complications of bleeding, infection, recurrent surgical debridements and limb amputation. They found that conservative treatment as per the above-mentioned recommendations has superior results. Fasciotomy was recommended in the case of imminent gangrene when the distal pulses are absent in a patient for whom both vascular injury and systemic hypotension have been ruled out.

The use of mannitol and hyperbaric oxygen for reducing compartment pressure and tissue oedema has been reported with good results, but still questionable and not fully experimented.

Further reading

Greaves I, Porter K, Smith JE. Consensus statement on the early management of crush injury and prevention of crush syndrome. J R Army Med Corps 2003; 149:255–259.

Michaelson M. Crush injury and crush syndrome. World J Surgery 1992; 16:899–903.

Reis ND, Better OS. Mechanical muscle crush injury and acute muscle-crush compartment syndrome: with special reference to earthquake casualities. J Bone Joint Surg Br 2005; 87:450–453.

Related topics of interest

- *Topic 1* Amputations – mangled extremities and decision making
- *Topic 14* Compartment syndrome
- *Topic 17* Damage control orthopaedics and trauma physiology

17 Damage control orthopaedics and trauma physiology

Key points

- Trauma is a significant cause of mortality and can lead to complications such as systemic inflammatory response syndrome (SIRS), acute respiratory distress syndrome (ARDS), multiple organ distress syndrome (MODS) and sepsis
- Surgery soon after trauma can itself constitute a fatal 'second-hit': careful decision-making is required regarding early definitive fixation versus an approach that applies damage control principles
- Resuscitation measures such as lactate, base excess and pH are useful tools in this process

Epidemiology

Injuries are responsible for over 5 million deaths worldwide each year according to data from the World Health Organization. Road traffic accidents are the main cause of death in those aged between 15–29 years and in 2012 resulted in 3500 deaths each day. Tens of millions more sustain injuries that do not result in mortality. Estimates for the year 2030 show that these figures will continue to rise.

Mortality following trauma occurs in one of three phases. The first consists of those who die immediately or soon after their injuries. The second phase occurs in the hours following the injury, namely from causes such as hypovolaemia and hypoxia. Thirdly a significant proportion of deaths occur in the days to weeks following admission due to complications such as disseminated intravascular coagulation (DIC), ARDS, MODS and sepsis. As clinicians, we are in a position to have the biggest impact in reducing morbidity and mortality resulting from the latter two phases.

The last half a century has seen significant shifts in the management of the multiply injured patient. The popularity of internal fixation techniques such as intramedullary nailing in the 1970s and 1980s superseded the use of prolonged periods of traction and gave rise to the concept of 'early total care.' Subsequently it became apparent that a group of patients could not withstand the 'second-hit' of early definitive surgery and the principle of 'damage control orthopaedics' (DCO or 'do no more harm') was born. This focussed on the early stabilisation of the patient with a view to proceeding to definitive fixation or treatment when the patient is medically stable. More recent evidence has demonstrated that early definitive treatment may be suitable in patients who are adequately resuscitated, a concept termed 'early appropriate care.'

Pathophysiology

Inflammation

Trauma creates a 'first-hit' leading to an inflammatory response within the body. This results from the product of cytokines including interleukins (IL) from the locally damaged tissues. These activate cells such as neutrophils and macrophages. The central response involves the release of hormones including catecholamines and growth hormone which react with the cytokine cascade. This systemic activation of inflammation can be beneficial when mild in helping recover from the traumatic insult. When exaggerated, however, this leads to SIRS (**Table 17.1**).

Table 17.1 Definition of SIRS

- Temperature >38°C or <36°C
- Heart rate >90/min
- Respiratory rate >20/min or $PaCO_2$ <32 mmHg
- White cell count >12 × 10^9 L or <4 × 10^9 L or >10% immature forms

Two or more criteria are necessary for a diagnosis

Acute respiratory distress syndrome

SIRS can lead to ARDS. ARDS is defined by the 'Berlin definition', which was produced by a consensus group comprising of The European Society of Intensive Care Medicine, The American Thoracic Society and Society of Critical Care Medicine. The Berlin definition defines ARDS as the acute onset (<1 week) of bilateral pulmonary oedema not fully explainable by cardiac failure. Neutrophil migration and activation in the lungs produce cytotoxins which damage lung endothelium, increasing permeability and causing the accumulation of proteins in the alveoli. Fluid follows as a result of the osmotic gradient leading to oedema and alveolar collapse. Lung function is compromised from the ventilation-perfusion mismatch and reduced lung compliance.

Multiple organ distress syndrome

SIRS contributes to the development of MODS which is defined as the potentially reversible deterioration in two or more organ systems not involved in the original insult. It is best viewed as a spectrum of progressive deterioration and typically begins with the lungs. Hypoperfusion resulting from hypovolaemia and/or coagulation abnormalities adds to this problem.

Sepsis

Paradoxically certain cytokines have been described as anti-inflammatory. The presence of either a pro-inflammatory or an anti-inflammatory state depends on the particular balance of cytokines at a given time. The latter predisposes to post-traumatic immunosuppression and sepsis. The migration of gut flora across a dysfunctional intestinal wall may explain the bacteraemia and sepsis seen in MODS in the absence of an obvious focus of infection.

Coagulation

Coagulation abnormalities are common. DIC arises through activation of both intrinsic and extrinsic pathways. This leads to microthrombosis and further organ hypoperfusion and dysfunction whilst also predisposing to bleeding due to the depletion of clotting factors. Pulmonary emboli can develop and the fat emboli produced as a result of long bone fractures further compromises lung function.

Second hit

Surgery acts a 'second hit' through the same mechanisms as above and can worsen the clinical picture. Definitive fixation while in a pro-inflammatory state with aggressive soft tissue dissection and multiple reamed intramedullary nailing increases systemic inflammation and fat emboli production. DCO is a solution to this problem in expediently stabilising long-bone fractures through minimally invasive external fixation techniques, thereby reducing the release of cytokines and fat emboli and the resulting inflammatory load.

Treatment

The initial aim is to adequately resuscitate the multiply injured patient. This includes the control and treatment of life-threatening haemorrhage, favouring blood products over crystalloid solutions and managing the patient according to established trauma protocols (see chapters 'Major trauma – Advanced Trauma Life Support principles' and 'Resuscitation and massive transfusion').

'Early appropriate care' is then instituted with either early definitive fixation or stabilisation by DCO principles. Various factors have been proposed to help guide decision-making. Measures of injury such as the Injury Severity Score (ISS) and IL-6 levels are either unhelpful in predicting patient outcome or are not easily available. Our shift in focus to measures of resuscitation has led to more widespread use of markers of hypoperfusion. Initially a lactate of <2.5 mmol/L or less was generally accepted as safe to proceed with early definitive fixation. Recent evidence suggests that a lactate of <4 mmol/L, a base excess >5.5 mmol/L or a pH >7.25 are indicators of an adequate resuscitation.

If resuscitation is unsatisfactory then the orthopaedic injuries are managed by external fixation techniques as per DCO principles and the patient is medically optimised in an intensive care setting. This includes the reversal of any coagulopathy, acidosis and hypothermia (the 'lethal triad'). Once resuscitated the patient can proceed to definitive fixation. Decision-making is multi-disciplinary and in conjunction with intensive care colleagues. To avoid contamination and infection when converting to definitive fixation it is generally recommended that this occur within 2 weeks of placement of the external fixator. The treatment process is illustrated in **Figure 17.1**.

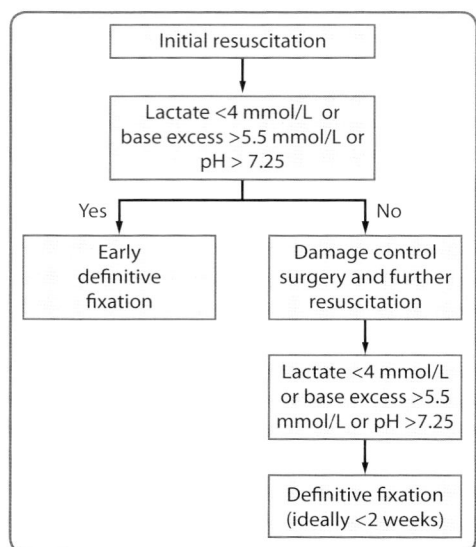

Figure 17.1 Algorithm for the management of major trauma patients.

Further reading

Giannoudis PV. Current concepts of the inflammatory response after major trauma: an update. Injury 2003; 34:397–404.

Tasker A, Kelly MB. Managing trauma: the evolution from 'early total care'/'damage control' to 'early appropriate care.' J Trauma Orthop 2014; 2:66–70.

Vallier HA, Wang X, Moore TA, et al. Timing of orthopaedic surgery in multiple trauma patients: development of a protocol for early appropriate care. J Orthop Trauma 2013; 27:543–551.

Related topics of interest

- *Topic 62* Major trauma – Advanced Trauma and Life Support principles
- *Topic 86* Resuscitation and massive transfusion
- *Topic 99* Trauma scoring systems

18 Elbow – dislocations and associated fractures

Key points
- Elbow dislocation, whether simple or complex, results in significant stiffness and functional disability
- Elbow dislocation is usually provoked by significant forces applied to it

Epidemiology
Despite the fact that the elbow joint is one of the most stable joints in body, it is the second most common joint dislocation in adults, with a prevalence of 0.6–1.3%. Elbow dislocation accounts for 25% of elbow injuries, and posterior dislocation is the most prevalent (80–90%). Half of the dislocations are sports-related, hence it occurs mostly in the younger population. High impact injury often results in elbow fracture-dislocation.

Pathophysiology
The elbow is commonly dislocated when subjected to combination of axial and posteriolateral valgus forces with a forearm that in is supination-external rotation position, e.g. a gymnast falling on outstretched hand (FOOSH).
Posterior elbow dislocation occurs in three stages:
- Stage 1: complete tear of the lateral ulnar collateral ligament (LUCL) with partial/total disruption of lateral collateral ligament (LCL)
- Stage 2: failure of the anterior capsule
- Stage 3: medial collateral ligament (MCL) disruption

Anatomy and biomechanics
The elbow is a hinge joint. It includes the humeroulnar and the capitulo-radial joints which in combination have a high range of motion; extension, flexion, supination and pronation. The elbow has two types of stabilisers:

1. Static and primary (bone and ligaments):
   - Trochlea: main stabilisation factor in varus/valgus stress
   - Capitulum, coronoid and olecranon: limits flexion/extension
   - Radial head: stabilises valgus external rotation
   - Medial ulnar collateral ligament (MUCL): composed of 3 bundles: anterior, posterior and oblique. It provides valgus stability
   - LCL complex: composed of the LUCL, radial collateral ligament and annular ligament. It gives varus stability
2. Dynamic and secondary (muscles that cross the joint)
   - Anconeus, brachialis and triceps

Posteriolateral rotation stability relies on the LCL and dynamic stabilisers. Posterior dislocation results from compressive forces. Anterior dislocation results from a direct posterior impact to a flexed elbow. Divergent dislocation usually is a component of high-energy trauma.

Clinical features
The dislocated elbow is swollen, painful and deformed. Neurovascular assessment should be clearly documented because vascular and neurological injuries are frequently associated with an elbow dislocation. Common sites of injury are the brachial artery, ulnar nerve (14%) and median nerve (20% have neuropraxia). Assessment of soft tissue is important to identify open fracture or skin tenting. Compartment syndrome should always be considered in patients with persistent pain or neurovascular compromise.

Investigations
Plain anteroposterior and lateral radiographs should be taken pre- and postreduction (Figure 18.1). A CT scan can be used for the diagnosis of complex injuries and

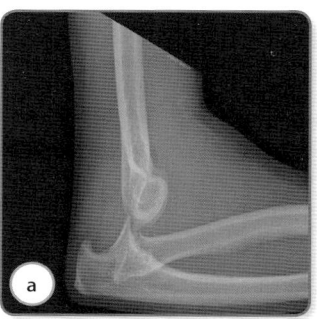
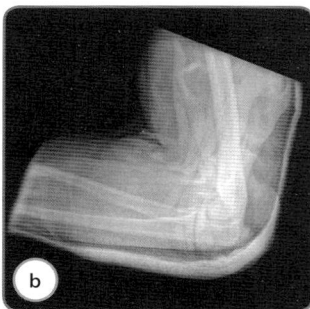

Figure 18.1. (a) Lateral view of a stable posterior elbow dislocation. (b) Post reduction.

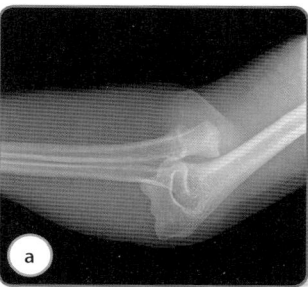
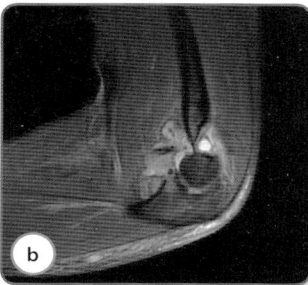

Figure 18.2. (a) Anteroposterior view of unstable elbow dislocation with no obvious fracture. (b) Coronoid fracture with suspected LCL and MCL tear.

preoperative planning. Ligamentous injuries are usually evaluated by evaluation under anaesthesia (EUA) or MRI (**Figure 18.2**).

Classification is based on the direction of dislocation and associated fractures, and whether the fracture is stable or unstable.

1. According to direction: either posterior, anterior or divergent. The position of the forearm is described in relation to the arm. Divergent elbow dislocation is a high impact injury that separates the ulna from the radius and involves disruption of the interosseous membrane and annular ligament.
2. According to associated fractures:
   I. Simple: dislocation with no associated fracture
   II. Complex: fracture dislocation, subdivided into:
      a. Elbow dislocation with radial head fracture: radial head fracture originally classified by Mason and modified by Hotchkiss (**Table 18.1**).
      b. Elbow dislocation with coronoid process fracture: coronoid fracture has been classified according to Regan and Morrey (**Table 18.2**). Sometimes CT scan or MRI identify the fracture (**Figure 18.2**).
      c. Terrible triad: is a combination of elbow dislocation, coronoid process and radial head fractures.

Table 18.1 Mason classification as modified by Hotchkiss for radial head fracture

Type	Description
I	Minimally displaced fracture; <2 mm, no rotational block or instability
II	Displaced fracture >2 mm, or any rotational block
III	Comminuted fracture, or radial head fracture with elbow dislocation

Table 18.2 Regan and Morrey classification for coronoid fracture

Type	Description
I	Coronoid process tip avulsion
II	Fracture of 50% or less
III	Fracture of more than 50%

d. Transolecranon fracture-dislocation: most of the time is associated with anterior elbow dislocation. It has two subtypes: dislocation with simple olecranon fracture and one with comminuted olecranon fracture.
e. Posterior Monteggia fracture-dislocation: involves fracture of the proximal ulna with radial head dislocation. The radial head is dislocated dorsal to the ulnar distal fragment.
3. According to stability: either stable or unstable. Identification of elbow stability is difficult in the acute setting. However, EUA is the mainstay method of diagnosis.

Treatment

The goals of treatment are to restore stable reduced joint, function, and avoid complications: infection, vascular compromise and compartment syndrome. Early range of mobility is important to prevent stiffness. Treatment can be nonoperative or operative depending on the severity of injury and patient factors (**Table 18.3**). However, elbow stability should be checked after reduction for all treatments.

Nonoperative

1. Simple posterior elbow dislocation (stable): stage 1 and 2 are usually treated by traction and flexion. Then, stability is assessed in 30° and the cast is applied to the forearm in supination (LCL disruption) or pronation (MCL disruption) and in 90° flexion. Early range of motion is recommended. There are different protocols according to the injury. Generally, adjusted motion depends on the type of injury and starts at week 1 or 2.
2. Simple posterior elbow dislocation (unstable): in stage 3 the elbow is not stable in extension; the cast should be applied at 110°. Surgical stabilisation follows within 1–2 weeks.

Operative

Operative treatment is indicated for unstable elbow fractures. It is the case for most elbow fracture-dislocations. Indications and treatment options can be summarised as the following:

1. Elbow dislocation with a radial head fracture: this applies for type II and III Mason radial head fracture. It results in posteriolateral instability due to the associated LCL complex injury. Treatment options are:
   a. reconstruction of the radial head with LCL repair
   b. Radial head arthroplasty for unfixable head
2. Terrible triad: very unstable injury. It has complications of recurrent dislocation, chronic instability, and post-traumatic pain and stiffness. Surgery includes utilisation of posterior approach and:
   a. Radial head open reduction and internal fixation (ORIF), if unfixable then should be replaced. If the fractured fragment is <25% it can be excised.
   b. Coronoid process reattachment: type I can be repaired by suturing the anterior capsule to the ulna. Type III

Table 18.3 Summary of management of elbow dislocation				
Type	Radial head/neck fracture	Coronoid	LCL	Treatment
Simple posterior elbow dislocation	No	No	Yes	Nonoperative
Terrible triad	Yes	Yes	Yes	Operative
Dislocation with radial fracture	Yes	–	Yes	Operative (except Mason I)
Anterior transolecranon dislocation	Rare	Often	Rare	Operative
Posteriomedial instability	Rare	Yes	Common	Operative
Criteria for nonoperative treatment to be met are: 1. joint alignment restoration. 2. Radial head fracture Mason I. 3. Coronoid process fracture type I. 4. Stable joint				

can be managed by ORIF using either cannulated screws or plating. Type II management is controversial and can be addressed by either way
   c. LCL repair +/− MCL repair
3. Elbow dislocation with an isolated coronoid fracture: the repair of the coronoid depends on the degree of injury as mentioned above. Anteriomedial, lateral (Kocher), or posterior approach can be used. Hinged external fixator is used for fragile bone or instability post repair.
4. Chronic instability: this is a challenging issue. Most common types are posteriomedial (coronoid fracture) and posteriolateral (LCL and dynamic stabilisers). Failure to repair ruptured collaterals can result in painful compensation of the extensor mechanism. There are various methods described depending on the underlying pathology which range from ligament reconstruction and triceps lengthening to osteochondral grafting and elbow replacement.

Complications

Acute
- Neurovascular injury
- Compartment syndrome

Chronic
- Chronic instability
- Restricted motion: the most common complication post elbow dislocation. It is estimated that there is 8° loss of extension by 1 year
- Stiffness (5–10%). Increased risk with radial head fracture and prolonged period of immobilisation
- Heterotrophic ossification range between 1.6% to 50%

Further reading

Chan K, King G, Faber K. Treatment of complex elbow fracture dislocations. Curr Rev Musculoskelet Med 2016; 9:185–189.

Englert C, Zellner J, Koller M, Nerlich M, Lenich A. Elbow dislocations: a review ranging from soft tissue injuries to complex elbow fracture dislocations. Adv Orthop 2013; 2013: 951397.

Lee DH. Treatment options for complex elbow fracture dislocations. Injury 2001; 32:SD41–69.

Related topics of interest

- *Topic 32* Forearm – distal radial fractures
- *Topic 34* Forearm – radius and ulna fractures
- *Topic 85* Principles of operative management of fractures

19 Elbow – olecranon fractures

Key points
- Olecranon fractures occur mostly due to direct trauma
- Whilst undisplaced fractures of the olecranon can be managed conservatively, displacement of the fracture fragments is better treated with reduction and internal fixation
- In elderly frail patients, particularly with comorbidities, even displaced fractures could be managed nonoperatively. Extension of the elbow is still possible, as this movement is aided by gravity

Epidemiology
Olecranon fractures comprise 10% of all upper limb fractures. Over 80% of these fractures are displaced at presentation.

Pathophysiology
Most of these fractures are in the elderly and occur as a result of direct trauma. Indirect trauma is usually caused by a fall on an outstretched arm. The triceps tendon is attached to the olecranon process. Pull of the triceps tendon results in the displacement of the fracture fragments. High-energy injuries result in comminution at the fracture site. As the olecranon articulates with the distal humerus these fractures are intra-articular fractures. A proportion of these fractures are open fractures, particularly in high-energy injuries.

Clinical signs and symptoms
Patients present with swelling and pain around the point of the elbow. Patients will have difficulty in extending the elbow. Clinical examination may reveal a palpable gap at the fracture site due to the displacement of the fragments. Patients have inability to extend the elbow against gravity.

Investigations
Plain radiographs of the elbow in two views, anteroposterior and lateral, may be the only investigation required in most cases. However in patients with more complex injuries and multiple injuries CT scan may give more information about the fracture anatomy.

Classification
Mayo classification is commonly used.
Type I
- Undisplaced or nondisplaced fracture
- IA: Undisplaced noncomminuted fracture
- IB: Undisplaced comminuted fracture

Type II
- Displaced but stable fracture. The ligaments of the elbow are not damaged.
- IIA: Displaced noncomminuted fracture
- IIB: Displaced comminuted fracture

Type III
- Displaced unstable fracture associated with dislocation
- IIIA: Displaced unstable noncomminuted fracture
- IIIB: Displaced unstable comminuted fracture

Treatment
The aims of the treatment are to restore the anatomy, repair the extensor mechanism of the elbow, restore stability of the elbow joint, early mobilisation to prevent elbow stiffness and prevent any complications (**Figure 19.1**).

Nonoperative treatment is the preferred treatment of choice in nondisplaced fractures or minimally displaced fractures, where the extensor mechanism is not disrupted. Conservative treatment may also be used for elderly patients with displaced fractures who cannot have surgery due to medical reasons.

Surgical treatment is reserved for displaced fractures, with incongruity of

Topic 19

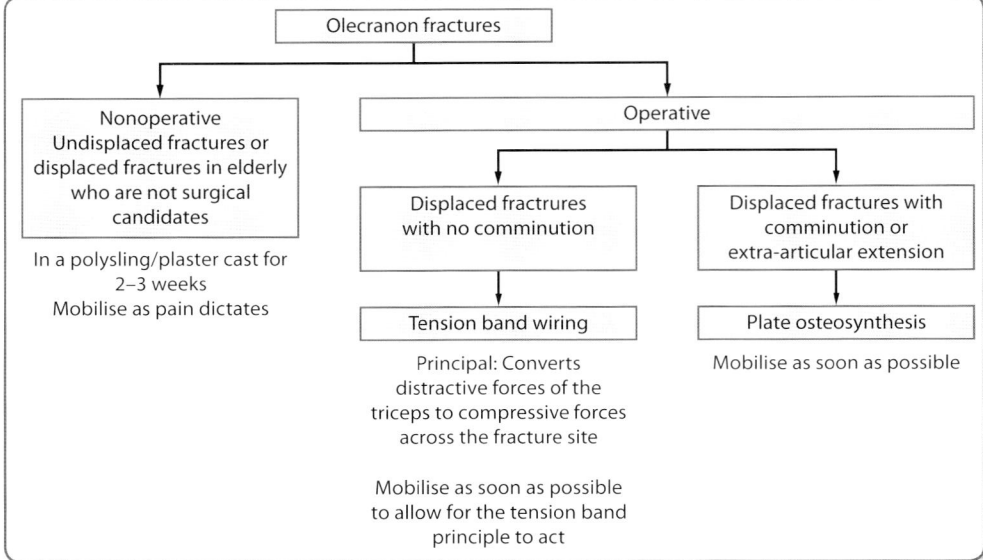

Figure 19.1. Management of olecranon fractures.

the articular surface and disruption of the extensor mechanism.

Tension band technique is used for displaced fractures with little or no comminution. The principle of tension band technique is to convert distractive forces to compressive forces across the fracture site. There are a few important surgical tips:
- It is better to have the 'K'-wires engage the anterior cortex of the distal fragment to prevent wire migration or back out.
- It is important to bury the 'K'-wires to prevent skin complications and wire pull-out.
- The circlage wire is placed underneath the triceps tendon to prevent wire back out and to be more effective in converting the distractive forces to compressive forces.

Comminuted displaced fractures are best treated with plate osteosynthesis (**Figure 19.2**).

Complications

Resulting from the fracture

Painful nonunion and weakness of elbow extension against gravity. Instability and loss of function may occur. Post-traumatic arthrosis may occur due to articular incongruity.

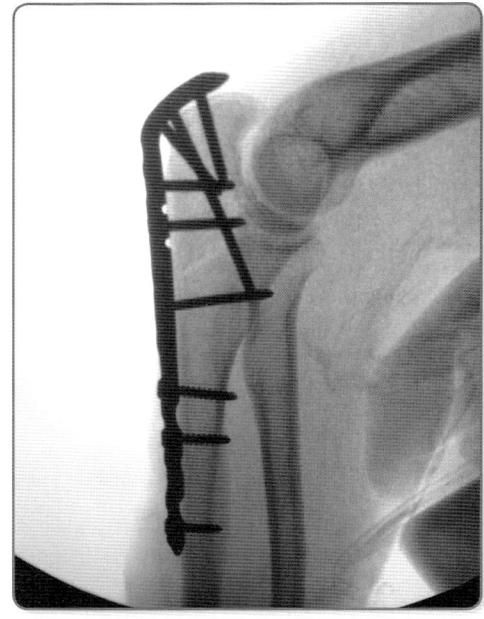

Figure 19.2. Plating of olecranon fracture with metaphyseal extension.

Arising due to surgery

Metal work prominence could lead to pain. The incidence varies from 3–80%. Wire back out is a common complication.

Risk of infection is 0–6%. Neurological symptoms related to ulnar nerve is reported to be between 2% and 5%.

Further reading

Hak DJ, Golladay GJ. Olecranon fractures: treatment options. J Am Acad Orthop Surg 2000; 8:266–275.

Wiegand L, Bernstien J, Ahn J. Fractures in brief: Olecranon fractures. Clin Orthop Relat Res 2012; 470:3637–3641.

Related topics of interest

- *Topic 18* Elbow – dislocations and associated fractures
- *Topic 20* Elbow – radial head and neck fractures

20 Elbow – radial head and neck fractures

Key points
- Most fractures of the radial head and neck are either nondisplaced or minimally displaced and can be managed conservatively
- Classification of radial head and neck fractures can guide the treatment and predict the outcome
- Treatment options for displaced fractures can be either fixation, excision, or replacement of the radial head

Epidemiology
Fractures of the radial head account for 4% of all fractures and approximately 20% of elbow fractures. These fractures can be a part of a more complex elbow injury and can affect elbow stability as the radial head is a secondary stabiliser of the elbow.

Radial neck fractures are less common; their incidence increases with age and they are usually less complex.

Pathophysiology
The most common mechanism of injury is falling onto the out-stretched hand while the forearm is in pronation, which results in axial loading and fracture. Due to this mechanism of injury, other associated fractures can occur such as carpal fractures, distal radioulnar joint injury and Monteggia's fracture-dislocations.

Ligamentous injuries to the elbow can be also associated with radial head fractures and if these are suspected a MRI should be performed for further evaluation.

When the radial head fracture is associated with other injuries such as elbow dislocation and/or coronoid fracture, it can result in elbow instability and the elbow must be examined carefully to check for signs of instability.

Clinical features
The patient typically has pain and tenderness around the lateral aspect of the elbow. They will also have a painful range of motion of the elbow in flexion/extension and pronation/supination.

Careful examination of the wrist should be performed to exclude injury and instability at the distal radioulnar joint. The forearm must also be examined for tenderness and signs of interosseous membrane injury or Essex–Lopresti lesion.

If there is pain and bruising around the medial side of the elbow this can mean there is injury to the medial collateral ligament.

Investigations
Plain radiographs in both the anteroposterior and lateral view of the elbow should be obtained routinely. Radial head views can be helpful with the forearm at different degrees of supination and pronation. Other views include the radiocapitellar view, which is performed by taking a lateral view to the elbow with the tube tilted 45° to the shoulder.

Undisplaced fractures of the radial head can be diagnosed radiologically by elevation of the anterior and posterior fat pads (Sail sign).

If there is a clinical suspicion of other associated , e.g. wrist or forearm, appropriate radiographs should be obtained.

For comminuted fractures a CT scan can be useful for preoperative planning. MRI can be used to evaluate the ligamentous structures around the elbow, especially in the case of a radial head fracture with associated elbow dislocation.

Classification
The Mason classification is the most commonly used classification system (**Figure 20.1**).

Elbow – radial head and neck fractures

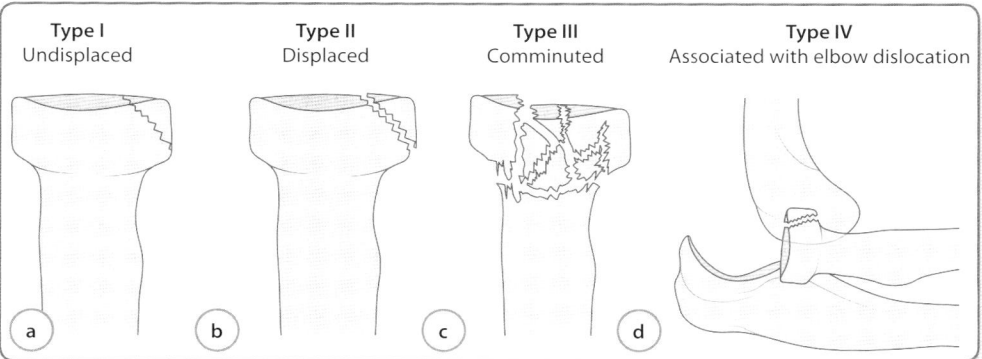

Figure 20.1 Mason classification of radial head fracture.

There are other less commonly used classification systems, such as Hotchkiss, which determines the suitability of the radial head for fixation.

Treatment

Nonoperative treatment

Most radial head fractures are nondisplaced and conservative management usually results in a satisfactory outcome.

Early mobilisation is the key to avoid stiffness which can result from capsular contracture. Most patients who have an extension lag following conservative treatment respond well to a stretching program.

Aspiration of the haematoma in a stable nondisplaced radial head fracture can help with pain relief and to check the range of motion of the elbow, but this is not routinely performed.

Operative treatment

Indications for surgery include:
- Mason type II fracture with mechanical block
- Mason type III fracture
- Associated injuries affecting elbow stability

The operative treatment can be either fixation of the radial head, excision or radial head replacement, depending on the complexity of the fracture pattern and the presence of any associated injuries.

Fixation of the radial head has a superior outcome to the radial head excision, when it is technically feasible.

A summary of treatments is shown in Table 20.1.

Open reduction and internal fixation of the radial head

This is performed by a lateral approach to the elbow (Kocher), and the fixation options include screws, plates and K-wires.

The hardware must be placed in the safe zone in the radial head so it does not affect elbow rotation. Any implants applied outside this zone should be countersunk.

Radial head replacement

Radial head replacement is an option in comminuted fractures which are not suited for surgical fixation. Implant designs include unipolar and bipolar designs, silicon and metal implants. Care should be taken not to oversize the radiocapitellar joint.

Radial head excision

This can be offered to the low demand patients or in the delayed setting of pain after isolated comminuted fracture of the radial head. It is contraindicated in the presence of forearm or elbow instability as the radial head is a secondary stabiliser to the elbow laterally.

When excision is indicated a push–pull test should not show >2 mm movement of the radius.

Table 20.1 Summary of the management of radial head fracture

Fracture type	Management
Mason (I)	Conservative treatment
Mason (II)	Conservative treatment unless: • Mechanical block (ORIF) • Instability (ORIF + ligament reconstruction)
Mason (III)	Surgical: • ORIF • Replacement • Excision
Mason (IV)	Reduce and treat as type (III)

ORIF, open reduction and internal fixation

Complications

- Pain at the radiocapitellar articulation and secondary arthritis
- Joint instability
- Proximal radial migration when there is associated interosseous membrane injury
- Decreased strength and elbow range of motion
- Cubitus valgus
- Complications related to surgery as infection, posterior interosseous nerve palsy

Further reading

Aktselis I, Zahid Saeed M, Ahrens P, et al. Radial head fractures – an instructional review of current concepts of management. Internet J Orthop Surg 2014.

Duckworth AD, McQueen MM, Ring D. Fractures of the radial head. Bone Joint J 2013; 95B:151–159.

Related topics of interest

- Topic 18 Elbow – dislocations and associated fractures
- Topic 19 Elbow – olecranon fractures
- Topic 33 Forearm – Galeazzi's and Monteggia's fractures

21 Fat embolism and acute respiratory distress syndrome

Key points

- Fat embolism is the presence of fat globules in circulation or lung parenchyma. It is usually asymptomatic, but when symptomatic it can cause fat embolism syndrome (FES)
- FES symptoms comprise respiratory changes, petechial rash and neurological manifestations. Respiratory changes of FES produce a clinical picture similar to acute respiratory distress syndrome (ARDS)
- ARDS is the acute onset of lung inflammation that impairs gaseous exchange at alveolar level

Incidence and causes

Fat embolism is mainly caused by trauma after a long bone or pelvic fracture, or as a result of surgical interventions such as joint reconstruction, intramedullary nail fixation and liposuction.

The incidence increases with the number of fractures involved (1–3% in single long bone fractures rising to 33% in bilateral femoral fractures) and is more common in closed as opposed to open fractures. Nontraumatic causes of fat embolism include sickle cell disease, pancreatitis, diabetes mellitus and steroid therapy.

Pathophysiology

The description of fat embolism dates back to 1873, but it is still challenging for clinicians to diagnose. It is not clearly understood how fat emboli produce clinical symptoms, though this can be explained by biochemical and mechanical theories.

The mechanical theory focuses on obstructive mechanism when fat globules enter the circulation through torn venules following a long bone fracture or disrupted adipose tissues. With the increase in pulmonary artery and right heart pressure they can pass through the patent foramen ovale to cause systemic manifestation. Studies have demonstrated the appearance of embolic material even in the absence of a patent foramen ovale, which suggests that an increase in right intraventricular pressure forces emboli to pass through the pulmonary capillaries and into the systemic circulation, causing a systemic effect. This theory is supported by transoesophageal echocardiography showing echogenic material passing into the right heart during orthopaedic surgery, which is related to an increase in intramedullary pressure.

The bio-chemical theory focuses on the production of toxic intermediates. Fat globules in circulation are hydrolysed over time to several products including free fatty acids (FFAs), which in turn cause clinical manifestation. This theory is supported by the delay in development of symptoms as it takes time to produce toxic intermediates.

Clinical features

The FES usually presents 12–72 hours after the initial injury with the triad of respiratory changes, cerebral manifestations and petechial rash. Respiratory changes are usually the first to develop, including hypoxaemia, tachypnoea, dyspnoea, haemoptysis, chest discomfort and crepitation. The severity of these symptoms can progress to respiratory failure and may require mechanical ventilation.

Cerebral features result from cerebral emboli and can cause a wide spectrum of changes from diffuse cerebral abnormality to focal neurological signs. Clinical features include confusion, agitation, restlessness, seizures, hemiparesis, hemiplegia, aphasia, apraxia and visual field disturbance.

A petechial rash usually develops 24 hours after respiratory and cerebral symptoms and results from embolisation of the small dermal capillaries causing extravasation of erythrocytes. The characteristic petechial rash appears bilaterally in the axilla, neck, front of the chest, mouth, palate and conjunctiva. It never appears on the face or posterior aspect of body and it rarely occurs on legs.

Other systemic features include pyrexia, tachycardia, right heart strain, ECG changes, oliguria, proteinuria, coagulation abnormalities, Purtscher's retinopathy (consisting of cotton wool exudates), macular oedema and haemorrhage.

Diagnosis

An unexplained anaemia (70% of patients) and thrombocytopaenia (platelet count <150,000/mm^3) are often found. Hypocalcaemia (due to binding of FFAs to calcium) and elevated serum lipase have also been reported. Blood gas analysis usually shows hypoxia and hypocapnia.

A chest X-ray is normal at the time of injury but later signs of generalised pulmonary interstitial and alveolar shadowing occur with no cardiomegaly (See **Figure 21.1**). A chest CT will demonstrate ground glass opacities with interlobular septal thickening.

Fat droplets can be found in urine, blood, sputum and macrophages of bronchoalveolar lavage, although their presence does not necessarily mean FES as they can also be detected in asymptomatic cases.

The most common diagnostic set based on major and minor criteria was published by Gurd and Wilson. Major criteria are based on the classic triad of respiratory changes, neurological manifestation, and petechial rash. Rash is often pathognomic though it is not present in every case. For diagnosis of FES to be made at least one major and four minor criteria must be present.

Gurd's and Wilson's criteria

Major criteria:
- Axillary or subconjunctival petechiae
- Hypoxaemia (PaO_2 <60 mmHg; FiO_2 = 0.4)
- Central nervous system depression disproportionate to hypoxaemia
- Pulmonary oedema

Minor criteria:
- Tachycardia >110 bpm
- Pyrexia >38.5°C
- Emboli present in the retina on fundoscopy
- Fat present in urine
- A sudden inexplicable drop in hematocrit or platelet values
- Increasing erythrocyte sedimentation rate (ESR)
- Fat globules present in the sputum

Lindeque's criteria are based on respiratory features of sustained PaO_2 <8 kPa, sustained PCO_2 > 7.3 kPa or pH <7.3 and sustained tachypnoea > 35/min despite sedation with increased work of breathing (dyspnoea, tachycardia, accessory muscle use and anxiety). Schonfield's criteria are based on a semi-quantitative means of diagnosing FES with a score >5 required for positive diagnosis (**Table 21.1**).

Treatment

There is no specific treatment for FES, so prevention, early diagnosis and adequate symptomatic treatment are of paramount importance.

Early intervention to immobilise fractures reduces the risk of developing FES, as fracture

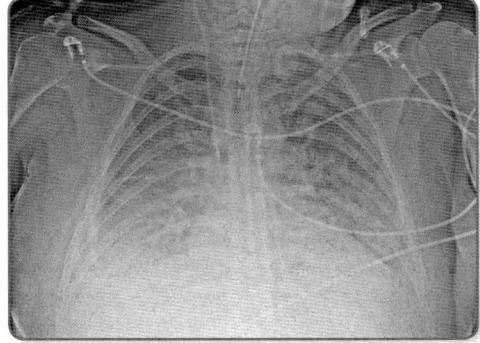

Figure 21.1 Portable anteroposterior chest radiograph showing widespread bilateral pulmonary infiltrates with no cardiomegaly. The changes are consistent with acute respiratory distress syndrome (ARDS), endotracheal tube and right internal jugular central venous catheter (CVC) can also be seen.

Fat embolism and acute respiratory distress syndrome

Table 21.1 Schofield's criteria	
Criteria	Score
Petechiae	5
X-ray chest diffuse infiltrates	4
Hypoxaemia	3
Fever	1
Tachycardia	1
Tachypnoea	1
Confusion	1

mobility continues to liberate fat globules into the circulation through venous sinusoids. Another strategy to prevent FES is to limit elevation of intraosseous pressure during orthopaedic procedures, particularly hip arthroplasty and intramedullary nail fixation.

Symptomatic treatment is aimed at maintaining adequate pulmonary exchange and follows the same principle as management of ARDS which includes spontaneous ventilation with oxygen inhalation using a face mask and high flow gas delivery system (with the aim of delivering 50–80% FIO_2). Continuous positive airway pressure (CPAP) is also used to improve PaO_2 without increasing FIO_2. Mechanical ventilation and positive end expiratory pressure (PEEP) should be considered if the patient requires $FIO_2 >60\%$ and CPAP >10 cm of Hg to maintain $PaO_2 > 60$ mmHg.

Prophylactic treatment with albumin has been recommended for volume resuscitation in cases of hyperproteinaemia because it not only restores volume but also binds FFAs and may decrease the extent of injury. Studies have shown a mixed response on the use of corticosteroids and it is currently not recommended for prophylaxis or treatment.

Further reading

Bernard GR, Artigas A, Brigham KL, et al. The American-European Consensus Conference on ARDS. Definitions, mechanisms, relevant outcomes, and clinical trial coordination. Am J Respir Crit Care Med 1994; 149:818–824.

Johnson MJ, Lucas GL. Fat embolism syndrome. Orthopedics 1996; 19:41–48.

Wofe WG, DeVries WC. Oxygen toxicity. Annu Rev Med 1975; 26:203–214.

Related topics of interest

- *Topic 17* Damage control orthopaedics and trauma physiology
- *Topic 24* Femoral fractures – shaft
- *Topic 52* Implants – nails
- *Topic 86* Resuscitation and massive transfusion
- *Topic 98* Tibial shaft fractures

22 Femoral fractures – distal

Key points
- Distal femoral articular fractures often need surgical treatment
- Intra-articular fractures are most often unstable and lead to loss of limb alignment
- Very comminuted fractures can require limb salvage procedures including endoprosthetic replacement

Epidemiology

Distal femoral fractures are those which include the distal femoral metaphysis (supracondylar) and the articular surface fractures. These are much less common than hip fractures.

These fractures have a bimodal distribution. They are more common in the elderly who have osteoporotic bone, but in the young distal femoral fractures are high energy injuries often with unrecognised associated injuries to the knee itself. Complicating factors include pre-existing arthritic change within the knee, which may change management in the older population considerably.

Pathophysiology

These fractures can result from severe varus or valgus with axial loading. Rotational forces can also be involved. The amount of energy transferred at the time of fracture will be reflected in the fracture pattern, particularly in young patients with good bone quality. Comminuted fractures in this group of patients should raise the possibility of associated neurovascular injury. In this population, these often occur in motor vehicle accidents or falls from heights. In the elderly population fractures result from minor slips and falls, particularly onto a flexed knee.

The deforming forces are produced by the hamstring muscles which cross the knee posteriorly and cause posterior displacement of the distal fragment and shortening as well as angulation. Depending on the level of the fracture adductor muscle action on the more proximal segment can increase the amount of angulation at the fracture site.

Clinical features

History of the mechanism of injury, particularly in the young patient, should alert one to the presence of associated injuries. Initial assessment should be done according to the Advanced Trauma Life Support guidelines. Injuries to the ipsilateral femur, especially of the femoral neck should also be ruled out, especially in dashboard injuries where the flexed knee has met with a large deforming force.

Examination will reveal swelling and extreme discomfort, even on light palpation. If the fracture is intra-articular a large haemarthrosis is inevitably present. If reliable documentation of intact neurology and vascular status is not available, the distal neurovascular status of the limb should be assessed. Often, by the time trauma assessment of the patient is to be performed the limb has been immobilised in a long leg back slab. If treatment is not imminent in theatre, the immobilisation should be split and the limb examined thoroughly.

Soft tissue injuries should be documented carefully because they may delay treatment. Compartment syndrome is uncommon in these injuries.

Investigations

Routine radiographic evaluation with an anteroposterior and lateral radiographs often show enough detail to plan treatment. If a fracture in the supracondylar region is thought to extend into the joint and this is not obviously evident, then a CT scan may be required for further evaluation to plan treatment. One may need a CT scan in comminuted fractures to aid joint reconstruction planning. If doubts are present about vascularity of the distal part of the limb, arteriography should be performed and a vascular surgery referral will need to be made.

Femoral fractures – distal

Classification

The most widely accepted classification of supracondylar fractures is that developed by Muller and refined by (Arbeitsgemeinschaft für Osteosynthesefragen (AO)/Orthopaedic Trauma Association (OTA) classification systems) (**Table 22.1**). This separates these fractures into three general types. Type A are extra-articular, type B are partial articular or unicondylar and type C are complete articular, which are bicondylar. In each of the three types A, B and C, three sub groups are present.

Treatment

Treatment principles are based on fracture morphology:
- Extra-articular
- Intra-articular – reconstructable
- Intra-articular – not reconstructable

Extra-articular fractures can be treated with retrograde nailing, particularly in transverse fracture patterns. The nailing procedure can be done through a minimally invasive approach with a support under a flexed knee on a radiolucent table. The nail can be passed through the patellar tendon, just below the inferior pole of the patella. Satisfactory fixation may be obtained with medial and lateral distal locking and in very portoic bone there are systems available where bolts can be used to lock the nail distally. Proximal locking can be achieved with jigs if nail length is short. If a longer nail is used, this will need to be freehand. Proximal locking is best done in orthogonal planes with two screws at 90° to each other. Nontransverse fracture patterns are often better treated with plate fixation (**Figure 22.1**). The plate can help act as a buttress to aid reduction or prevent loss of position. Anatomically contoured locking plates to deal with distal femoral anatomy have been a major advance in the treatment of these fractures. A combination of compression screws and locking screws can be inserted, both distally and proximally to help reduce the fracture and obtain a stable construct (**Figure 22.2**). These plates can be very stiff and as a result the construct can be

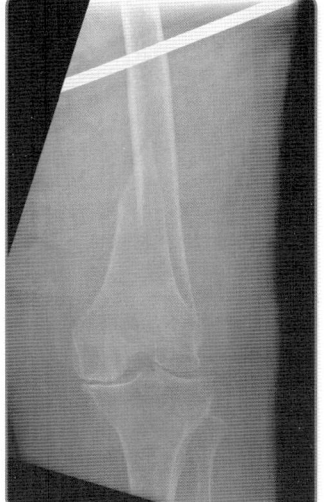

Figure 22.1 Type 1A distal femoral fracture with long spiral fragment.

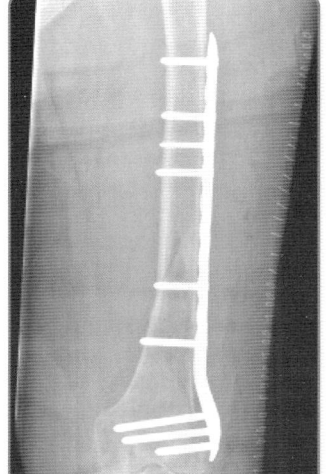

Figure 22.2 Same fracture fixed using a long distal lateral femoral locking plate.

Table 22.1 AO/OTA classification of distal femoral fractures

Type A	Type B	Type C
Simple two-part fracture	Lateral condyle (sagittal plane) fracture	Articular simple and metaphyseal (T or Y configuration)
Metaphyseal wedge	Medial condyle (sagittal plane) fracture	Articular simple and metaphyseal comminuted
Metaphyseal complex	Frontal (coronal plane) fracture; Hoffa's fracture	Multifragmentary articular

too rigid leading to nonunion as a result of loss of micro motion. They are applied as an internal 'external fixator' and so a reasonable working length of the plate is needed to allow compression at the fracture site and yield satisfactory healing before metal fatigue and fixation failure occurs.

In intra-articular fractures locking plate fixation can still be used. However, first the articular fragments should be converted into a single distal fragment through reduction manoeuvres. Compression screws may be required anterior to where the plate is to be later placed or from anterior to posterior (as in the case of Hoffa fractures). The plate can then be applied as for extra-articular fractures as described above.

In severely comminuted fractures where it is felt that the fracture is unreconstructable, one may have to make a decision about whether to treat the fracture nonoperatively (where comorbidities preclude operative management) or operatively using a distal femoral endoprosthesis while performing a knee replacement.

Complications

Intraoperative complications includes neurovascular injury and care must be taken to avoid this when reducing the fracture and also when inserting the metalwork. Penetration of metalwork into the joint is to be avoided at all costs. This will result in pain and early degeneration if not recognised. When using locking plates, penetration of the intercondylar notch can result in damage to the cruciate ligaments and lead to excessive stiffness.

Infection can result, particularly if operating through a soft tissue envelope which is injured. Compartment syndrome is an unusual complication in this type of fracture, but should be kept in mind if there is unexplained pain and/or neurovascular compromise postoperatively. Early failure of fixation can occur if there is poor bone stock or poor compliance with postoperative care. Unfortunately, failure of fixation can indicate technically deficient surgery in terms of obtaining a satisfactory reduction and poor fixation, so it is generally better to extend fixation proximally when there is doubt about a quality of bone.

Nonunion is uncommon as these are metaphyseal fractures and usually heal quite readily. Malunion is a result of failure of a reduction, failure of fixation, or both. These can lead to a poor functional result with excessive knee stiffness and predispose the knee to early osteoarthritis. Knee stiffness can occur even with satisfactory fixation and early active mobilisation should be encouraged. Metalwork protrusion can be a problem, particularly if the screws are long on the medial side and may require removal. Post-traumatic osteoarthritis unfortunately is common with intra-articular fractures, especially with those fractures where there has been poor reduction and resultant joint surface incongruence.

Further reading

Appleton P, Moran M, Houshian S, Robinson CM. Distal femoral fractures treated by hinged total knee replacement in elderly patients. J Bone Joint Surg Br 2006; 88:1065–1070.

Collinge CA, Wiss DA. Distal femoral fractures. In: Rockwood and Green's Fractures in Adults 8th edn. Wolters Kluwer 2015:2229–2268.

Ehlinger M, Ducrot G, Adam P, Bonnomet F. Distal femur fractures. Surgical techniques and a review of the literature. Orthop Traumatol Surg Res 2013; 99:353–360.

Related topics of interest

- *Topic 24* Femoral fractures – shaft
- *Topic 61* Knee dislocations – multiligament injuries
- *Topic 97* Tibial plateau fractures

23 Femoral fractures – periprosthetic

Key points
- Periprosthetic fractures can involve the proximal femur around a total hip replacement or the distal femur around a knee replacement
- Stability of the prosthesis is key to decision making
- These can be challenging injuries which may require referral to a specialist treatment centre

Epidemiology

There is an increase in prevalence of periprosthetic fractures in the proximal and distal femur. This is related to the growing number of arthroplasties being performed every year. Patients are more active following arthroplasty surgery and live longer. A periprosthetic fracture is more common following a revision surgery, and is the third most common reason for reoperation on a total hip replacement, accounting for approximately 1 in 10 reoperations. One in 20 revision hip replacements are done for periprosthetic fracture.

The mortality following periprosthetic fracture is very similar to that for a primary hip fracture at 1 year. It is approximately five times as high as that for primary hip arthroplasty. Proximal periprosthetic fractures are associated with high complication rates and reoperation in up to 50% of cases. Risk factors predisposing individuals to periprosthetic fracture are osteoporosis, increased age and obesity. Poor surgical technique in the primary procedure can also contribute. High-energy injuries tend to occur in younger patients.

Periprosthetic fractures around the knee are associated especially with poor bone quality and occur commonly in older patients with minimal trauma, particularly in those who have rheumatoid arthritis and previous steroid use. Neurological conditions predisposing patients to falls such as Parkinson's disease can also contribute to increasing incidents in the older population.

Pathophysiology

Fractures around a hip replacement occur more easily in patients with poor bone quality or loosening. They are more commonly associated with instability following primary joint replacement as this predisposes the patient to falls. High-energy injuries are noted in younger patients with well-fixed prostheses. The fracture pattern reflects the mechanism of loading. Torsional loading will lead to complex fracture patterns and increase the risk of instability of the prosthesis, necessitating revision procedure. Low-energy injuries can occur in simple falls in patients with loosening or where there is poor bone stock, often when there has been osteolysis surrounding an old hip replacement.

Mechanisms of injury in distal femur periprosthetic fractures around a knee replacement are similar to those for supracondylar fracture of the femur. High-energy injuries are seen in relatively younger patients with good quality bone and low-energy injuries are seen in patients with poor quality bone. Loosening of the prosthesis in this area is more likely to occur in a patient with poor quality bone as the fracture is likely to extend to the bone cement interface.

Clinical features

With occult proximal femoral fractures around a hip prosthesis, patients will complain of pain and being unable to weight bear. Straight leg raise is often absent. These fractures may require a high index of suspicion and additional investigation. Displaced fractures will cause shortening and deformity with swelling and localised tenderness. The patient is unlikely to be able to actively move the hip to a large degree. Dislocation in association with fracture of the femur around a femoral stem is unusual.

Neurovascular injury is also unusual, but must still be assessed for.

Clinical features of periprosthetic fractures around a knee replacement will be pain with associated swelling and deformity. Recurvatum at the fracture site is common due to muscle action and the effect of gravity. One must be aware of the risk of neurovascular damage at the level of the fracture due to the deformity and angulation.

In both these groups of injuries open fractures are relatively uncommon.

Investigations

Plain anteroposterior and lateral radiographs of the proximal or distal femur usually are sufficient in diagnosing the fracture. However, in preoperative planning oblique views may be required. In addition, CT scan is useful for seeing fracture lines which are not evident on plain X-rays due to superimposition of in situ metalwork. CT scans are invaluable in allowing one to plan appropriate surgery.

If periprosthetic fracture is associated with an osteolytic lesion, a skeletal survey or bone scan may also be required. MRI is less useful because of artefact, but metal artefact reduction sequences (MARS) can provide useful information.

Where vascular injury is suspected, urgent arteriography may be required.

Classification

For periprosthetic fractures around the femoral stem, the most widely accepted classification is the Vancouver grading system (**Table 23.1**). Type A fractures occur in the trochanteric region and require internal fixation if displaced. Type B fractures can be subclassified into three further sub types: B1 fractures are around the stem or just below where the stem itself is well fixed. B2 fractures are those around the stem, but with a loose stem and good proximal bone. B3 fractures are those around the stem or just below, but with poor quality or severely comminuted proximal bone. Type C fractures are those which are well below the prosthesis.

Distal femur periprosthetic fractures have various classification systems. Lewis and Rorabeck classification helps guide treatment (**Table 23.2**). Type 1 fractures are nondisplaced with the component fixation intact. Type 2 fractures are those which are displaced with the component fixation intact. Type 3 fractures are displaced with the component loose or failing. The latter often have significant comminution and are present in osteoporotic bone which contributes to the component loosening and failure.

Treatment

Proximal femoral periprosthetic fracture treatment is challenging to plan and execute.

Table 23.2 Lewis and Rorabeck classification of distal femur periprosthetic fractures

Type	Description
1	Undisplaced fracture, component intact
2	Displaced fracture, component intact
3	Displaced fracture, component loose or failing

Table 23.1 Vancouver classification of periprosthetic proximal femoral fractures

Type	Description	Treatment
A	Trochanteric region fracture	ORIF if significantly displaced
B1	Fracture around well fixed stem	ORIF
B2	Fracture around loose stem, good bone stock	Revision
B3	Fracture around loose stem, poor bone stock	Revision
C	Fracture well below prosthesis	ORIF

ORIF, open reduction and internal fixation

Femoral fractures – periprosthetic

It is generally accepted that significantly displaced type A and type C fractures can be treated with internal fixation. Type C fractures are treated with plating. A single lateral plate or one used in combination with an anterior plate can be used. An alternative construct of a single lateral plate with strut grafts fixed using cerclage wires may also be used if it is felt that bone stock is compromised. At the proximal end of the plate cerclage wires can be used, though more recently blunt tipped periprosthetic screws and locking plates have become available to fix these fractures. Distally, the plate can be fixed with standard screws, both in nonlocking and locking configurations.

B1 fractures are most challenging to plan treatment. It is now becoming recognised that 'true' B1 fractures are relatively uncommon and in the majority of cases the stem is loose because of loss of fixation of uncemented stems or compromise of the cement mantle in cemented hips. In these cases wherever possible a revision is likely to be needed which bypasses the fracture by at least two cortical widths. Decision making for B2 and B3 fractures is more straightforward since femoral prosthesis is unstable (**Figure 23.1**). In Vancouver B2 and B3 fractures, my preference is to remove the stem and cement where needed and use a distal fit (cone conical) stem to restore femoral integrity. Proximal bone can be cerclaged around the body of this prosthesis and in time this bone reconstitutes remarkably well (**Figure 23.2**). Nonweight-bearing is recommended for 8 weeks until stable in growth is likely to have occurred. Where it is felt that cortical fixation using a cone conical stem will not be possible due to bone loss, a distal locked femoral stem may be necessary. In these cases, protected weight-bearing will also be needed for a period of approximately 8 weeks.

There are occasions where Vancouver B fractures occur with relatively good bone stock in patients with advanced age and significant comorbidities. In these cases, fixation with a combination of plate, screws and cerclage wires may yield a satisfactory clinical result, avoiding risky surgery. In these cases, the patient and relatives will need to accept a lower level of mobility than before the injury.

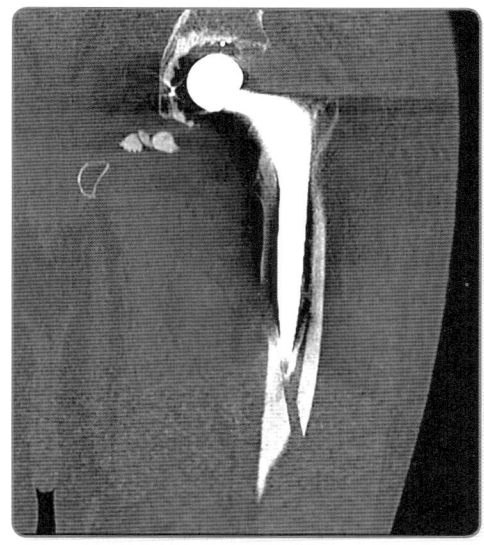

Figure 23.1 Vancouver type B2 periprosthetic femoral fracture.

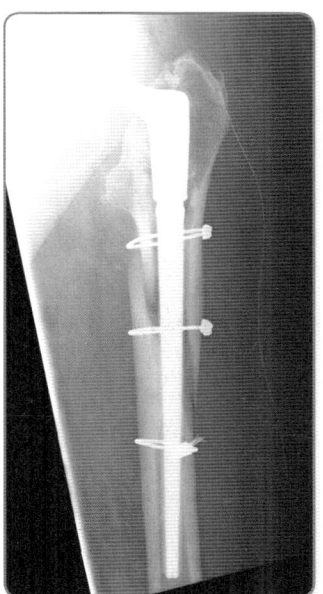

Figure 23.2 Vancouver type B2 periprosthetic femoral fracture with revision of the femoral component using a distal fit cone conical stem (cup revised with dual mobility component).

In distal femoral periprosthetic fractures, Lewis & Rorabeck type 1 and 2 fractures with the component intact should be fixed wherever possible. Preferred method of fixation is to use a lateral distal femoral locking plate as this avoids the need to violate the knee joint and lowers the incidence of prosthetic infection. Supracondylar nailing can be done with cruciate retaining femoral prosthesis as the femur can be accessed through the intercondylar notch. Unfortunately, during the reaming procedure and nail insertion, the femoral component can dislodge, thus considerably complicating operative management. Type 3 fractures, where the femoral prosthesis is loose, need stable fixation of the femoral condyles where possible and revision with a stemmed femoral implant. In some cases the distal femur cannot be reconstructed due to comminution and bone loss (**Figure 23.3**). In these cases distal femoral replacement and hinged revision knee replacement may be required (**Figure 23.4**).

Complications

Complications of treatment around fractured femoral stem are as of those for a primary hip replacement. Infection is more common than in primary hip replacement. Venous thromboembolism remains a risk and local guidelines should be followed. Extension of the fracture intraoperatively can also occur requiring the use of longer stems than was initially expected. Leg length discrepancy can occur and careful intraoperative reconstruction should be done. The trochanter when reconstructed correctly is a useful guideline for femoral length and intraoperative X-rays may be required to avoid excessive shortening or lengthening, and therefore preventing later instability. Dislocation can be common following these procedures and often the acetabular component is also revised in these cases. Where the soft tissue envelope has been compromised and the patient is having revision surgery, the use of dual mobility cups can reduce the risk of postoperative dislocation considerably.

In distal femoral periprosthetic fracture management, infection and venous thromboembolism are unfortunately also risks and local guideline should be followed for antibiotic prophylaxis and postoperative deep vein thrombosis prevention.

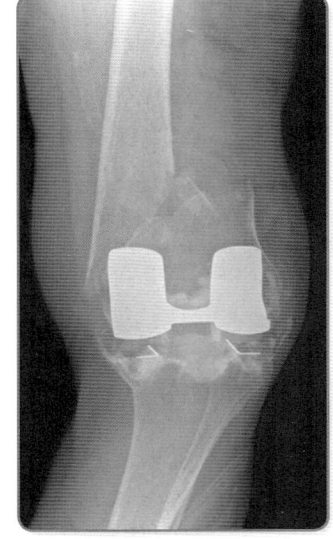

Figure 23.3 Severely comminuted type 3 distal femoral periprosthetic fracture with distal femoral bone loss.

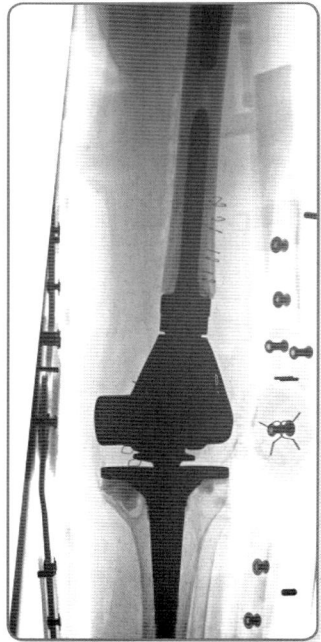

Figure 23.4 Severely comminuted type 3 distal femoral periprosthetic fracture with distal femoral bone loss treated with distal femoral replacement.

In both proximal and distal fractures, poor compliance can lead to loss or failure of fixation requiring a further revision procedure.

Further reading

Fleischman AN, Chen AF. Periprosthetic fractures around the femoral stem: overcoming challenges and avoiding pitfalls. Ann Transl Med 2015; 3:234.

Fink B. Revision arthroplasty in periprosthetic fractures of the proximal femur. Oper Orthop Traumatol 2014; 26:455–468.

Kancherla VK, Nwachuku CO. The treatment of periprosthetic femur fractures after total knee arthroplasty. Orthop Clin North Am 2014; 45:457–467.

Related topics of interest

- Topic 22 Femoral fractures – distal
- Topic 24 Femoral fractures – shaft
- Topic 25 Femoral fractures – subtrochanteric

24 Femoral fractures – shaft

Key points
- With fractures of the shaft of the femur associated injuries are not uncommon and increase the risk of complications
- Timing and type of surgery depend on patient's physiological condition
- Intramedullary nailing is the gold standard treatment for most femoral shaft fractures (FSFs)

Epidemiology
The annual incidence of FSFs ranges between 10 and 37 fractures per 100,000 population. The frequency of open and bilateral FSF is 12–16% and 7.3–9.6%, respectively. Ipsilateral neck of femur fractures have a reported incidence of 2.5–10% and are missed on initial assessment in 20–30% of the cases. Ipsilateral knee injuries coexist in 5–30% of FSF with some studies raising the incidence of arthroscopically confirmed findings to 50%. High energy fractures occur in young adults and low energy ones in the elderly (mostly women).

Pathophysiology
The considerable amount of force required to fracture the femur causes soft tissue damage which may affect the fracture healing biology. The average blood loss following an isolated FSF is 1250 mL. The location of the fracture in relation to the thigh muscles insertions determines the occurring deformity. The proximal fragment is typically flexed, abducted and externally rotated, whereas the distal fragment is translated medially or angulated in varus and can also be flexed in distal FSF.

Fat globules may enter the bloodstream through disrupted venules and cause acute respiratory distress syndrome (ARDS) or affect the brain and other organs. The overall physiological condition of the patient will dictate the timing and type of definitive fracture treatment.

Clinical features
Clinical assessment follows the Advanced Trauma Life Support priorities. FSF are not infrequently associated with life-threatening head and chest injuries, shock, and pelvis, spine or lower limb fractures. Clinical examination should always include the spine and the whole lower extremity. Concomitant hip fractures should be diagnosed preoperatively. Knee ligament injuries are better assessed under anaesthesia following the FSF fixation.

A FSF will invariably cause significant thigh pain, inability to bear weight, swelling, bruise and deformity. The affected leg is usually shortened and rotated. The thigh is tense and tender. Abnormal thigh motion should be prevented. Symptoms and signs of compartment syndrome should be sought and monitored closely.

Open wounds, especially those on the medial and posterior aspect of the thigh, may be related to vascular or neurological injuries. The presence of bruit, thrill or expanding hematoma mandates the exclusion of vascular injury. An ankle-brachial index of <0.9 indicates arterial damage. Thorough examination of the peripheral nerves should be conducted on the alert and cooperative patient.

Investigations
Adequate plain anteroposterior (AP) and lateral X-rays should allow visualisation of the entire length of the femur including the hip and the knee. Dedicated hip and knee X-rays should be obtained if there is suspicion of ipsilateral hip and knee injuries. CT scans are requested if the X-rays are inconclusive. They are also helpful in establishing the diagnosis of nonunion. Occult stress or insufficiency fractures are best investigated by means of MRI or bone scans. Periosteal reaction, bone marrow changes (oedema) or a visible fracture line on the MRI determine the grade

of the stress fracture and provide information about its chronicity.

Classification

The AO/OTA classification is based on fracture configuration and has good interobserver reliability only for the type but not for the groups of the fractures. In type A (simple) fractures (spiral, oblique or transverse) the circumference of the main proximal and distal fragment can appose by at least 90% after adequate reduction. Partial or no apposition is maintained in type B (wedge) and type C (complex) fractures, respectively. Winquist and Hansen classified FSF according to the cortical contact between the main proximal and distal fragments and the degree of stability following intramedullary nailing (**Table 24.1**).

Treatment

Nonoperative

Nonoperative treatment is only indicated for patients who are unfit for surgery or when resources for operative treatment are not available. Temporary immobilization for pain relief and prevention of further soft tissue injury and bleeding is achieved with traction splints, skin or skeletal traction. Skin traction is poorly tolerated, is correlated with skin problems and only allows application of light weight (3–4 kg), which is not enough for adequate fracture control. Thomas splints should be applied with care to prevent pressure sores in the groin and kept for as short time as possible. Skeletal traction can be applied through centrally threaded 5 mm or 6 mm pins at the distal femur or the proximal tibia. Distal femoral pins have better control on the fracture and don't affect the knee function. Proximal tibial pins are contraindicated in case of knee injuries. When traction is the definitive treatment it is maintained for at least 5–6 weeks or until there is no tenderness or movement at the fracture site.

Operative

External fixators

The role of external fixators as definitive treatment is limited. They can be used in patients who are managed according to the damage control orthopaedics (DCO) principles (see Topic 17). External fixators have the advantages of being minimally invasive, quick application and implant-free fracture site. They are indicated in polytrauma patients, open or significantly comminuted fractures or when transfer to another facility is contemplated. Conversion to definitive treatment is decided after the inflammatory response to trauma has settled, usually after 5 days.

Open reduction internal fixation

Fixation of FSF with plates has been considered for reducing the incidence of ARDS but has not been proven superior to nailing. The inevitable violation of the soft tissue envelope may affect healing. Indications for plating are recalcitrant nonunions, contamination of the nail entry point or anatomic limitations for nailing, intramedullary sequestrum and open fractures with vascular injury. Minimally invasive plate osteosynthesis (MIPO) has better outcomes in fracture healing; lower infection rate and risk of re-fracture or need for bone grafting. Partial weight-bearing is advised for 6–8 weeks.

Intramedullary nails

Intramedullary nailing is the gold standard for most FSF as it prevents fracture shortening, angulation and rotation, and allows early weight-bearing. Even though reaming can affect endosteal perfusion it promotes

Table 24.1 Winquist–Hansen classification of femoral shaft fractures	
Grade 0	No comminution
Grade I	Minimal comminution or a small butterfly fragment <25% of the width of the femur
Grade II	Comminution with a butterfly fragment <50% of the width of the femur
Grade III	Comminution with a large butterfly fragment >50% of the width of the femur
Grade IV	Segmental comminution
Grade V	Segmental bone defect

perfusion within the soft tissues and increases the serum levels of growth factors. Additionally, reamings act like an inner bone graft. Unreamed nails have a four-fold higher nonunion rate. The risk of fat embolism and activation of the systemic inflammatory response system (SIRS) should not be overlooked. The nails are usually locked statically. Dynamic locking is recommended for delayed unions or primarily in transverse fractures. Nails can be inserted in an antegrade or retrograde fashion. Retrograde nailing can be complicated with knee septic arthritis (0.5–1%), knee pain, reduced range of motion and retropatellar arthritis. Weight-bearing is commenced immediately postoperatively as tolerated although local symptoms usually prevent it.

Hip dislocations and acetabular or neck of femur fractures are reduced and fixed prior to the FSF fixation. Cephalomedullary nails are the implants of choice for the fixation of ipsilateral femoral shaft and neck of femur fractures. Ipsilateral femur and tibia fractures (floating knee) are treated with retrograde nailing in the femur and antegrade nailing in the tibia through the same approach (**Figure 24.1**). Pathological metastatic fractures, stress or fatigue fractures and atypical fractures related to biphosphonates are usually subtrochanteric and treated with cephalomedullary nails (**Figures 24.2a** and **24.2b**) (see Topic 25). Atypical fractures have a high nonunion rate after IM nailing.

Complications

Nerve injury – The peroneal division of the sciatic nerve and the pudendal nerve are most commonly injured.

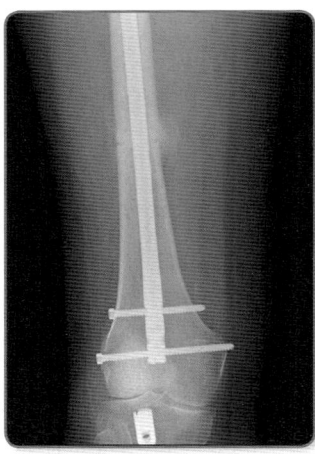

Figure 24.1 Anteroposterior radiograph of the right femur with a retrograde nail in situ. There is callus formation mainly medially. Note the presence of an intramedullary nail in the tibia. The patient sustained ipsilateral femoral and tibial fractures which were treated with IM nails in one stage.

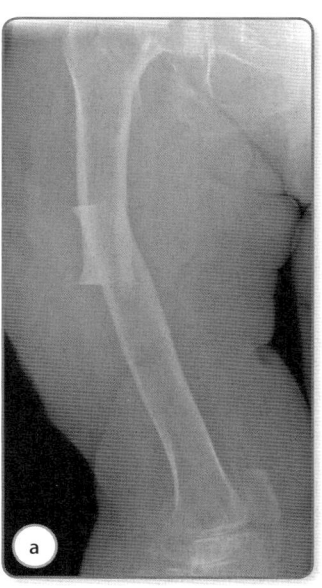
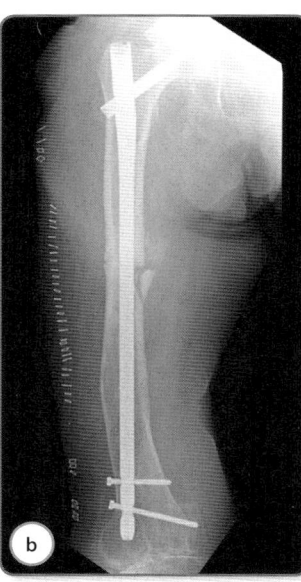

Figure 24.2 (a) Transverse fracture of the midshaft of the right femur with significant shortening. The patient sustained the injury after a fall from standing height. (b) The fracture was fixed with cephalomedullary nail. Note the distal femur deformity which was consequent to osteomyelitis.

Femoral fractures – shaft

Vascular injury – The reported incidence is approximately 2%. It is usually related to distal femoral fractures or the proximal sagittal locking of retrograde nails.

Compartment syndrome – The anterior compartment is most commonly affected.

Fat embolism and ARDS – The incidence is much higher in patients with coexisting thoracic or pulmonary injuries. The contribution of reaming to the development of the syndrome is controversial.

Tromboembolic disease – The incidence of deep vein thrombosis has been reported up to 40% when subclinical cases are included.

Iatrogenic fracture – Neck of femur fractures can occur during antegrade nailing if the entry point is incorrect.

Malunion – Malrotation can alter foot orientation and walking and should be corrected as soon as it is detected. The threshold for angular malalignment is 5°.

Nonunion – The reported rate is 3–5%. Principle risk factor is the degree of damage to the bone vascularity and the soft tissue envelope. Other factors are occult infection, fixation in distraction and inadequate stability. Only 50% of the fractures unite after isolated nail dynamisation. Exchange nailing with a larger implant (usually by 2 mm) and bone grafting with or without biological enhancement is the surgical method of choice. Unicortical locking plates can be considered, especially in the presence of a retrograde nail to avoid further violation of the knee joint.

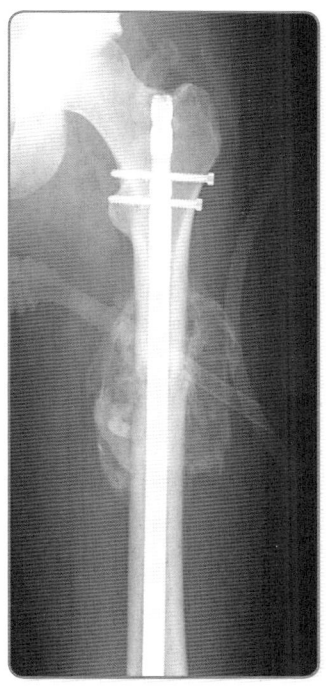

Figure 24.3 Femoral shaft fracture treated with intramedullary nail. The patient was intubated and admitted to intensive care unit for severe head injury and pulmonary contusions. Note the abundant callus formation despite the patient was not mobile and the heterotopic ossification at the nail entry point.

Infection – Infected nonunions are treated with debridement and exchange nailing in one or two stages. Antibiotic impregnated beads can be used initially.

Muscular weakness – Abductors should be protected in antegrade nailing.

Heterotopic ossification – Risk factors are male sex, intubation for >4 days and nailing >2 days after the injury (**Figure 24.3**).

Further reading

Bone LB, Giannoudis P. Femoral shaft fracture fixation and chest injury after polytrauma. J Bone Joint Serg Am 2011; 93:311–317.

Hak DJ, Mauffrey C, Hake M, Hammerberg EM, Stahel PF. Ipsilateral femoral neck and shaft fractures: current diagnostic and treatment strategies. Orthopedics 2015; 38:247–251.

Madhuri V, Dutt V, Gahukamble AD, Tharyan P. Interventions for treating femoral shaft fractures in children and adolescents. Cochrane Database Syst Rev 2014; 29:CD009076.

Related topics of interest

- *Topic 17* Damage control orthopaedics and trauma physiology
- *Topic 21* Fat embolism and acute respiratory distress syndrome
- *Topic 52* Implants – nails

25 Femoral fractures – subtrochanteric

Key points
- Subtrochanteric fractures are often among the most challenging of the femoral fractures to treat
- High energy injuries in young people with good quality bone and low energy injuries in weakened bone
- Accurate reduction is key to success

Epidemiology

Fractures in the subtrochanteric region of the femur account for <1% of all fractures and include a wide spectrum of fracture patterns. They have a bimodal age distribution, with the majority occurring in persons older than 50 years of age. In the older age group, they tend to occur from simple falls. In the younger age group high energy mechanisms predominate. Although there is soft tissue damage, in displaced fractures early intervention is preferable as this allows early mobilisation of the patient and prevents further complications.

Pathophysiology

In younger patients, the usual mechanism of injury is high energy to the proximal femur. The most common cause in developed countries is motor vehicle accidents, including those involving pedestrians, motor cycles and falls from heights. The fracture pattern often indicates the amount of energy transferred to the bone at the time of the injury and one must therefore be aware of other injuries in widely displaced fracture patterns.

In the older population, those over 50 years of age, high energy injuries do still occur, but there is a predominance of low energy injuries related to falls. One should be aware of the presence of osteoporosis or other pathological process (primary bone disease or metastatic deposits) which can predispose the femur to fracturing in this region with relatively low levels of energy transfer.

The proximity of femoral neurovascular structures and the sciatic nerve places them at risk in these fractures, although overt injury to these structures is relatively uncommon.

Clinical features

Initial management of patients who are likely to have suffered a high-energy injury should be in accordance with Advanced Trauma Life Support guidelines. There can be considerable blood loss from these fractures (500–1000 mL) and fluid replacement should be initiated as part of the initial assessment. For older patients with low energy mechanisms of injury pathologic aetiologies should be investigated. Bone pain in the days or weeks before the fracture occurring may indicate a pathological fracture.

Clinical findings will include thigh pain, swelling and deformity with significant shortening in displaced fractures. The iliopsoas muscle causes flexion of the proximal segment, and the combination of the abductors acting on the proximal segment and adductor action on the distal fragment, result in a varus deformity of the femur. Whenever possible, the distal limb should be assessed for neurovascular injury preoperatively and documented.

Investigations

It is important to fully visualise the injury as well as the joint above and below. In high-energy injuries this helps detect associated fractures, but does not guarantee that all will be found during initial evaluation. The majority of these fractures require only plain X-rays. Anteroposterior and lateral views of the entire femur should be obtained as a bare minimum though oblique views may also be required. Commonly in major trauma centres, CT scans are done as part of the initial evaluation and whilst these are useful in showing extension of the fracture into the piriform fossa, it can be difficult to appreciate the overall anatomy of the injury and so 3D reconstructions may be required if plain X-rays cannot be obtained before treatment is needed.

In patients where a pathologic process is suspected, such as metastatic disease, a skeletal survey or bone scan may be required to complete assessment.

Classification

Unfortunately, with subtrochanteric fractures no universal classification system exists, and unusual fracture patterns are often seen which do not fit any classification. Many systems have been used to try and classify subtrochanteric fractures. More useful ones are by Russell and Taylor, and Seinsheimer. The Russell–Taylor classification disregards the degree of comminution on the basis that an intramedullary device should address this problem. This classification divides the injuries into those that have an intact piriform fossa and those with extension into this region, and takes lesser trochanter involvement into account (**Table 25.1**).

Also useful classification is that of Seinsheimer (**Table 25.2**), although this is more complex. The main advantage of this classification is that it allows one to visually compare X-ray findings with the described fracture patterns and therefore helps in assessing fracture severity and stability.

In combination, these two classification systems help guide treatment. Extension into the piriformis fossa was felt to preclude intramedullary nailing but more recent studies have shown that these fractures can be successfully treated this way. In my opinion, Seinsheimer type V fractures (where there is extension of the fracture through the greater trochanter in combination with loss of the medial buttress) should be treated with alternative means such as a 95° angle device or proximal femoral locking plate. This is especially true if the proximal femoral lateral wall has a coronal plane split.

Treatment

The ultimate purpose of treatment of these fractures is to restore alignment, length and rotational axis of the femur. Operative treatment also allows early mobilisation and whenever possible, weight-bearing. For injuries where there is minimal comminution length can be restored on the basis of intraoperative image intensifier films. However, when there is comminution it may be useful to X-ray the opposite leg before commencing the procedure and measuring this with a ruler to compare with the injured leg.

Whilst the first option in fracture care should always be to consider conservative management, in the case of subtrochanteric femoral fractures in adults, most require surgical intervention. This is because of the deforming forces influencing this injury which make it very difficult to control the fracture with closed means. Closed treatment can result in malunion or late displacement, which can complicate later operative intervention.

Table 25.1 Russell–Taylor classification of subtrochanteric fractures

Type	Description
1	A – below lesser trochanter extends distally to isthmus
	B – includes lesser trochanter and extends distally to isthmus
2	A – lesser trochanter intact, extends to piriform fossa
	B – lesser trochanter disrupted, extends to piriform fossa

Table 25.2 Seinsheimer classification of subtrochanteric fractures

Type	Description
1	Displacement less than 2 mm, regardless of fracture pattern
2	A – 2-part transverse
	B – 2-part, lesser trochanter attached to proximal fragment (reverse oblique)
	C – 2-part, lesser trochanter attached to distal fragment
3	A – 3-part, lesser trochanter detached from proximal fragment
	B – 3-part, lesser trochanter attached to proximal fragment
4	Comminuted, 4 or more fragments
5	Subtrochanteric, extending up through greater trochanter

The patient should be placed on the fracture reduction table as for intertrochanteric fractures. Initially, if there is no injury to the contralateral leg, the opposite hip can be flexed and externally rotated to allow for intraoperative image intensifier screening (radiographs) to be performed.

Because of the deforming forces on the fracture one should have a low threshold for opening the fracture site if closed reduction is not easily obtained. Often there is soft tissue interposition which will prevent passage of the intramedullary guidewire into the distal fragment. Correct entry point using the awl for the guidewire introduction is crucial. Once the fracture has been reduced it is essential that varus deformity remains corrected during intramedullary reaming, preventing lateral wall breach (**Figure 25.1**). If the lateral wall is found to be compromised when the fracture is opened to obtain reduction, or during intramedullary reaming careful consideration should be given to using an extramedullary device (**Figure 25.2**). Most cephalomedullary nailing systems do not control such fractures with adequate stability and failure of fixation may occur. For subtrochanteric fractures the use of short cephalomedullary devices is not recommended as there is fracture extension into the distal fragment which will cause fixation failure.

If using a 95° angle device, care must be taken to introduce this into the inferior half of the femoral head and on the lateral view, the hip screw or blade should be as central as possible (**Figure 25.3**). Care should be taken to obtain X-rays and prevent penetration of the joint as the screw is inserted inferiorly in femoral head. The plate must extend two cortical widths or more below the level of the extension of the fracture. Since one has to dissect the femur to apply the plate, fracture lines can be seen or palpated in order to assess for optimal length of the plate.

Complications

Immediate complications can be divided into soft tissue injuries and bony injuries. Vascular and neurological injuries are relatively uncommon, but one must take care when passing any instruments over the femur medially or behind the femur in order that prolonged compression or penetration of neurological and vascular structures does not occur. Unfortunately, when using cephalomedullary nail for such fractures during reaming and also during drilling for the hip screw in a 95° angle device, it is not unusual to note that extension of the fracture has occurred and the lateral wall of the proximal fragment of

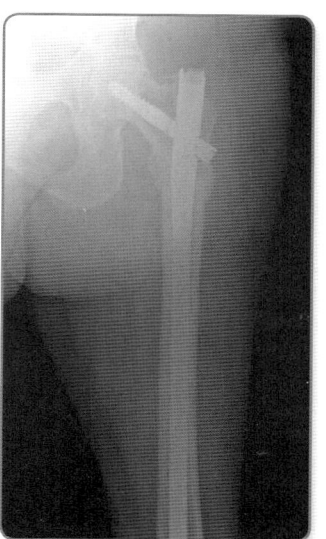

Figure 25.1
Two-part transverse subtrochanteric fracture treated with intramedullary nail.

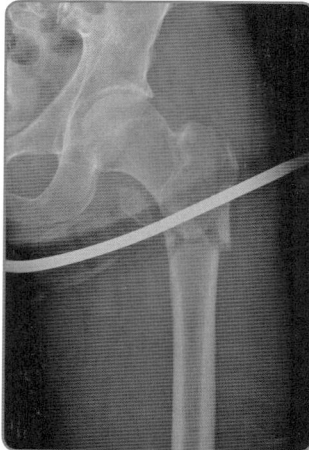

Figure 25.2
Comminuted subtrochanteric fracture with proximal extension through greater trochanter (Seinsheimer type 5).

Femoral fractures – subtrochanteric

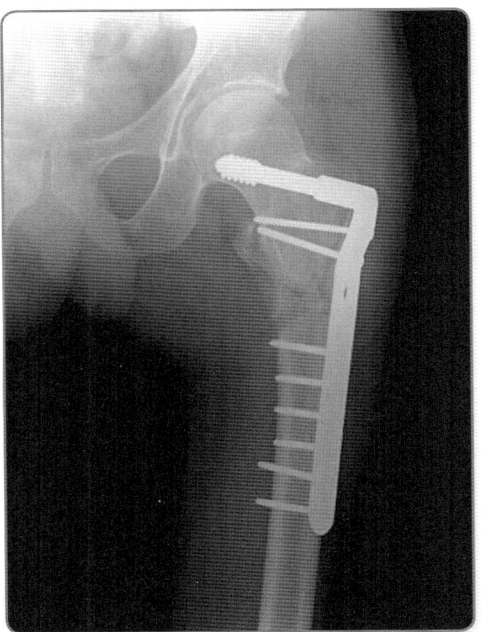

Figure 25.3 Comminuted subtrochanteric fracture treated with 95° angle device.

the femur is compromised. If this occurs the overall fracture pattern has to be considered carefully, as well as the fixation likely to be obtained. If it is felt that the lateral wall has been significantly compromised it may be necessary to switch to a proximal femoral locking plate to obtain stability.

Infection is usually detected in the days following surgery. Early aggressive debridement with use of targeted antibiotics helps eradicate infection. Preserving the metalwork whenever possible is useful as stability will help infection treatment.

Late complications include loss of position and failure of metalwork, which are related to delayed nonunion. Delayed and nonunion are all too common in this type of injury. If significant healing is not noted on serial X-rays after 4–6 months following fixation, consideration should be given to grafting the fracture site and/or dynamisation of the fracture. Avascular necrosis of the proximal femur is unusual in these fractures unless there is an associated ipsilateral femoral neck fracture.

Further reading

Hu SJ, Zhang SM, Yu GR. Treatment of femoral subtrochanteric fractures with proximal lateral femur locking plates. Acta Ortop Bras 2012; 20:329–333.

Jiang LS, Shen L, Dai LY. Intramedullary fixation of subtrochanteric fractures with long proximal femoral nail or long gamma nail: technical notes and preliminary results. Ann Acad Med Singapore 2007; 36:821–826.

Sassoon AA, et al. Subtrochanteric fractures. In: Tornetta P, et al. Rockwood and Green's Fractures in Adults (8th edn). Philadelphia: Lippincott Williams and Wilkins, 2014.

Related topics of interest

- *Topic 24* Femoral neck fractures – shaft
- *Topic 26* Femoral fractures – extracapsular
- *Topic 62* Major trauma – Advanced Trauma and Life Support principles

Femoral neck fractures – extracapsular

Key points

- A holistic approach is required to optimise outcomes, with early involvement of the elderly care team
- Dynamic hip screw (DHS) fixation with a tip–apex distance (TAD) of <25 mm has good results for stable fractures
- Reverse oblique fractures should be managed with a cephalomedullary nail rather than DHS

Epidemiology

Most commonly, extracapsular fractures are caused by a fall from standing height in an individual with osteoporosis. Patients are typically older than those who sustain intracapsular fractures and often there will be X-ray evidence of osteoarthritis; the stiffened hip joint in these individuals concentrates the stress outside the capsule, meaning fractures occur here instead of across the femoral neck. Young adults with high-energy injuries and those with bone metastases may also present with femoral neck fracture.

Presentation

Usually there is a clear history of fall, followed by groin pain. Fracture would be suspected if there was pain on passive internal or external rotation of the leg, pain on attempting to perform straight leg raise and inability to bear weight on the affected leg. Usually, X-rays clearly show a fracture. However, if the fracture is undisplaced it may be difficult to visualise on plain radiography. In this situation MRI or fine slice CT scanning will help lead to early recognition and treatment.

The patient should be examined thoroughly, including the head and cervical spine, for evidence of any associated injuries. Medical assessment should also seek to establish the cause of the fall. There may be a urine or chest infection present, arrhythmia, or it may be the result of a medication side effect or due to problems with vision or balance. Often dementia, delirium or the effects of pain medication preclude a full history from the patient in which case a collateral history from family or care home staff is useful. Early involvement of elderly care physicians cannot only prevent further falls in the future but also help to optimise these patients for theatre.

Classification

Generally fractures are described according to the number of parts. AO classification (**Figure 26.1**) also takes into account whether the fracture line is pertrochanteric (running through the trochanters) or intertrochanteric (between). This consideration of the primary fracture line angle is important in determining fixation – the reverse oblique fracture has a high tendency to shorten and failure rates of conventional DHS for A3 type fractures are greater than type A1 fractures.

Management

Extracapsular hip fractures occur through cancellous bone. Compared to fractures through the neck there tends to be increased blood loss but a lower nonunion rate of 1–2% when treated by fixation. Patients admitted with hip fracture are usually frail with limited physiological reserve. Survival at 1-year is improved in patients who receive surgery within 48 hours. In order for this to be achieved, early identification and correction of medical problems is required.

Nonoperative treatment consists of skin traction until the initial pain has settled, followed by touch weight-bearing transfers to sit in a chair as soon as pain permits. Touch weight-bearing is recommended over nonweight-bearing as the forces across the hip joint are less. Due to a high-incidence of urinary and chest infections, pressure ulcers and venous thromboembolism, nonoperative management is not recommended if patients are deemed fit enough to undergo surgery.

Femoral fractures – extracapsular

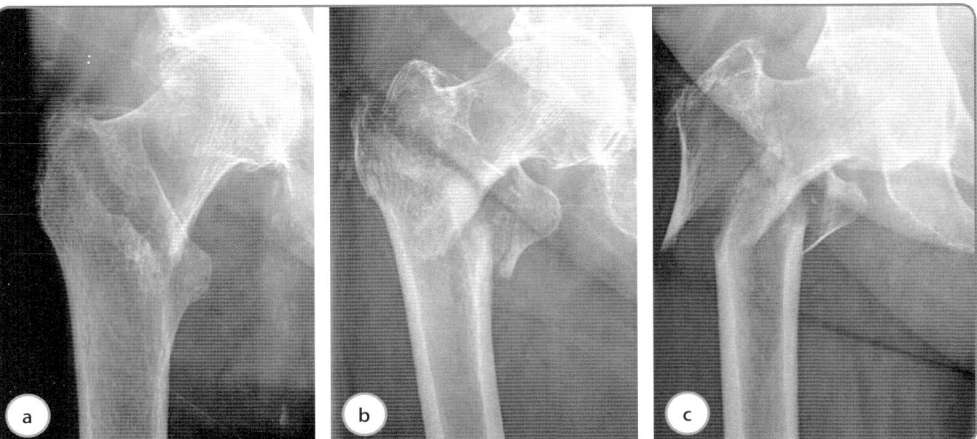

Figure 26.1 AO classification. (a) 31-A1 are two part fractures with the fracture line running through the greater trochanter laterally. They are relatively stable after reduction. (b) 31-A2 are comminuted fractures with the fracture line running through the greater trochanter laterally. They may be stable or unstable. (c) 31-A3 fractures are unstable. Laterally the fracture line exits distal to the greater trochanter, medially it exits proximal to the lesser trochanter. The fracture angle may run transversely or in a reverse oblique direction.

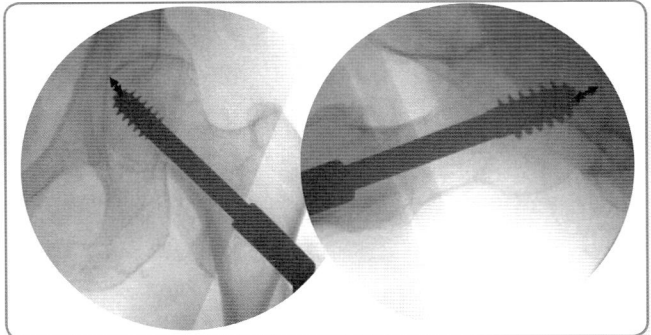

Figure 26.2 The sum of the tip–apex distance (sum of the distance on anteroposterior and lateral films between the tip of the lag screw and the apex of the femoral head) should be <25 mm.

Dynamic hip screw

Closed reduction on the traction table is usually possible. Commonly slight internal rotation of the foot is required so that the patella is uppermost. Fracture reduction is important; fixing a hip fracture in varus increases the bending moment and failure rates are greater. Similarly excessive internal rotation should be avoided as it will affect gait. The principle of a DHS is to allow compression during weight-bearing. Type A1 and A2 fracture lines are perpendicular to the sliding screw allowing this to happen. Compression helps to ensure bone apposition and reduces rotation and shear movements between fragments, promoting healing. Use of a DHS to fix type A3 fractures allows uncontrolled shearing across the fracture site. This is contrary to bone healing and high failure rates are reported.

To minimise the risk of screw cut-out the TAD should always be <25 mm (**Figure 26.2**). If the screw is not perfectly central within the femoral head, a slightly inferior position, or inferior-anterior position is better than a superior or posterior position. The entry point for the lag screw on the lateral femur should not fall below the lesser trochanter as this creates a stress riser, predisposing to subtrochanteric fracture. The angle between the plate and the barrel is commonly 135°. Greater angle plates are available and have a greater biomechanical propensity to slide, giving fracture site compression. However, it can be difficult to place the guidewire in a central position within the femoral head without the entry point being below the lesser trochanter.

Cephalomedullary nail

The cephalomedullary nail offers the advantage of a minimally invasive approach with superior biomechanics compared to plate fixation. For unstable fractures, such as the reverse obliquity fracture, the biomechanical advantage is important: cephalomedullary nails are recommended for AO type 31-A3 fractures as there is a lower failure rate compared to DHS. For pertrochanteric fractures which extend no more than 2 cm distal to the lesser trochanter a short nail may be used. Long nails, locked in the distal metaphysis of the femur should be chosen if there is a greater extension of the fracture distally and also for pathological fractures. Lag screw placement is important; superior positioning of the screw predisposes to cut-out (**Figure 26.3**). In addition, the screw should not be too short as the lateral end of the lag screw should be well engaged with the lateral femoral cortex for optimum stability. For stable fractures, research has failed to show an advantage to fixation with a cephalomedullary device.

Fixed angle plate

The 95° dynamic condylar screw or a fixed angle blade plate can be used for extracapsular fractures AO type 31A-3 if there is contraindication to intramedullary nailing. The blade plate utilises the area of the femoral head where he tension and compression trabeculae intersect to achieve strong purchase in the femoral head. An open approach to the proximal femur is required and the procedure is technically challenging. Results are inferior to those offered by intramedullary nailing.

Arthroplasty

Total hip replacement (THR) may be appropriate if the patient is fit and has an extracapsular fracture in a severely arthritic hip joint with secondary avascular necrosis: In severe cases, collapse of the femoral head can leave insufficient bone to achieve satisfactory fixation. Also the lack of movement at the hip joint puts additional stress on the fracture site, increasing the risk of fixation failure. Arthroplasty is also valuable as a salvage procedure where there has been failure of internal fixation.

Surgery is complicated by loss of the calcar and compromise of the abductor muscles where the greater trochanter has fractured. To minimise the dislocation risk it is important to

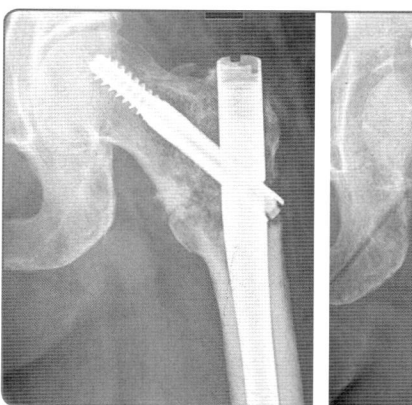
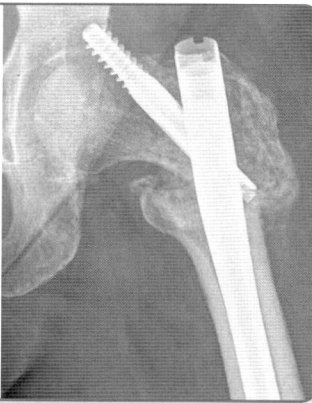

Figure 26.3 A lag screw situated high in the femoral head with a combined anteroposterior and lateral tip–apex distance of >25 mm is at increased risk of cut out.

preserve abductor function by re-attaching the greater trochanter; specifically designed plates exist for this purpose. Although outcomes can be good it is a more major operation compared to fracture fixation with longer operating times and increased blood loss. Dislocation rates are also higher than for elective THR.

Greater trochanter fracture

An isolated fracture of the greater trochanter is uncommon. When it does occur it tends to be due to strong abductor contraction in a young adult. In an older person there is frequently either an undisplaced extension of the fracture through the femoral neck or underlying bone pathology such as metastatic disease. MRI is useful to confirm the diagnosis. An undisplaced fracture of the greater trochanter in healthy bone can be managed nonoperatively with early weight-bearing mobilisation.

Prognosis

In elderly patients who sustain hip fractures, the 1-year mortality is as high as 33%. Factors associated with a higher mortality include male gender, age over 90 years, nursing home residents and those with dementia and other medical co-morbidities.

Further reading

Al-Ani AN, Samuelsson B, Tidermark J, et al. Early operation on patients with a hip fracture improved the ability to return to independent living. A prospective study of 850 patients. J Bone Joint Surg Am 2008; 90:1436–1442.

Baumgaertner MR, Curtin SL, Lindskog DM, Keggi JM. The value of the tip-apex distance in predicting failure of fixation of peritrochanteric fractures of the hip. J Bone Joint Surg Am 1995; 77:1058–1064.

Brinker M. Review of orthopaedic trauma. Philadelphia, PA: Lippincott Williams and Wilkins; 2013.

Haidukewych GJ, Berry DJ. Salvage of failed treatment of hip fractures. J Am Acad Orthop Surg 2005; 13:101–109.

Matre K, Havelin LI, Gjertsen JE, et al. Sliding hip screw versus IM nail in reverse oblique trochanteric and subtrochanteric fractures. A study of 2716 patients in the Norwegian Hip Fracture Register. Injury 2013; 44:735–742.

Reliability of predictors for screw cutout in intertrochanteric hip fractures. De Bruijn K et al. J Bone Joint Surg Am 2012; 94:1266–1272.

Sadowski C, Lübbeke A, Saudan M, et al. Treatment of reverse oblique and transverse intertrochanteric fractures with use of an intramedullary nail or 95 degrees screw-plate: a prospective randomised study. J Bone Joint Surg Am 2002; 84:372–381.

Related topics of interest

- *Topic 9* Bone structure and physiology
- *Topic 25* Femoral fractures – subtrochanteric
- *Topic 27* Femoral neck fractures – intracapsular
- *Topic 37* Guidelines in trauma

27 Femoral neck fractures – intracapsular

Key points
- Management of femoral neck fractures in the elderly requires multidisciplinary input to achieve optimum outcomes
- Total hip replacement (THR) should be considered for individuals who live in their own home and walk independently if they are cognitively unimpaired and fit for surgery
- Femoral head salvage should be attempted for displaced fractures in younger, fit patients, with the understanding that delayed THR may be required

Epidemiology

Intracapsular femoral neck fractures are usually seen after falls from standing height in elderly, osteoporotic patients. Fractures in younger adults represent higher energy injuries such as a fall from a height. Approximately 2.5% of femoral shaft fractures have an ipsilateral femoral neck fracture; anteroposterior (AP) and lateral radiographs of the entire bone should be obtained.

The femoral neck is a relatively common site for tumour metastases and this should always be considered, particularly in the presence of pre-existing symptoms and in patients with a history of malignancy. Stress fractures are uncommon but are an important differential diagnosis in young adults presenting with atraumatic groin or thigh pain that is associated with weight-bearing activity. Metabolic disease such as Paget's can predispose patients to a fracture or may be an incidental finding. Identification of Paget's is important as increased bleeding can be expected.

Presentation

Undisplaced fractures may result in subtle clinical findings; pain is often minimal and some patients will maintain the ability to straight-leg-raise. This is particularly the case in impacted fractures which are relatively biomechanically stable. Likewise, radiographs may be nondiagnostic, especially if taken with the femur in an externally rotated position. MRI is highly sensitive, although if timely MRI is unavailable (ideally it should be performed within 24 hours) fine slice CT scan will identify most fractures.

With displaced fractures the patient's leg tends to be shortened, abducted and externally rotated. The iliopsoas contributes to the deformity by pulling the posteriorly sited lesser trochanter in an upwards and anterior direction; without the fulcrum of the hip joint to cause flexion, this externally rotates the leg. The gluteal muscles also contribute to the shortening.

Stress fractures of the femoral neck

Stress fractures of the femoral neck typically occur in individuals who have had a sudden increase in weight-bearing physical activity. Plain radiographs are initially normal but MRI is highly sensitive for diagnosis. Stress fractures affecting the lateral (tension) cortex are at high risk of propagating and cannulated screw fixation should be considered, whilst those affecting the medial (compression) cortex are more stable, and may be managed nonoperatively.

Classification

Intracapsular femoral neck fractures can be broadly classified into subcapital fractures which occur at the head-neck junction, and transcervical fractures where the fracture line runs across the neck. Fracture displacement is of importance in determining management as the blood supply to the femoral head (**Figure 27.1**) is disrupted with displaced fractures.

Garden's classification (**Figure 27.2**) has been commonly used over the past 50 years. He described four stages of femoral neck fracture, with increasing energy. Although

Femoral neck fractures – intracapsular

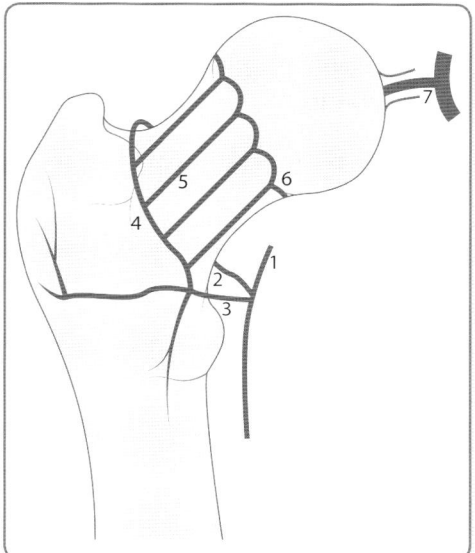

Figure 27.1 The blood supply of the femoral head. The profunda femoris artery (1) gives rise to the medial (2) and lateral (3) femoral circumflex arteries. Of these the medial is the most important. The ascending branch of the medial femoral circumflex artery anastamoses with the medial circumflex femoral artery to give the extracapsular arterial ring. From the ring arise the retinacular branches (4), which ascend the femoral neck and anastamose again to make the intracapsular subsynovial ring (5). There are also contributions from the intramedullary vessels and a small amount from the artery of the ligamentum teres (6), a branch of the obturator artery.

Management

The surgical goal in older people is to perform one operation which firstly relieves pain and secondly allows early mobilisation. Most elderly people will not tolerate partial weight-bearing, and this should be considered when planning surgery. Holistic care should include assessment as to why the fall occurred and implementation of measures to prevent further falls. In addition, bone health should be considered and osteoporosis treatment started unless there are contraindications.

Nonoperative management is associated with a high rate of medical complications due to immobility. However, if someone is in the very last days of life, nonoperative treatment may be appropriate. In this situation, a nerve block or catheter with local anaesthetic can be very useful to maintain comfort and allow nursing care.

Displaced fractures in older adults

Hemiarthroplasty is recommended for displaced femoral neck fractures in elderly patients who have a poor level of mobility preoperatively and no pre-existing acetabular wear. These patients are unlikely to experience problems with acetabular erosion and benefit from undergoing a shorter operation with a smaller dislocation risk compared to THR. Use of a cemented stem does increase the early mortality, but this can be reduced to some extent by cleaning and venting the canal before cementing. Use of an uncemented stem avoids this increased mortality but there is a higher incidence of periprosthetic fracture. Patients receiving an Austin Moore prosthesis have higher rates of residual pain and reduced mobility compared to those receiving a cemented Thompson hemiarthroplasty at 6 months.

Bipolar hemiarthroplasty was hoped to reduce acetabular wear but after implantation the prosthesis tends to function mainly as a unipolar hemiarthroplasty. Meta-analysis of randomised controlled trials has shown that although there was a slight reduction in acetabular wear at 1 year, this difference did not persist at 2 and 4 years follow-up.

widely used there is poor intraobserver reliability with Garden's classification. It is recommended to instead split intracapsular fractures into either undisplaced (Garden stages I and II) or displaced (Garden stages III and IV). This is more reliable and remains an effective guide to treatment and prognosis.

Pauwels' classification (**Figure 27.3**) is based on the orientation of the fracture line relative to the horizontal plane. Depending on the fracture angle, joint reaction forces have a compressive or shearing effect on the fracture. Pauwels type III fractures are the least stable with a poorer prognosis if treated by internal fixation.

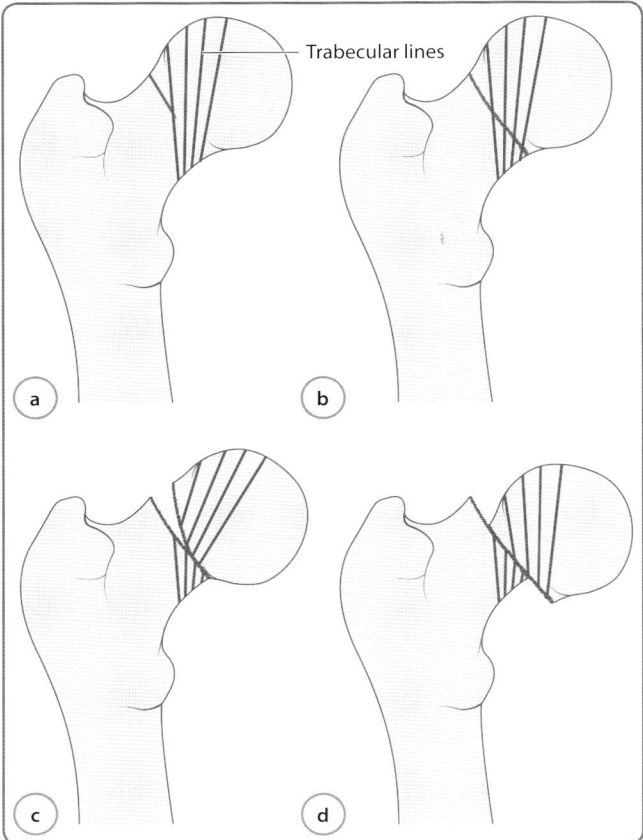

Figure 27.2 Garden classification of intracapsular femoral neck fractures. (a) Stage I is an incomplete fracture with posterolateral impaction. The impaction gives the fracture some stability but still at least 15% will displace if treated nonoperatively. (b) Stage II is a complete fracture without displacement, it lacks the impaction seen in stage I fractures and is consequently less inherently stable. (c) Stage III is a complete fracture that is partially displaced. (d) Stage IV is a complete fracture with displacement, allowing the femoral head to realign itself to a neutral position within the acetabulum.

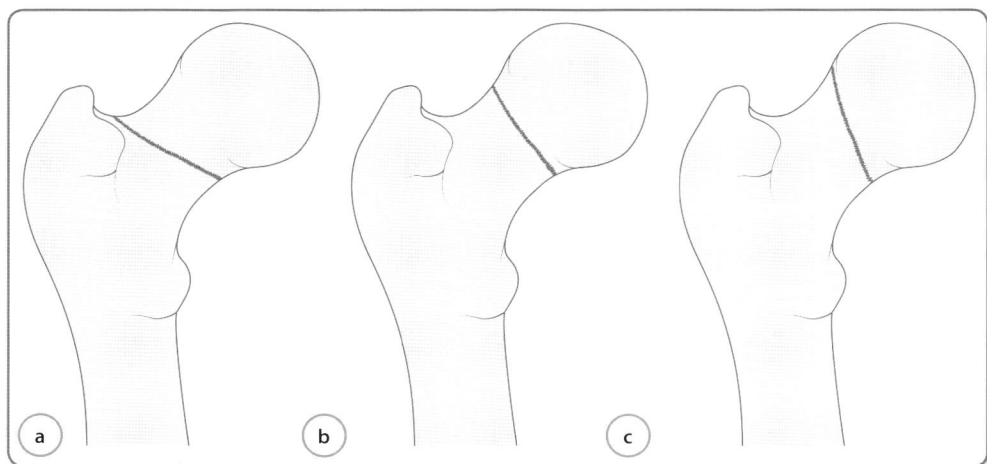

Figure 27.3 Pauwels' classification. Fractures that are orientated near to the horizontal are relatively stable but as the angle increases the shear stress across the fracture site increases. (a) Type I fractures are orientated at 0–30° to the horizontal. (b) Type II fractures 30–50°. (c) Type III fractures >50° from the horizontal.

Total hip replacement for trauma has higher dislocation rates compared to both hemiarthroplasty and elective THR. However, for people who are mobile and live independently, THR offers better walking distance and overall function compared to hemiarthroplasty [National Institute for Health and Care Excellence (NICE) guidelines, therefore recommend THR over hemiarthroplasty for people with displaced intracapsular fractures who were able to walk outdoors independently or with one stick, who are cognitively unimpaired and who are medically fit for a THR]. Patients with pre-existing osteoarthritis have stiff hip joints and tend to sustain extracapsular fractures, but occasionally intracapsular fractures are sustained. When there has been significant acetabular wear THR should be offered.

Undisplaced fractures

Nonoperative treatment for undisplaced fractures will lead to displacement in about one-third of cases. However, undisplaced fractures tend to do well with internal fixation; compared to hemiarthroplasty the operation time, perioperative complication rate and 1-year mortality are reduced. Femoral head blood supply is likely to be preserved and as such avascular necrosis rates are less than 8% in Garden type I and II fractures. There is a greater incidence of re-operation in these patients, but 1-year pain and mobility are shown to be better than in a matched group of people receiving hemiarthroplasty. The entry point of the screws should not be distal to the lesser trochanter as this will lead to a stress riser and is a risk factor for subtrochanteric fracture.

Displaced intracapsular fractures in younger adults

For younger adults, the benefits of keeping a native hip joint outweigh the risks associated with re-operation and attempts to salvage the femoral head should be made. Closed reduction is performed where possible, using the Leadbetter manoeuvre to correct displacement. Reduction is assessed on image intensifier: Garden's alignment index describes the angle between the compression trabeculae and the femoral shafts on AP and lateral views, it should lie between 155° and 180° on both views. Where closed reduction is not achieved easily, repeated efforts should not be made as this can cause damage to the femoral head vasculature. Instead, open reduction should be performed. Use of either a Smith Peterson (anterior) or Watson Jones (anterolateral) approach allows access whilst the patient remains on the traction table, facilitating insertion of screws across the fracture.

Some studies have shown an improved outcome with surgery undertaken within 12 hours, but good results have been reported with delays of >48 hours so delay to diagnosis alone is not a contraindication to fixation. Some advocate capsular decompression to help reduce the risk of avascular necrosis, particularly in undisplaced fractures which are less likely to have caused a capsular tear at the time of the injury. There is no evidence that decompressing the joint helps but it is generally regarded as a quick procedure with minimal additional morbidity for the patient. The presence of co-morbidities, such as liver or renal disease is a predictor of outcome and fixation is contra-indicated in individuals who have abnormal underlying bone or arthritis of the hip due to increased failure rates.

Patients should be followed-up with radiographs as the avascular necrosis rate after displaced intracapsular fractures is at least 30%. Femoral neck shortening of > 5 mm is associated with a worse functional outcome. THR performed as a salvage procedure for failed cannulated screws has a similar revision rate to if it is performed as a primary procedure following trauma, however, this is greater than the revision rate of elective THR (4.4% at 7 years compared to 2.9%).

Further reading

Baker RP, Squires B, Gargan MF, Bannister GC. Total hip arthroplasty and hemiarthroplasty in mobile, independent patients with a displaced intracapsular fracture of the femoral neck. J Bone Joint Surg Am 2006; 88:2583–2589.

Blomfeldt R, Törnkvist H, Eriksson K, et al. A randomised controlled trial comparing bipolar hemiarthroplasty with total hip replacement for displaced intracapsular fractures of the femoral neck in elderly patients. J Bone Joint Surg Br 2007; 89:160–165.

Gjertsen JE, Lie SA, Vinje T, et al. More re-operations after uncemented than cemented hemiarthroplasty used in the treatment of displaced fractures of the femoral neck. An observational study of 11 116 hemiarthroplasties from a national register. J Bone Joint Surg Br 2012; 94B:1113–1119.

Leonardsson O, Rogmark C, Kärrholm J, Akesson K, Garellick G. Outcome after primary and secondary replacement for subcapital fracture of the hip in 10 264 patients. J Bone Joint Surg Br 2009; 91B:595–600.

Papakostidis, Panagiotopoulos A, Piccioli A, Giannoudis PV. Timing of internal fixation of femoral neck fractures. A systematic review and meta-analysis of the final outcome. Injury 2005; 46:459–466.

Parker MJ, White A, Boyle A. Fixation versus hemiarthroplasty for undisplaced intracapsular hip fractures. Injury 2008; 39:791–795.

Watson JT, Moed BR. Ipsilateral femoral neck and shaft fractures: complications and their treatment. Clin Orthop Relat Res 2002; 399:78–86.

Related topics of interest

- *Topic 26* Femoral neck fractures – extracapsular
- *Topic 37* Guidelines in trauma

28 Foot – calcaneal fractures

Key points
- Calcaneal fractures are high-energy injuries commonly associated with long bone and spine fractures
- Displaced fractures treated non-operatively have poor outcomes, including symptomatic subtalar arthritis
- Operative treatment has a benefit in certain subgroups

Epidemiology
Calcaneus fractures account for 2700 and 17,000 patient admissions per year in the UK and USA respectively, representing 2% of all fractures. Typically, they are high-energy injuries, of which 17% are open. Up to 75% of calcaneal fractures are intra-articular extending into the subtalar joint. Associated injuries are common. Approximately 25% of patients have other associated lower leg injuries including long bone fractures and 10% have lumbar spine fractures.

Pathophysiology
The calcaneus functions as a lever arm for the gastrocnemius–soleus complex, supports body weight and maintains lateral column length. It is composed of:
- An extra-articular calcaneal tuberosity
- Three articular facets (anterior, medial and posterior) articulating with the talus
- An anterior process articulating with the cuboid
- A lateral wall in close proximity to the peroneal tendons, sural and superficial peroneal nerves
- The sustentaculum tali projecting medially to support the talar neck, with flexor hallucis longus immediately inferior to it

Extra-articular fractures (25%)
Avulsion fractures of the anterior process occur following an inversion mechanism, due to pull of the bifurcate ligament. Calcaneal tuberosity avulsion fractures occur secondary to the pull of the Achilles tendon.

Intra-articular fractures (75%)
The Essex-Lopresti classification divides intra-articular fractures into:
- Tongue type fractures (**Figures 28.1** and **28.2**)
- Joint depression fractures

The primary fracture line crosses obliquely through the posterior facet, generated by the lateral talar process pile driving into the calcaneus, dividing the lateral wall and body. With continued force, a secondary fracture line occurs in two distinct patterns: a posterior directed force creates a joint depression fracture, the fracture exiting on the superior surface of the calcaneus posterior to the posterior facet; an inferior force produces a tongue-type fracture (**Figures 28.1** and **28.2**).

The Eastwood–Atkins classification (**Table 28.1**) provides a practical classification. Three major fragments are described in the coronal plane (**Figure 28.3**):
- Sustentaculum tali

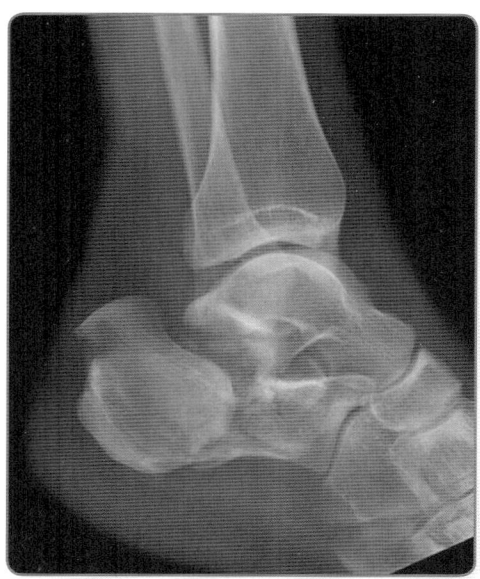

Figure 28.1 Plain radiograph showing an intra-articular depressed calcaneal fracture.

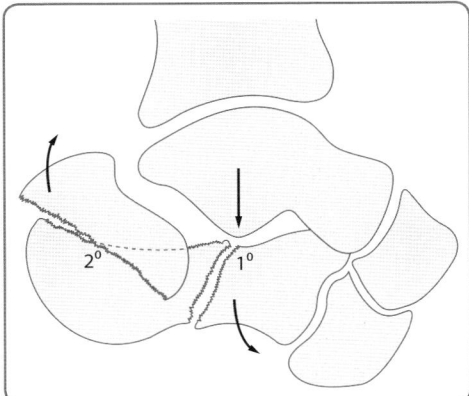

Figure 28.2 Mechanism showing forces responsible for tongue type calcaneal fracture shown in Figure 1. The lateral process of the talus drives into the calcaneum, creating a primary fracture. With continued inferior force, the secondary fracture is produced.

Table 28.1 Eastwood–Atkins classification calcaneus fractures, describing the composition of the lateral wall

Type	Lateral wall composition	Frequency (%)
1	Lateral wall formed by lateral joint fragment alone	37
2	Lateral wall formed by both lateral joint fragment and body	45
3	Lateral wall formed by body fragment only	18

- Lateral wall
- Body

The sustenatculum tali often rotates into varus, the lateral joint fragment into valgus and body fragment impacts and displaces laterally into varus. The sustenaculum fragment is known as the 'constant' fragment because it is often held in its approximate relation with the talus by the deltoid ligament complex and interosseous ligament. Knowledge of the major fracture fragments is useful when planning open reduction and internal fixation.

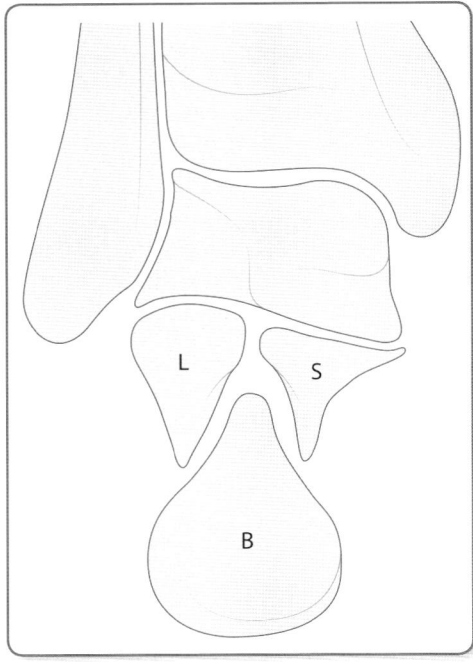

Figure 28.3 The Eastwood–Atkins classification describes three calcaneal fracture components which are the sustentaculum (S), lateral wall (L) and body (B).

Clinical features

Advanced Trauma Life Support protocols should be followed, including assessment for spine, pelvis and long bone injuries. Soft tissue swelling is often significant and compartment syndrome occurs in 10% of cases. Skin can be threatened in association with avulsion fractures of the calcaneal tuberosity. Displaced intra-articular fractures cause loss of height, a shortened and widened heel, and varus malalignment.

Investigations

Plain radiographs should include:
- An anteroposterior view of the foot
- Lateral view of the hindfoot (**Figure 28.4**)
- A mortise ankle view
- A Harris axial view of the heel

If the posterior facet has detached from the sustentaculum tali and is depressed, the Böhler angle (normal 20–40°) flattens and crucial angle of Gissane (normal 130–145°) increases (**Figure 28.4**). The Harris axial view may show increased width, varus malalignment and the articular surface of the posterior facet.

Sanders classification

Computed tomography is the gold standard investigation. The fracture is assessed in a 30° semi-coronal plane taken at the widest part of the talus (**Figure 28.5**). The Sanders classification describes the number of fracture fragments and whether the fractures are medial (sustentaculum tali), central, lateral (**Table 28.2**). A step of <2 mm is defined as undisplaced.

Treatment

Initial management

Initial management of the limb includes patient admission, limb elevation, ice and a removable splint or back slab. Intermittent pneumatic compression devices applied to the foot can reduce swelling.

Nonoperative management

Undisplaced fractures (<2 mm) are treated nonoperatively, with nonweight-bearing for 6–10 weeks. Displaced fractures are often managed nonoperatively in noncompliant patients or those with high-risk co-morbidities such as diabetes mellitus, smoking, peripheral vascular disease, alcohol dependence and peripheral neuropathy.

Operative management

Indications for surgery include:
- Displaced intra-articular fractures >2 mm (Sanders type 2 and 3)
- Displaced extra-articular calcaneal tuberosity fractures (surgical emergency if threatened skin)
- Significant varus deformity causing subtalar impingement
- Anterior process fractures with >25% calcaneocuboid joint involvement

Timing

Surgery should not be performed until the soft tissue swelling has decreased to the extent that the lateral skin wrinkles. Optimal timing is 7–14 days.

Patient positioning and surgical approach

The patient is positioned in the lateral decubitus position, allowing easy access to the lateral hindfoot.

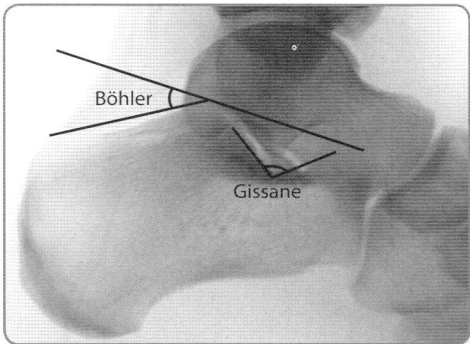

Figure 28.4 Plain radiograph allows assessment of the Böhler angle and the crucial angle of Gissane.

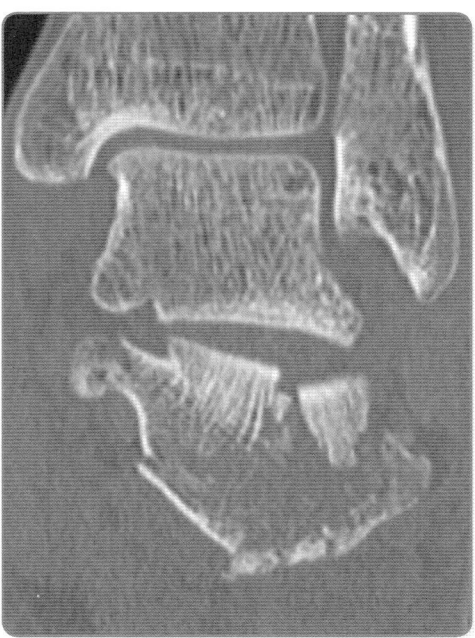

Figure 28.5 Plain CT showing a 30° semicoronal view through the posterior facet of the talus, showing a multifragmentary calcaneal fracture (Sanders type IV).

Table 28.2 Sanders classification – based on coronal CT image of the posterior facet taken at the widest point of the talus	
Type I	All articular fractures <2 mm displaced
Type II	2 part fractures of the posterior facet
Type III	3 part fractures of the posterior facet
Type IV	4 part fractures

An extended lateral transcalcaneal approach is performed through an incision made approximately 2 cm proximal to the tip of the lateral malleolus, just lateral to the Achilles tendon (**Figure 28.6**). The vertical limb extends towards the sole of the foot. The horizontal limb extends from the base of the 5th metatarsal towards the heel, along the upper border of the thick specialised heel skin, meeting the vertical limb at an angle of 100°. A full thickness flap is elevated subperiosteally, so that the sural nerve and blood supply are contained and preserved within the flap. The sural nerve, peroneal brevis and peroneal tertius tendons remain at risk at the distal extent of the incision. Three Kirschner (K) wires are then inserted into the fibula, talus and cuboid (**Figure 28.7**), allowing safe retraction of the flap, which avoids repetitive grasping of the skin edges.

The lateral wall usually has to be opened up allowing access to the medial sustentaculum fragment. This is elevated and reduced, and if necessary bone graft used to fill any defect. The lateral wall is then reduced and a calcaneal plate applied.

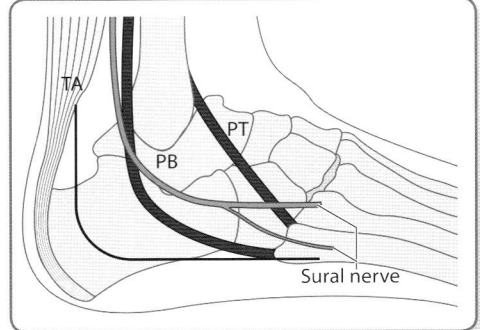

Figure 28.6 Lateral transcalcaneal approach. The tendo Achilles (TA), peroneal brevis (PB) and peroneal tertius (PT) tendons are shown.

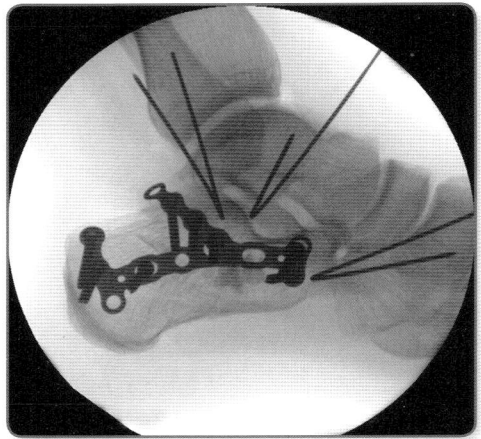

Figure 28.7 Intraoperative fluoroscopy following open reduction internal fixation of the calcaneum using a low profile lateral plate. K wires have been inserted to retract the soft tissue flap.

Complications

Initial

Early complications include severe swelling leading to compartment syndrome. Treatment is controversial. According to the British Orthopaedic Association, no consensus exists on whether foot compartment syndrome should be nonoperatively or by urgent fasciotomies.

Early

Early operative complications include infection in approximately 16% of patients, even when surgery is delayed until skin wrinkling occurs. Skin necrosis in particular may develop for significantly displaced tongue-type fractures that threaten the posterior skin.

Late

Long term complications of displaced fractures include significant functional impairment. The heel typically is short, widened and in varus. Loss of height causes the talus relatively dorsiflexed in the ankle mortise. Symptoms include subtalar stiffness and pain. A depressed Böhler's angle predicts a worse outcome. A nonoperatively treated patient with a displaced calcaneus fracture is 5.5 times more likely to require subtalar arthrodesis compared with nonoperative treatment.

Anatomic reduction and fixation of displaced fractures improves clinical outcomes in comparison to nonoperative treatment of displaced fractures. For moderately displaced fractures (Sanders type II), Buckley et al. showed that patients did well with operative care if female, <29 years old, in moderate workload jobs and not on workers' compensation. However, older male patients with severe injury patterns (Sanders type IV), bilateral calcaneal fractures, and on Workers' compensation did not benefit from operative treatment. In contrast, the recent UK Heel Fracture Study controversially failed to show a significant difference in outcomes between operative and nonoperative treatment.

Further reading

Buckley R, Tough S, McCormack R, et al. Operative compared with nonoperative treatment of displaced intra-articular calcaneal fractures. A prospective randomised controlled multicentre trial. J Bone Joint Surg Am 2002; 84A:1733–1744.

Eastwood DM, Gregg PJ, Atkins RM. Intra-articular fractures of the calcaneus. Part I: Pathological anatomy and classification. J Bone Joint Surg Br 1993; 75:183–188.

Sanders R, Fortin P, DiPasquale T, Walling A. Operative treatment in 120 displaced intra-articular calcaneal fractures. Results using a prognostic computed tomography scan classification. Clin Orthop Relat Res 1993; 290:87–95.

Related topics of interest

- *Topic 14* Compartment syndrome
- *Topic 62* Major trauma – Advanced Trauma and Life Support principles
- *Topic 68* Open fractures

29 Foot – Lisfranc's fracture–dislocations

Key points

- For Lisfranc's injuries anatomical reduction and internal fixation is required in most cases
- Delayed treatment leads to significant morbidity – 20% of Lisfranc's injuries are missed at initial assessment
- Secondary midfoot arthritis is common, especially following ligamentous only injuries

Epidemiology

Tarsometatarsal joint ligament injuries and fracture-dislocations account for approximately 0.2% of all limb injuries. Such injuries are referred to as Lisfranc's injuries, attributed to the French gynaecologist who described surgical amputation through the midfoot of Napoleonic soldiers who had sustained severe twisting injuries in horse stirrups.

Pathophysiology

Midfoot stability is important for efficient gait, allowing transmission of force from forefoot to hindfoot. The tarsometatarsal complex is stabilised by unique bony architecture and strong capsuloligamentous attachments. In the coronal plane, the metatarsal bases are arranged similar to a Roman arch. The second metatarsal base extends more proximal than the other metatarsal bases to link with the cuneiforms, acting as a 'keystone' (**Figure 29.1**). The Lisfranc's ligament originates from the medial cuneiform and inserts into the second metatarsal base, organised as weak dorsal and strong interosseous and plantar components. Strong intermetatarsal ligaments connect each metatarsal base, apart from between the 2nd and 1st metatarsals, which explains why Lisfranc's ligament is so important to midfoot stability.

According to Myerson, the tarsometatarsals are organised into three functional units. The medial cuneiform-first metatarsal make up the medial column, allowing approximately 3.5 mm of sagittal plane motion. The middle column consists of the 2nd and 3rd metatarsals and their respective cuneiforms, and is virtually rigid allowing only 0.6 mm of motion. The 4rth and 5th tarsometatarsal joints make up the lateral column and are highly mobile in comparison to the medial and middle columns.

Classification

The mechanism of injury can be direct or indirect. Indirect injuries are more common and usually occur when an axial load is applied through the heel of a fixed hyperplantarflexed foot. Direct injuries are high-energy crush injuries associated with motor vehicle accidents, industrial accidents or falls from a height.

Injuries can be purely ligamentous or involve fracture and dislocations. The Myerson classification is shown in **Figure 29.2**. Type A involves complete (homogenous) displacement of all the metatarsals. Type B is

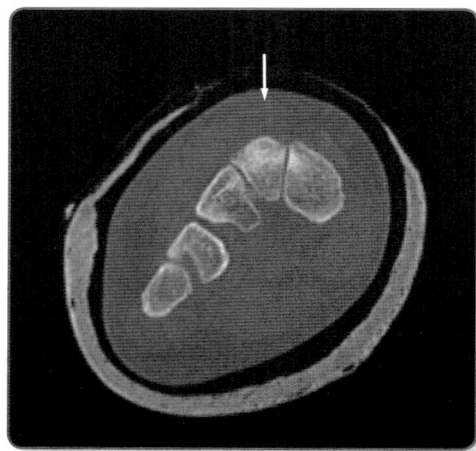

Figure 29.1 Coronal CT demonstrating the roman arch configuration of the tarsometatarsal complex. The 2nd metatarsal acts as a keystone (arrow).

Foot – Lisfranc's fracture–dislocations

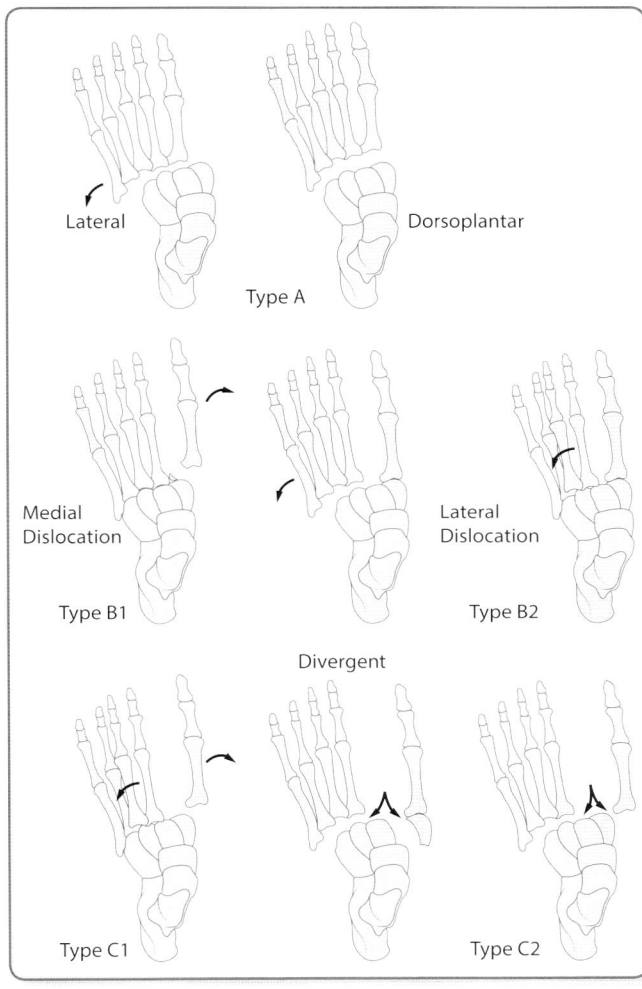

Figure 29.2 Myerson classification of Lisfranc's fracture–dislocations.
(a) Type A; total incongruity.
(b) Type B1; partial incongruity.
(c) Type B2; partial incongruity.
(d) Type C1; partial displacement.
(e) Type C2; total displacement.

partial incongruity divided into medial (B1) and lateral (B2) dislocations. Type B2 injuries are the most common Lisfranc's injury patterns. Type C is a divergent pattern in which the medial and lateral metatarsals are displaced in opposite directions.

Clinical features

Delayed diagnosis of even subtle Lisfranc's injuries can lead to significant long-term dysfunction. Up to 20% of injuries are missed during initial assessment, hence the clinician should have a high-index of suspicion. The foot is often significantly swollen. Plantar ecchymosis is considered pathognomonic of a midfoot fracture-dislocation. Deformity may be apparent in severe injuries. Pain upon application of abduction and pronation of the foot is the most sensitive clinical test for Lisfranc's injuries. Compartment syndrome and injury to the dorsalis pedis artery should be excluded, more common following high-energy crush injuries.

Investigation

Initial anteroposterior (AP), lateral and 30° internal oblique radiographs of the foot should be taken initially. Congruence of the midfoot is assessed using lines drawn along the cuneiform and cuboid bones, which should line up with their respective metatarsals. The space at the Lisfranc's joint between the medial cuneiform and 2nd metatarsal base should be the same as the medial-intermediate cuneiform space. A fleck sign (flake of bone seen in the Lisfranc's joint) is consistent with a bony avulsion and a predominantly ligamentous injury. On the lateral view, the dorsal cortex of the metatarsals should line up perfectly with the dorsal cortex of the tarsal bones. If subtle Lisfranc's injuries are suspected, weight-bearing stress views may reveal collapse of the longitudinal arch or diastasis at the medial cuneiform-second metatarsal base (**Figure 29.3**). CT reformatted in the plain of the tarsometatarsal joints allow detailed assessment of fracture displacement, subluxation and show occult fractures not seen on plain radiographs. Pronation-abduction fluoroscopic stress views performed under anaesthesia can be useful if stability of the tarsometatarsal complex is uncertain.

Treatment

Initial management

Primary aims of treatment are to provide a stable, plantigrade foot, by restoring normal tarsometatarsal joint anatomy.

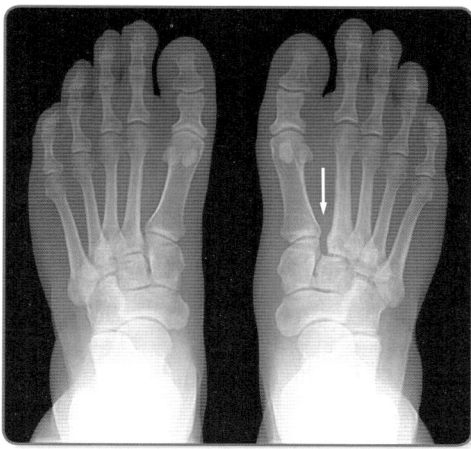

Figure 29.3 Weight-bearing AP views of both feet. A diastasis at the Lisfranc joint is consistent with a ligamentous injury (arrow).

Initial management should include hospital admission for splinting in a below-knee backslab, elevation and ice. The patient should be closely monitored for signs and symptoms of compartment syndrome. A pneumatic calf pump incorporated into the backslab may improve swelling. Surgery should be deferred until the swelling has subsided enough to allow the skin to wrinkle.

Nonoperative treatment is rarely appropriate, although undisplaced fractures can be treated in a nonweight-bearing below-knee cast for 6–12 weeks.

Operative treatment

Displacement at the tarsometatarsal joints is poorly tolerated and leads to long-term dysfunction. Open reduction internal fixation (ORIF) is the recommended treatment in order to restore normal anatomy and optimise outcome. Percutaneous reduction and fixation is a described technique but risks malreduction because fluoroscopy is not always reliable enough to assess joint reduction.

Medial and middle column injuries are approached via a dorsal longitudinal incision centred over the 2nd metatarsal base, ensuring protection of the deep peroneal nerve and dorsalis pedis artery. A medial approach may be utilised for more extensive foot injuries that require a medial bridging plate.

Internal fixation is performed using 4 mm screws or dorsal locking plates. Screws can be fully or partially threaded, used as placement screws rather than in compression. Screw placement should be tailored according to the injury pattern. The priority is anatomical reduction of the 2nd metatarsal base (the 'keystone') using a bone reduction clamp (**Figure 29.4**). This joint is subsequently stabilised with a Lisfranc's screw, which is placed in the same orientation as the Lisfranc's ligament (**Figure 29.5**). The first tarsometatarsal joint is often involved, usually adequately stabilised with a single retrograde screw. The middle column can be stabilised with a dorsal locking plate or retrograde screws placed from the 2nd and 3rd into the cuneiforms (**Figure 29.6**).

Following stabilisation of the medial and middle columns, the stability of the more mobile lateral column is assessed. The 4th

Foot – Lisfranc's fracture–dislocations

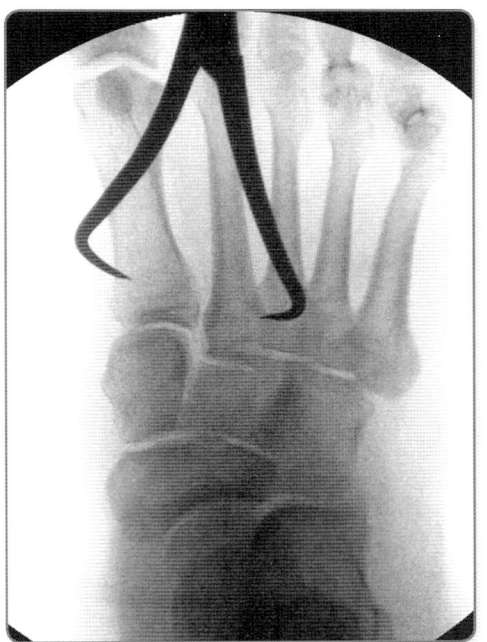

Figure 29.4 A large bone reduction clamp facilitates reduction of the 2nd metatarsal base, the 'keystone' to the tarsometatarsal bony architecture.

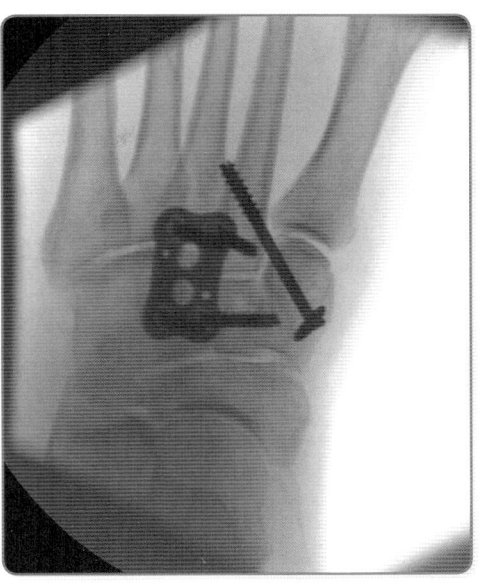

Figure 29.6 Radiograph showing internal fixation of a ligamentous Lisfranc's injury involving the medial and middle columns.

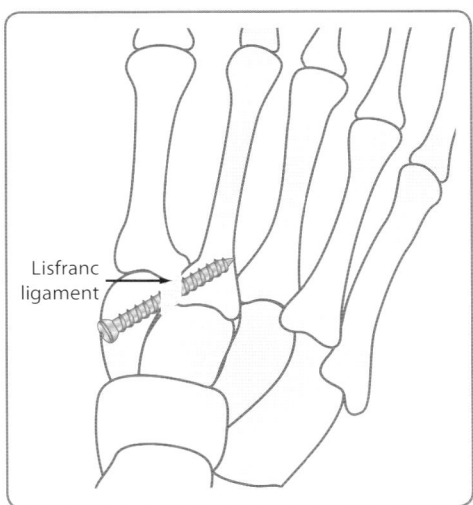

Figure 29.5 An illustration showing the orientation of the Lisfranc's ligament and the optimal placement of a screw to stabilise the Lisfranc's joint.

and 5th metatarsal bases tend to move as one unit. If unstable, retrograde Kirschner (K) wire fixation across the metatarsals into the cuboid or cuneiforms is usually sufficient.

Controversy continues regarding the treatment of primarily ligamentous injuries. Most commonly internal fixation is performed using screws. Dorsal locking plates avoid penetration of the joint surface, potentially reducing the risk of subsequent arthritis. A novel suture button technique has been described but may not adequately control sagittal plane motion.

Primary fusion tends to be reserved as a salvage procedure for Lisfranc's injuries, especially for severe crush injuries of the midfoot or if diagnosis has been delayed. Interestingly, Ly and Coetzee reported that outcomes are so poor following ligamentous only injuries that primary fusion has better clinical outcomes than ORIF. A subsequent systematic review has however shown equivalent results comparing primary arthrodesis with ORIF.

Complications

Early complications

Degloving or open fracture-dislocations are associated with high-energy crush injuries. Severe crush injuries have a reported compartment syndrome rate of 41%. Management of foot compartment syndrome remains controversial and there is currently no consensus from the British Orthopaedic Association comparing urgent fasciotomies (two dorsal incisions, one medial) versus nonoperative treatment. Acute vascular injury to the dorsalis pedis artery is rare and usually associated with a late development of neglected compartment syndrome.

Skin necrosis complicating surgery occurs in 12.5% of patients. Timing of surgery is therefore important, deferred until skin wrinkling is apparent.

Late complications

Midfoot stiffness and symptomatic arthritis are common, occurring in up to 40% of patients. For patients treated with ORIF, up to 95% of patients report good to excellent function. Primarily ligamentous injuries have worse outcomes in comparison to fracture/dislocations, leading to debate regarding treatment. In the series reported by Ly and Coetzee, only 65% of patients returned to their preoperative level of function following ORIF, in comparison to 92% of patients who had primary arthrodesis. 5 out of 20 patients (25%) in the ORIF group subsequently required secondary arthrodesis for painful midfoot arthritis.

Neglected Lisfranc's injuries have reliably poor outcomes with over 70% of patients reporting significant dysfunction. Typical problems include collapse of the midfoot, pes planus deformity, a painful unstable midfoot during toe push off and early secondary arthritis. Significant deformity may lead to difficulty with shoe wear, requiring custom made orthoses. Arthrodesis is reserved for patients who fail nonoperative treatment, although only two thirds of patients have successful outcomes.

Further reading

Myerson MS. The diagnosis and treatment of injury to the tarsometatarsal complex. J Bone Joint Surg Br 1999; 81B:757–763.

Ly TV, Coetzee JC. Treatment of primary ligamentous Lisfranc joint injuries: primary arthrodesis compared with open reduction and internal fixation. A prospective, randomized study. J Bone Joint Surg Am 2006; 88:514–520.

Myerson MS, Fisher RT, Burgess AR, Kenzora JE. Fracture dislocations of the tarsometatarsal joints: end results correlated with pathology and treatment. Foot Ankle 1986; 6:225–242.

Related topics of interest

- Topic 14 Compartment syndrome
- Topic 16 Crush injuries and crush syndrome
- Topic 17 Damage control orthopaedics and trauma physiology

Foot – mid- and forefoot fractures

30

Key points

- The navicular is the keystone to the medial longitudinal arch; displaced navicular fractures therefore cause significant adduction deformity
- Displaced cuboid fractures cause lateral column shortening leading to foot abduction and pronation if not adequately reduced
- Jones type 5th metatarsal fractures (metaphyseal–diaphyseal junction) have up to a 33% nonunion rate when treated nonoperatively
- 'Turf toe' is disruption of the plantar plate of the 1st metatarsophalangeal joint, a career-threatening injury in elite athletes

Navicular fracture dislocations

The talonavicular articulation is a ball-and-socket type joint allowing midfoot rotation. The navicular is the keystone to the medial longitudinal arch, articulating with the talar head proximally, the three cuneiforms distally and the cuboid laterally. Up to 14% of the population have accessory navicular bones, often mistaken for fractures after a midfoot injury.

A navicular fracture–dislocation can result from either a direct crush injury or indirect trauma (**Figure 30.1**). The latter usually results from forced plantarflexion of the foot. A longitudinal force applied along the metatarsals compresses the navicular between the cuneiforms and talar head, producing shear forces in line with the intercuneiform joints (**Figure 30.2**). Tibialis posterior is the only muscle that inserts into the navicular and acts as a distracting force causing displacement of the fracture. 10% of navicular fractures are open, indicating a high-energy injury.

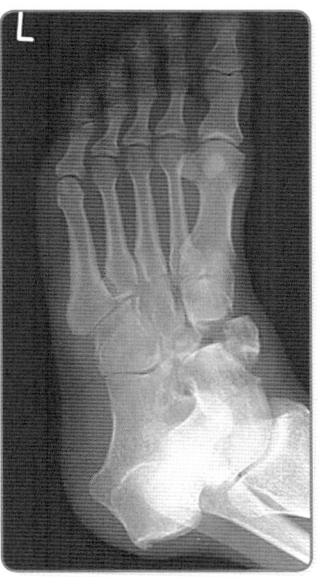

Figure 30.1 A navicular fracture–dislocation.

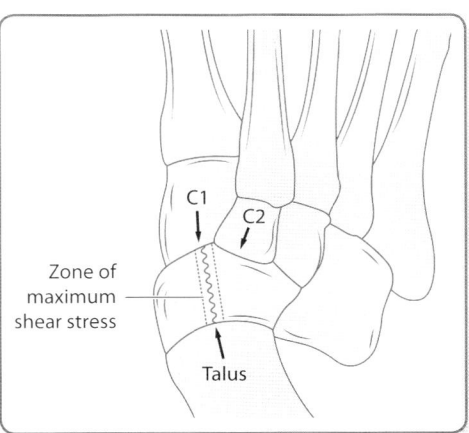

Figure 30.2 Typical direction of forces applied to the navicular leading to fracture as it is compressed between the tarsal head and medial (C1) and middle (C2) cuneiforms.

On clinical examination the midfoot is swollen. Displaced navicular fractures are often associated with varus deformity and the foot held in plantarflexion.

Plain radiographs of the foot are adequate to identify the fracture. CT imaging allows accurate assessment of the fracture pattern, fractures of adjacent bones and allows preoperative planning.

Anatomical reduction is the aim wherever possible in order to restore the medial longitudinal arch of the foot. The optimal surgical approach is dorsal, in between tibialis anterior tendon and extensor hallucis longus. The blood supply to the navicular is extra-articular; therefore, soft tissues attachments should be preserved. The extruded medial fragment is reduced ensuring a congruent articular surface. Depending upon the size of the fracture fragments internal fixation can be performed with small fragment AO screws or a small plate (**Figure 30.3**). Additional Kirschner wires may be needed to stabilise the talonavicular joint.

Navicular fractures are often associated with significant trauma, hence complication rates are high. In a series of 90 fractures, 49 were treated nonoperatively; secondary arthritis occurred in 62%. Persistent foot pain occurred in 43% and 31% were unable to wear normal shoes.

Cuboid fractures

Cuboid fractures are rare with only small series reported in the literature. Mechanism can be direct (crushing) or indirect, often resulting from jumping injuries. Cuboid fractures may occur in isolation or as part of a more significant midfoot injury. The calcaneocuboid (CC) joint is relatively immobile in comparison to the talonavicular joint. Therefore, cuboid fractures that lead to stiffness at the CC joint do not usually cause significant symptoms. The 4th and 5th metatarsal bases articulate distally, which have significant greater mobility.

The nutcracker fracture refers to a cuboid fracture resulting from forced plantar flexion and abduction of the foot, compressing the cuboid between the anterior process of the calcaneum and bases of the 4rth and 5th metatarsals. The articular surface of the lateral aspect of the cuboid is depressed at either the CC joint or the base of the 5th metatarsal. There may be an associated avulsion fracture of the navicular, fracture of the anterior process of the calcaneum or injury to the tibialis posterior tendon. Lateral column length is important for normal biomechanics. Displaced cuboid fractures with shortening leads to foot abduction

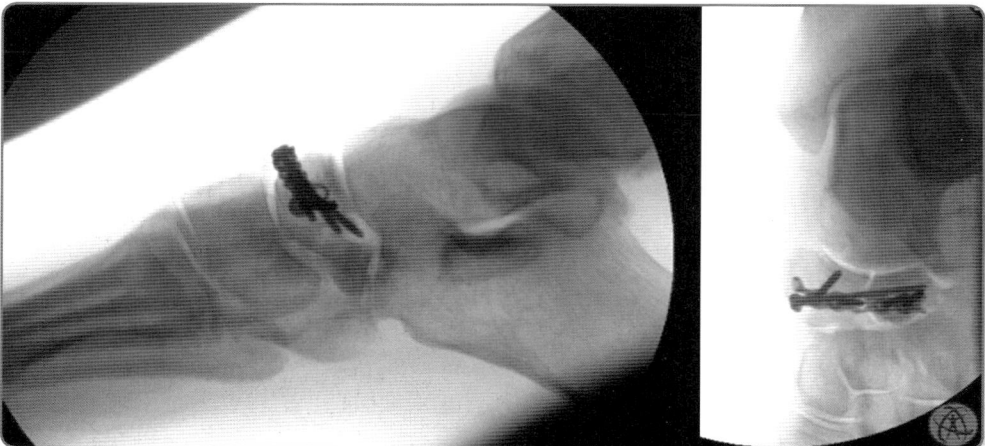

Figure 30.3 Intraoperative fluoroscopy following open reduction internal fixation of a navicular fracture–dislocation.

and pronation. Failure to restore normal lateral column length adequately can lead to significant long-term morbidity.

Undisplaced fractures can be treated nonoperatively in a nonweight-bearing cast or boot for 4–6 weeks. Displaced shortened fractures require open reduction internal fixation via a dorsolateral approach extending from 1 cm inferior to the sinus tarsi, to the base of the 4th metatarsal (**Figures 30.4** and **30.5**). Branches of the sural nerve are at risk. The extensor digitorum muscle belly is incised and elevated subperiosteally to expose the cuboid. Multifragmentary fractures may require application of a bridging plate across the CC joint or bone graft to fill significant defects. Small lateral external fixators can be used postoperatively to maintain reduction and lateral column length. Primary fusion of the CC joint is a salvage procedure and rarely indicated.

Only small case series exist so outcomes following cuboid fracture are unclear. Potential complications include stiffness, post-traumatic arthritis, abduction deformity, nonunion and osteonecrosis.

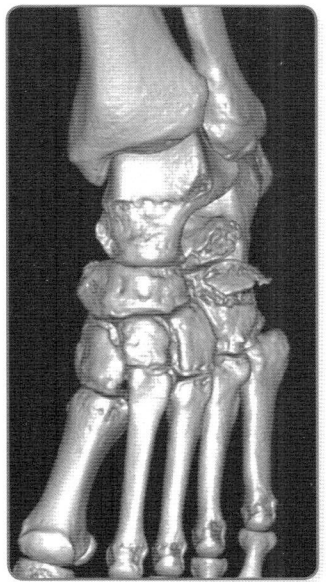

Figure 30.4 CT scans showing a displaced cuboid fracture.

Fifth metatarsal fractures

Fifth metatarsal fractures are the most common fracture of the foot. Base of 5th metatarsal fractures can be classified as tuberosity fractures (**Figure 30.6**), Jones fractures at the metaphyseal-diaphyseal junction, and diaphyseal fractures (**Figure 30.7**). The mechanism of injury is typically inversion of the foot leading to an avulsion fracture from the pull of peroneus brevis. Adduction mechanisms tend to lead to Jones type fractures.

Avulsion fractures can be successfully treated nonoperatively. Acute management using a slipper plaster is proven to provide better comfort in comparison to tubigrip. Early weight-bearing improves functional outcomes and 86% of patients are back to their usual activities by 6 months.

Jones fractures at the metaphyseal–diaphyseal junction continue to generate debate regarding the optimal management. The fracture occurs at a vascular watershed

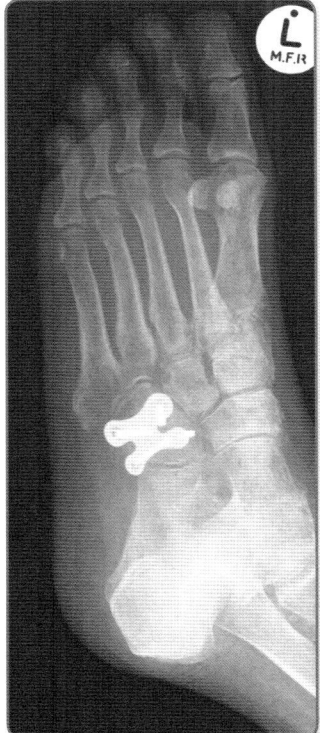

Figure 30.5 Postoperative radiograph following open reduction internal fixation of a cuboid fracture.

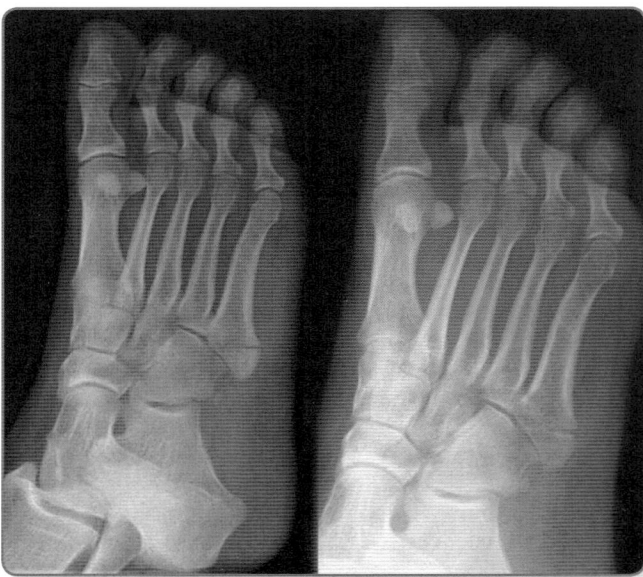

Figure 30.6 Type 1 base of 5th metatarsal fracture treated nonoperatively, which developed a painless nonunion at 8 months (note the sclerotic margins of the fracture margins).

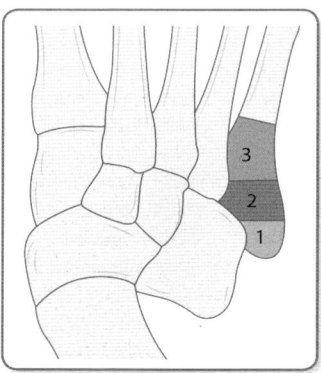

Figure 30.7 Base of 5th metatarsal fractures can be classified as tuberosity fractures (zone 1), Jones type fractures (zone 2) and diaphyseal fractures (zone 3).

contributing to an increased risk of nonunion. Nonoperative management is typically done using nonweight-bearing plaster or boot for 6–8 weeks, although such treatment has a non-union rate of approximately 21–33%. Mologne et al. demonstrated in a randomised controlled trial that for acute Jones' fractures screw fixation had a 95% union rate in comparison to only 67% in a cast group. Fixation is typically achieved with a single partially threaded 4.5 mm screw. Those patients in particular who benefit from acute fixation are elite athletes. Return to sport was 8 weeks in the operative group versus 15 weeks in the nonoperative group.

'Turf toe' – Hallux metatarsophalangeal joint dislocation

'Turf toe' is a common injury amongst athletes. In a study of intercollegiate football data in the USA, turf toe occurred at a rate of approximately 0.062 per 1000 athlete exposures, with a significantly higher risk in those athletes playing on artificial surfaces compared to grass pitches. Turf toe occurs following forced hyperextension of the toe, resulting in partial or complete rupture of the plantar plate, or sesamoid fracture. Turf toe can also be acute or chronic, the latter from repetitive hyperextension injuries.

Complete plantar plate rupture is a severe injury, which is potentially career threatening in elite athletes if not treated early and appropriately. Partial injuries can be treated nonoperatively with taping of the toe and a stiff soled shoe. For complete ruptures causing instability, the optimal treatment is plantar plate reconstruction done either arthroscopically or open.

Complications from turf toe relate to the severity of the initial injury. Delayed diagnosis worsens outcome. Sprains or partial ruptures treated appropriately cause a mean time away from sport for 10 days.

Such injuries are less likely to lead to long-term problems, but stiffness is common. Complete rupture can cause significant pain, stiffness and long-term instability limiting return to play.

Further reading

Coulibaly MO, Jones CB, Sietsema DL, Schildhauer TA. Results and complications of operative and non-operative navicular fracture treatment. Injury 2015; 46:1669–1677.

George E, Harris AH, Dragoo JL, Hunt KJ. Incidence and risk factors for turf toe injuries in intercollegiate football: data from the national collegiate athletic association injury surveillance system. Foot Ankle Int 2014; 35:108–115.

Hermel MB, Gersham-Cohen J. The nutcracker fracture of the cuboid caused by indirect violence. Radiology 1953; 60: 850–854.

Main BJ, Jowett RL. Injuries of the midtarsal joint. J Bone Joint Surg Br 1975; 57B:89–97.

Mologne TS, Lundeen JM, Clapper MF, O'Brien TJ. Early screw fixation versus casting in the treatment of acute Jones fractures. Am J Sports Med 2005; 33:970–975.

Related topics of interest

- *Topic 16* Crush injuries and crush syndrome
- *Topic 67* Nonunion of fractures
- *Topic 68* Open fractures

Foot – subtalar and Chopart's fracture-dislocations

Key points

- Subtalar dislocation includes disruption of both the talocalcaneal and talonavicular joints
- Associated osteochondral fractures of the talus are common
- Interposed soft tissues or failure to bend the knee to relax gastrocnemius-soleus complex may prevent closed reduction

Epidemiology

Isolated subtalar joint dislocation without an associated talar neck fracture is rare (<2% of all dislocations). The mean age of injury is 37 years, occurring far more commonly in men. Over 50% are high-energy injuries following a fall from height, or a road traffic accident, usually resulting in lateral dislocations. Less commonly, low energy inversion injuries can lead to medial subtalar joint dislocation during sport, hence the term 'basketball foot'. Associated injuries are common; approximately 40% of cases are open; osteochondral talar fractures occur in 47%; and foot fractures in >60%.

Pathophysiology

The subtalar joint comprises three articular facets through which the talus articulates with the calcaneus. Chopart's joint (also known as the transverse tarsal joint) refers to the talonavicular and calcanecuboid joints. Subtalar motion allows inversion and eversion of the foot. In subtalar inversion, the tibia externally rotates. In subtalar eversion, the tibia is driven to internally rotate. In normal gait, during heel strike the subtalar joint is in eversion, and mobile to accommodate uneven ground. The tibia is in relative internal rotation. During toe push off, the subtalar joint locks in inversion, the tibia now in external rotation, allowing forward propulsion. The subtalar joint therefore acts as an important 'torque converter', converting rotation of the foot to rotation of the tibia during normal gait.

Subtalar joint stability relies upon complex bony anatomy and soft tissue attachments. Ligamentous attachments include the strong talocalcaneal interosseous ligament in the sinus tarsi, medially the superficial deltoid ligament, and laterally the calcaneofibular ligament. All three ligaments must be disrupted for the subtalar joint to dislocate. The posterior process is comprised of the medial and lateral tubercles and allows insertion of the deep deltoid ligament and posterior talofibular ligament, respectively, with a groove for flexor hallucis longus. The tubercles, due to their soft tissue attachments, are subsequently prone to avulsion fractures during subtalar dislocation (**Figure 31.1**).

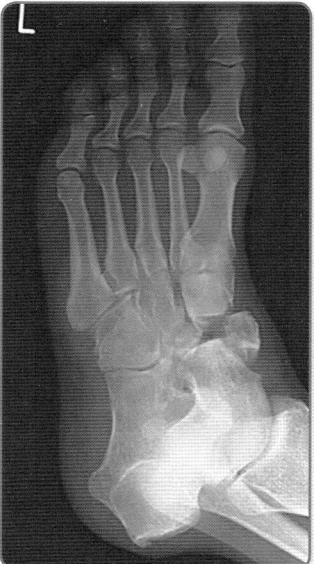

Figure 31.1 Medial subtalar joint dislocation.

Foot – subtalar and Chopart's fracture–dislocations

Table 31.1 Classification of subtalar dislocation

Direction	Frequency	Possible obstructions to reduction
Medial	80%	Talus button holed through extensor retinaculum Peroneal tendons
Lateral	17%	Tibialis posterior tendon Flexor digitorum longus tendon
Posterior	2.5%	–
Anterior	0.5%	–

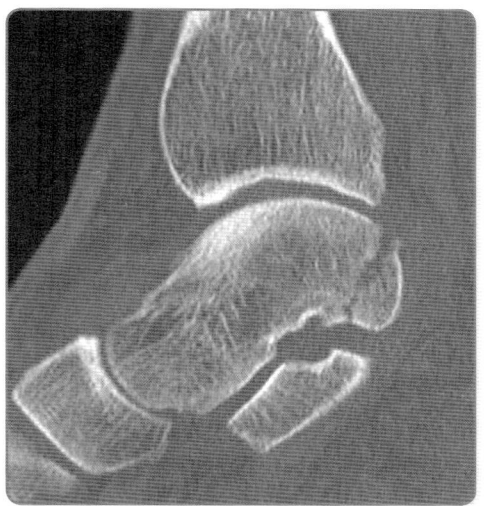

Figure 31.2 Post-reduction CT scan following subtalar joint dislocation, revealing an undisplaced posterior facet fracture.

Classification

Subtalar joint dislocations have been classified anatomically by Broca, modified by Malgaigne. In decreasing order of frequency, medial dislocations are most common (80%) followed by lateral (17%), posterior (2.5%) and rare anterior dislocations (**Table 31.1**).

Clinical features

Clinical deformity is usually obvious. In medial dislocations, the foot is plantar flexed, supinated and adducted. In lateral dislocations, the foot is pronated and abducted. Lateral dislocations are often more severe injuries because greater energy is required relative to a medial dislocation. Lateral dislocations have a higher incidence of associated fractures (72%), open injuries (25%). Almost 20% are irreducible by closed methods. Rare posterior dislocations occur with the foot in extreme plantar flexion. The foot may appear shorter in length compared with the normal foot. True anterior dislocations are incredibly rare, and thought to occur secondary to forcible distraction.

Investigations

Anteroposterior and lateral plain radiographs are required to distinguish an ankle fracture/dislocation from a subtalar joint dislocation. Following closed reduction, repeat radiographs are necessary to confirm joint congruence. CT scan is now readily available and is recommended to confirm reduction and identify occult fractures, such as posterior process fractures (**Figure 31.2**).

Treatment

The majority of subtalar dislocation can be managed with closed reduction and immobilisation. If performed promptly in the emergency department, reduction is usually possible under conscious sedation. The knee must be flexed prior to reduction to relax the gastrocnemius complex.

Medial dislocations

With the knee flexed to 90°, inline traction is applied via the heel. The deformity is accentuated, followed by abduction and dorsiflexion of the foot. Counter pressure should be applied by the clinician's thumb to the palpable talar head which is prominent dorsolaterally. A common cause of block to reduction is inadequate knee flexion. The talar head can button hole through the extensor retinaculum. Interposed peroneal tendons, or extensor digitorum brevis may also block reduction.

Irreducible medial dislocations can be approached via a longitudinal incision positioned over the talar head and neck. This allows access to the extensor retinaculum which is often button holed by the talar head.

Lateral dislocations

With the knee flexed, inline traction is applied. Further abduction is used to accentuate the deformity, followed by adduction and inversion, pivoting around the prominent talar head which is palpated medially. Failure to reduce closed occurs in 20% of cases, secondary to interposed posterior tibial tendon or flexor digitorum longus, which are displaced superolaterally over the talar neck.

For irreducible lateral dislocations, the talar neck can be approach via either a lateral incision over the sinus tarsi, or a medial incision from the medial malleolus to the prominent talar head.

Postreduction management

There is usually a palpable clunk upon reduction of the subtalar joint. It is then possible to determine stability of the joint, screened in both inversion and eversion if fluoroscopy is available. For unstable fracture/dislocations temporary Kirschner (K) wire fixation is usually sufficient (**Figure 31.3**), assuming that soft tissue interposition or a large intra-articular fracture fragment are not causes for the instability. If a displaced intra-articular fracture is the cause for instability, open reduction internal fixation is required. For more severe injuries, especially open injuries requiring soft tissue reconstruction and cover with a free flap, external fixation may be more appropriate.

Immobilization nonweight-bearing in a below knee cast for at least 6 weeks is the recommended management. Recurrent instability of the subtalar joint can occur in up to 60% cases according to the series by Zimmer and Johnson. Therefore, most authors recommend immobilisation for 6–12 weeks, nonweight-bearing for the first 6 weeks. Re-dislocation or subluxation can occur in plaster, especially during the first 2 weeks. Hence, screening radiographs are indicated at weeks 1 and 2.

Open subtalar joint dislocations

Open injuries require rapid administration of intravenous broad-spectrum antibiotics according to local microbiology protocols (usually co-amoxiclav). The subtalar joint should be reduced initially in the emergency department rather than await transfer to theatre as delays are frequent, and failure to reduce may cause further injury to tissues and neurovascular structures. Formal debridement and irrigation in theatre are necessary, with a second look and further debridement at 48 hours. During debridement, it is necessary to re-dislocate the joint in order to achieve adequate exposure.

Complications

Open injuries indicate high-energy trauma. Medial wounds can often be closed primarily, whereas one-third of open lateral dislocations require free flap soft tissue reconstruction. Up to one-third of open injuries are associated with posterior tibial artery injury. Tibial nerve injuries frequently lead to complex regional pain syndrome.

Secondary arthritis is apparent on radiographs in 40–75% of patients, and although subtalar joint stiffness is often apparent, pain is uncommon. The risk of developing secondary arthritis increases to 85% in the presence of intra-articular fractures. Symptomatic subtalar arthritis is treated with triple arthrodesis if nonoperative measures fail.

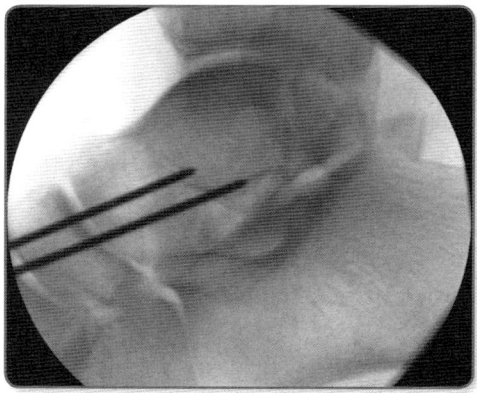

Figure 31.3 Temporary K wires inserted across the talonavicular joint following reduction of a subtalar joint dislocation.

Avascular necrosis (AVN) occurs in approximately 5% of subtalar dislocation and is more likely in severe subtalar joint dislocations. Subchondral lucency (Hawkins sign) seen on follow-up radiographs at 6–8 weeks indicates patent blood supply to the talar body. An absent Hawkins sign by 12 weeks, is associated with a 75% risk of developing subsequent AVN. If suspected, MRI is the gold standard investigation to confirm diagnosis. In most cases, AVN can usually be managed with protected weight-bearing to prevent subchondral collapse. In such cases, patients should be counselled that revascularization of talus is slow, potentially taking up to 5 years. In one series of 15 patients with severe subtalar dislocations, one-third of patients required subtalar fusion for AVN.

Factors that worsen prognosis include lateral dislocations, high-energy injuries and open injuries. Function following low energy medial dislocations is invariably reported to be excellent. Outcomes following high-energy dislocations, however, are far worse; in one series of severe open dislocations, all patients had ankle pain, 90% reported difficulty walking on uneven ground and 25% reported symptoms consistent with complex regional pain syndrome.

Further reading

Bohay DR, Manoli A 2nd. Subtalar joint dislocations. Foot Ankle Int 1995; 16:803–808.

DeLee JC, Curtis R. Subtalar dislocation of the foot. J Bone Joint Surg Am 1982; 64:433–437.

Goldner JL, Poletti SC, Gates HS 3rd, Richardson WJ. Severe open subtalar dislocations. Long-term results. J Bone Joint Surg Am 1995; 77:1075–1079.

Merchan EC. Subtalar dislocations: long-term follow-up of 39 cases. Injury 1992; 23:97–100.

Zimmer TJ, Johnson KA. Subtalar dislocations. Clin Orthop Relat Res 1989:190–194.

Related topics of interest

- *Topic 15* Complex regional pain syndrome
- *Topic 62* Major trauma – Advanced Trauma and Life Support principles
- *Topic 68* Open fractures

32 Forearm – distal radial fractures

Key points

- Fractures of the distal radius are common injuries affecting two disparate patient cohorts
- A degree of displacement is well tolerated in the low demand patient however in high demand patients with articular involvement anatomic reduction of the joint surface and restoration of radial length is essential
- Open reduction and internal fixation (ORIF) can restore anatomic alignment and permit early mobilisation at a cost of increased risk of surgical complications

Epidemiology

Fracture of the distal radius is one of the most common injuries presenting to emergency care. Some studies have suggested that this injury accounts for 2.5% of all emergency department visits and up to 20% of all fractures. The lifetime risk for women has been calculated at 36.8/10000 person-years whilst the lifetime incidence for males is 9/10000 person-years. There is a bimodal distribution with the most frequently affected demographic being females between the ages of 50 and 60 years with a second peak of males aged 10–30 years. These two cohorts are distinct in terms of biology and mechanism. The first group of fractures occur due to decreased mineral density and are a low-energy injury whilst the second group occurs following high-energy injury through normally mineralised bone. These differences dictate the variations in appropriate management strategies and explain the disparity in outcome.

Pathophysiology

In order to appreciate the pathophysiology it is important to understand the anatomical arrangement of the distal radius. This can be approximated to the rule of 11s. In a normal distal radius, there will be 11° of volar tilt, 11 mm of radial height compared to the ulna and 22° of radial inclination (**Figure 32.1**).

The pathophysiology reflects the bimodal distribution of the incidence. In the elderly osteoporotic patient the fracture occurs through the relatively weak metaphyseal bone. The mechanism is frequently a low-energy fall from standing. The position of the hand at the time of impact will dictate the direction of displacement. If the wrist is in extension the distal fragment will tend to angulate dorsally (**Figure 32.2**) and the wrist will adopt the classical dinner fork deformity. This is commonly referred to as a Colles' after Abraham Colles who described the deformity in 1814, long before the invention of radiograph imaging. If the wrist is in flexion the distal fragment will be volarly angulated. This is known as a Smith's fracture. Whilst

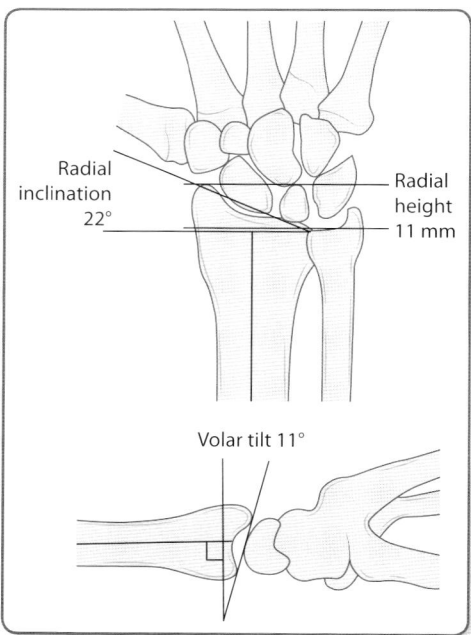

Figure 32.1 The normal anatomical relationship of the distal radius, the rule of 11s.

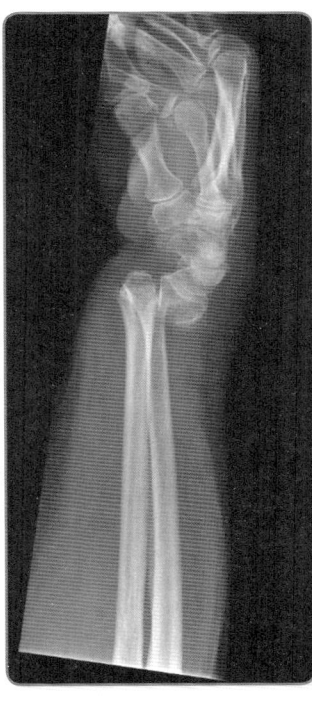

Figure 32.2 A lateral radiograph demonstrating the dorsal angulation seen in a Colles fracture.

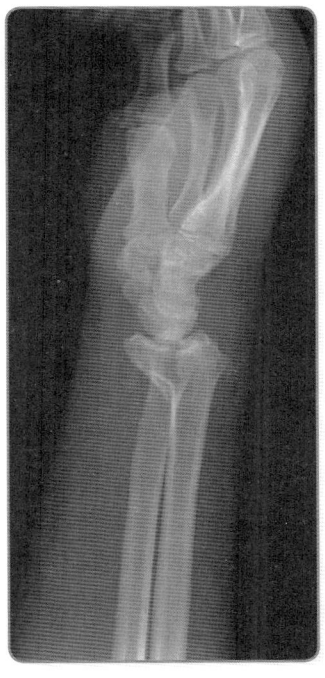

Figure 32.3 A lateral radiograph demonstrating the volar subluxation of the carpus seen in a volar Barton's fracture.

these two patterns are the most commonly seen intra-articular fractures also occur in this age group.

In the young adult patient fractures of the distal radius are high-energy injuries that are frequently of a complex intra-articular pattern. If an intra-articular split leads to subluxation of the carpus this is referred to as a Barton's fracture (**Figure 32.3**). The most common direction of subluxation is volar ward.

Clinical features

The patient will present with pain, swelling and loss of movement at the wrist following a fall onto an outstretched hand. If there is significant displacement then the deformity may be clinically detectable. Compromise to the neurovascular status of the hand can occur. The median nerve can be injured in severely angulated fractures. Assessment and documentation of neurovascular status is essential. Emergent reduction is indicated in the presence of median nerve symptoms.

Compartment syndrome is a rare but serious complication that can occur following distal radius fracture. Recognition and prompt decompression must occur in the presence of significantly raised compartment pressures.

Investigations

Plain radiographs are sufficient for diagnosis and management planning in most distal radius fractures. Angulation and shortening can be assessed and quantified using digital measurement tools. In complex intra-articular fractures CT scan may be required to assess the joint surface and plan surgical intervention.

Classification

Descriptive classification is frequently employed. Key distinctions are open or closed, degree of shortening, displacement, angulation and comminution. The Frykman classification (**Figure 32.4**) is an 8-stage classification based on joint involvement

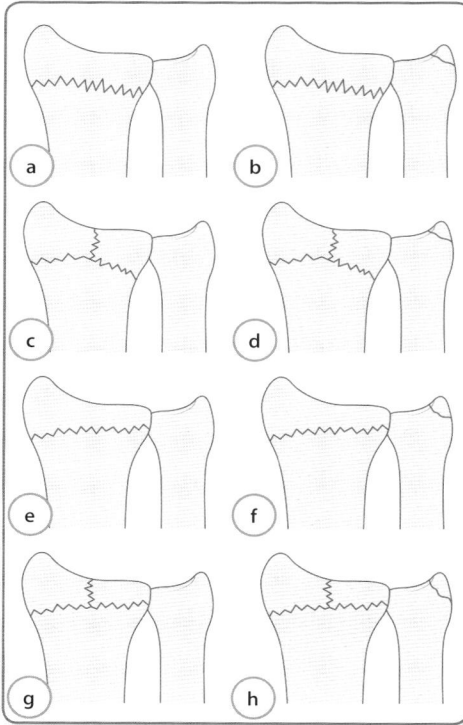

Figure 32.4 The Frykman classification of distal radius fractures. (a) I; extra-articular no ulnar styloid fracture. (b) II; extra-articular with ulnar styloid fracture. (c) III; radiocarpal involvement no styloid fracture. (d) IV; radiocarpal involvement with styloid fracture. (e) V; distal radioulna joint involvement no styloid fracture (f) VI; distal radioulna joint involvement with styloid fracture. (g) VII; radiocarpal and distal radioulna joint no styloid fracture. (h) VIII; radiocarpal and distal radioulna joint with styloid fracture.

Treatment

Undisplaced fractures can be treated in a below elbow backslab with completion of cast and check X-ray to ensure maintenance of position at 2 weeks. Cast is maintained for 4–6 weeks. Removable splint may be required for 3 weeks following removal of cast.

Displaced fractures should be reduced in the emergency department under appropriate anaesthesia and sedation. Haematoma block, Biers block or axillary block may be utilised. Alternatively, sedation may be required. Position should be maintained with a plaster splint on the side of the angulation (i.e. volar for Smith's type dorsal for Colles fracture). The extreme flexion and ulna deviation (Cotton-Loder) position traditionally used for the treatment of Colles fractures should be avoided as this can lead to unacceptable levels of post immobilisation stiffness and neurovascular compromise.

Acceptable alignment is dependent on the functional demands of the patient. In general, <2 mm of shortening, 10° of dorsal angulation and 30% of dorsal translation are regarded as acceptable in elderly osteoporotic fractures. The degree of deformity tolerated in younger patients is far less and anatomic reduction is desirable.

If acceptable alignment is not achieved or the position is lost at initial fracture clinic review then surgical intervention is indicated. If closed reduction is possible then the fracture can often be stabilised with Kirschner (K) wires and a plaster back slab applied. Check X-ray and clinical assessment is required at 7–10 days postoperative as position can still be lost. Wires are usually removed at 4 weeks followed by 2 further weeks in a plaster.

If open reduction is required then rigid internal fixation should be employed. Most commonly this is with a volar locking plate; however, the specific fracture pattern may dictate alternative approaches and fixation methods. If the fixation is sufficiently stable then the patient can be left out of cast and begin early supervised mobilisation.

In open fractures or in fractures so severely comminuted that they are

and presence or absence of an ulna styloid fracture. The Frykman classification brought attention to the importance of the ulnar styloid. The presence of this seemingly innocuous fracture is an indication that there has been a significant injury to the distal radioulna joint. The AO classification is detailed but somewhat cumbersome, so itsuse is usually reserved for research settings. Eponyms are frequently used to describe common fracture patterns as outlined above.

unreconstructable then spanning external fixators may be utilised with or without K-wire augmentation.

Complications

Early complications

- Vascular compromise – assess and document capillary refill, be prepared to split the cast/splint if blood supply compromised
- Nerve injury – compression of the median nerve in the carpal tunnel is common either by the deformity or by haematoma. Initial management should be reduction of the fracture and elevation. If the symptoms fail to settle then emergent carpal tunnel decompression should be performed. The fracture should be stabilised at the same sitting
- Triangular fibrocartilage complex injury. As the radius displaces, traction on the triangular fibrocartilage complex can lead to an ulna styloid fracture or soft tissue injury. This in turn leads to on-going ulna sided wrist pain and distal radioulna joint instability long after the initial fracture has healed

Late complications

- Malunion – this may occur secondary to inadequate initial reduction or subsequent loss of position in plaster. In the presence of shortening painful ulna carpal abutment may occur. Loss of the volar inclination can restrict flexion. Realignment osteotomy to restore length and volar inclination can be a successful salvage procedure in young patients
- Stiffness of the elbow wrist and fingers can occur following prolonged immobilisation or surgical insult to the soft tissues
- Degenerative change – failure to restore the articular surface of the distal radius to its anatomical position may lead to early degeneration and painful arthritis
- Tendon rupture – the extensor pollicis longus tendon may spontaneously rupture several weeks following a seemingly innocuous distal radial fracture. This may also occur following ORIF if the screw tips are left proud of the dorsal cortex. This may be treated with a simple tendon transfer however full retropulsion of the thumb will not be restored
- Complex regional pain syndrome can occur following wrist fracture

Further reading

Brogan DM, Ruch DS. Distal radius fractures in the elderly. J Hand Surg Am 2015; 40:1217–1219.

Costa ML, Achten J, Parsons NR, et al. Percutaneous fixation with Kirschner wires versus volar locking plate fixation in adults with dorsally displaced fracture of distal radius: randomised controlled trial. BMJ 2014; 349:g4807.

Ng CY, McQueen MM. What are the radiological predictors of functional outcome following fractures of the distal radius? J Bone Joint Surg British 2011; 93:145–150.

Related topics of interest

- *Topic 15* Complex regional pain syndrome
- *Topic 34* Forearm – radius and ulna fractures
- *Topic 44* Hand and wrist – tendon ruptures

33 Forearm – Galeazzi's and Monteggia's fractures

Key points

- Galeazzi's and Monteggia's fractures are fracture–dislocations of the forearm
- Failure to appreciate the associated ligamentous injury and consequent instability of the radioulna joints may lead to severe functional deficit
- Open anatomic reduction and rigid stabilisation of the fracture is essential to restore joint congruency in the adult

Definition

A Galeazzi's fracture is an isolated fracture of the distal or middle third of the radius with an associated dislocation of the distal radioulna joint (DRUJ).

A Monteggia's fracture is a fracture of the middle or proximal third of the ulna with an associated dislocation of the proximal radioulna joint.

Epidemiology

Galeazzi's fractures make up <6% of all forearm fractures whilst Monteggia's fractures are rarer still forming between 1% and 2% of all forearm injuries.

Pathophysiology

The relationship of the two bones of the forearm can be thought of as an osseoligamentous ring. Much like in the polo mint analogy for the pelvis, if there is a displaced fracture in one place there is almost certainly a second injury within this anatomical construct. In the Galeazzi's or Monteggia's fracture the second injury occurs as a dislocation of the radioulna joint rather than as a fracture of the second bone (**Figure 33.1**).

As discussed in the chapter 'Forearm – radius and ulna fractures', the complex anatomical relationship of the radius and ulna is critical if the ability to accurately position the hand in space is to be preserved.

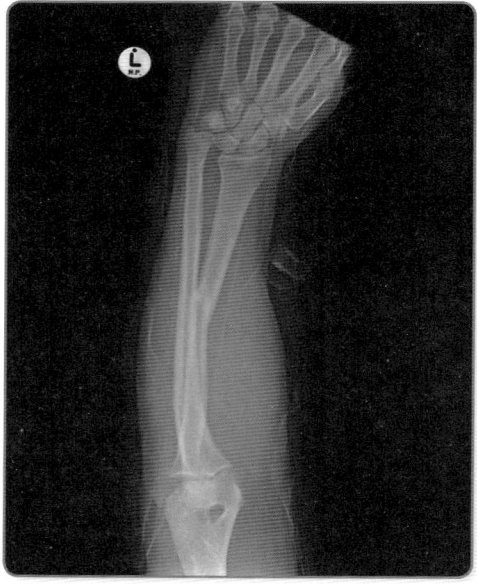

Figure 33.1 Posteroanterior radiograph demonstrating a Galeazzi's fracture–dislocation. Note the disruption to the DRUJ.

This relationship and the resulting kinematics are as reliant on the interconnecting joints as they are on the bony anatomy.

The ligamentous injury to the distal radioulna joint (DRUJ) in a Galeazzi's fracture may therefore lead to a severe functional deficit if left untreated. Failure to appreciate and adequately reduce the radial head dislocation in a Monteggia's injury will lead to significant compromise of elbow function.

Clinical features

As with any forearm fracture these two specific subtypes may present following a fall onto an outstretched hand or from a direct blow.

The Galeazzi's fracture will present with pain and deformity at the level of the radial fracture with associated wrist pain. The wrist

Forearm – Galeazzi's and Monteggia's fractures

discomfort may only be present on palpation, hence the diagnosis can be easily overlooked if the assessing clinician has not considered it in his/her differential.

Monteggia's fractures present as a painful deformed forearm following a fall onto a pronated outstretched arm or following a direct blow to the ulna. The injury to the proximal radioulna joint may equally be overlooked if one is distracted by the obvious painful deformity in the ulna.

Investigations

Anteroposterior and lateral radiographs of the forearm are essential. The elbow and distal radioulna joint must be included and the lateral in particular must be a true projection.

On the lateral view of the elbow a line drawn along the long axis of the radius should intersect the capitellum. If this is not the case then the radial head is dislocated (**Figure 33.2**). In paediatric fractures one must be particularly vigilant as the secondary ossification centres may not be apparent on radiographs making X-ray interpretation more challenging.

Ulna styloid fracture may be a radiological indication that the triangular fibrocartilage complex has been injured destabilising the DRUJ. Examination under anaesthesia with image intensification may be required to diagnose a dynamic instability of the DRUJ.

Classification

The Bado classification of Monteggia's fracture–dislocation describes the direction of displacement of the radial head. Type 1 is the most common and involves anterior dislocation, type 2 is posterior (**Figure 33.3**), type 3 lateral and type 4 involves a concurrent fracture of the proximal radius.

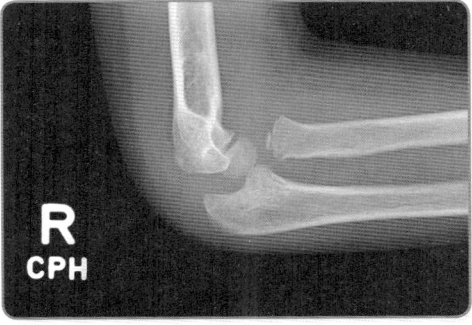

Figure 33.2 Lateral radiograph demonstrating at Bado type 1 Monteggia's fracture in a skeletally immature patient. Note that the radius does not line up with the capitellum.

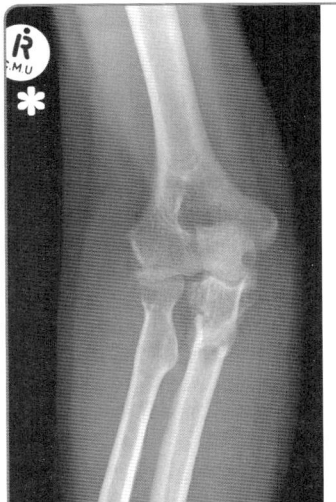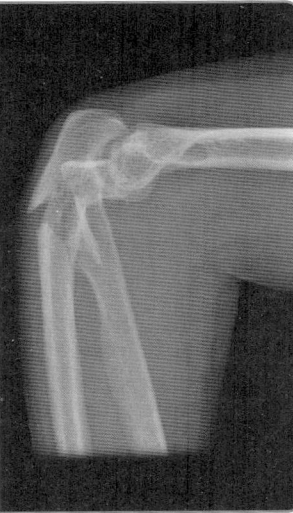

Figure 33.3 Lateral radiograph demonstrating a Bado type 2 Monteggia fracture in a skeletally mature patient.

Treatment

Nonoperative management of Galeazzi's fractures leads to severe functional compromise. Plaster cast immobilisation is insufficient to resist the deforming forces of the thumb extensors, pronator quadratus, brachioradialis and the weight of the hand. The consequent malalignment of the DRUJ compromises motion of the forearm and wrist.

Surgical management in the medically fit patient is therefore almost obligatory. Anatomic reduction and plate fixation of the radius is performed as for both bone forearm fractures (**Figure 33.4**). The approach and mode of fixation is dependent on the specific fracture location and configuration. Examination of the DRUJ is then performed. If instability persists then K-wire stabilisation in neutral rotation is required. Above elbow plaster cast is applied.

Failure to maintain anatomic reduction of the ulna in a Monteggia's injury will either prevent radial head relocation or lead to ongoing instability, both of which will compromise elbow and forearm mobility. Due to the thick periosteum surrounding paediatric bone, the ulna fracture in a skeletally immature Monteggia's fracture may be stable following closed reduction. The radial head will often simultaneously reduce and the fracture can be treated in an above elbow plaster cast. However in an adult maintenance of ulna reduction requires plate fixation. The radial head will reduce closed in 90% of cases and unless the radial head is completely stable at EUA plaster cast immobilisation is required to augment the fixation. If the radial head requires open reduction the decision to repair the annular ligament is controversial. Any increase in stability may lead to decreased range of movement.

Complications

Complications of Galeazzi's fractures occur as a consequence of failure to appreciate,

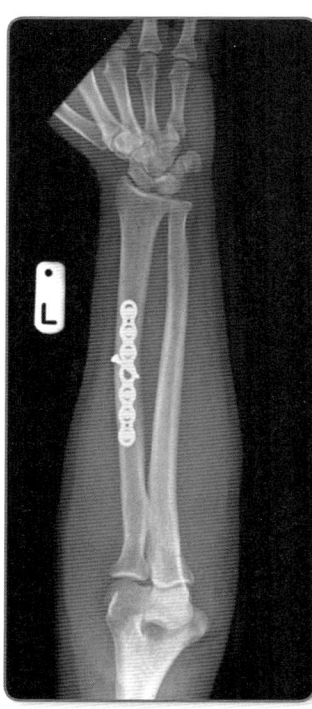

Figure 33.4 AP radiograph showing the postoperative appearance of a Galleazzi's fracture–dislocation. The radius has been fixed with a lag screw and compression plate.

appropriately reduce or maintain reduction of the DRUJ and the ensuing loss of mobility. Infection, neurovascular injury, nonunion, malunion and discomfort from the metal work may occur as a consequence of surgical treatment.

Nonunion and malunion may occur following surgical fixation of Monteggia's fractures. Accurate restoration of ulna length can be difficult in the comminuted fracture. Elbow movement is restricted by failure to relocate the radial head but is also seen in over-enthusiastic reconstruction of the annular ligament. Neurapraxia in particular of the posterior interosseus nerve may be seen. These should be managed expectantly in the main but nerve conduction studies and surgical exploration should be considered if no recovery is apparent by 2–3 months. Synostosis between radius and ulna can occur in high-energy fractures, particularly if there is concomitant head injury.

Further reading

Bulstrode C, Buchwalker J, Carr A, et al. Oxford: Oxford Textbook of Orthopaedics and Trauma. Oxford University Press; 2002.

Giannoulis FS, Sotereanos DG. Galeazzi fractures and dislocations. Hand Clin 2007; 23:153–163.

Kellam JF, Jupiter JF. Diaphyseal fractures of the forearm. In: Skeletal trauma, Browner BD, Jupiter JB, Levine AM, Trafton PG, (Eds). Philadelphia, PA: WB Saunders; 1992.

Rehim SA, Maynard MA, Sebastin SJ, Chung KC. Monteggia fracture–dislocations: a historical review J Hand Surg Am 2014; 39:1384–1394.

Related topics of interest

- *Topic 20* Elbow – radial head and neck fractures
- *Topic 34* Forearm – radius and ulna fractures
- *Topic 73* Paediatric forearm fractures

34 Forearm – radius and ulna fractures

Key points

- The radius and ulna have a precise anatomical relationship that allows pronation and supination of the forearm and the accurate positioning of the hand in space
- Multiple muscles insert on, or take their origin from, the radius and ulna. These deforming forces make controlling fractures in plaster almost impossible
- Open reduction with plate and screws leads to the optimal functional outcome

Epidemiology

Fractures of the radial and ulna diaphysis are relatively rare injuries in adulthood making up just 5% of upper limb fractures. Mechanism of injury is variable, the most common being a direct blow followed by a fall onto an outstretched hand. They frequently occur following high-energy injuries and predominantly effect young male patients.

Pathophysiology

The forearm serves to position the hand accurately in space. The laterally bowed radius rotates around the relatively straight ulna to allow pronation and supination. This precise bony anatomy and the five ligaments that link them in the interosseus membrane permit this complex multi-planar movement. It is for this reason that deformity in the adult forearm is so poorly tolerated. In fact the principles of treatment of an intra-articular fracture, namely anatomic reduction and absolute stability should be applied to the diaphyseal forearm fracture.

The pattern of fracture can be predicted from the mechanism of injury. A rotational force from a fall onto an outstretched hand produces a spiral pattern with fractures at different levels in each bone. An angular force will produce oblique or transverse fractures at the same level, while a transverse fracture of just one bone may occur following a direct blow.

Intrinsic deforming forces from the various muscle attachments occur in the forearm. The principle culprits are biceps and supinator in the upper one-third, pronator teres in the middle third and pronator quadratus and brachioradialis in the distal third.

Clinical features

Clinically apparent deformity is common and often quite distracting. The fracture is often highly mobile and abnormal motion may be seen or felt. The ratio of open to closed fractures is second only to that of the tibia hence the soft tissues must be closely inspected. Distal neurovascular status should be assessed and documented. Compartment syndrome may occur and requires prompt diagnosis and fasciotomy if severe disability is to be avoided.

Investigations

Anteroposterior (AP) and lateral radiographs can serve to diagnose the fracture and degree of displacement. Views of the wrist and elbow must be included. Pain and/or deformity may preclude true AP and lateral views in which case two orthogonal views should be acquired. Images will most commonly demonstrate fractures of both bones (**Figure 34.1**), either transverse at the same level or oblique at staggered levels depending on the deforming force. In the absence of a second fracture pay close attention to the proximal and distal radioulna joints (see **Chapter 33.4** for more details).

Displacement may occur in any plain and comminution may be present in proportion to the energy involved. Bone loss is not uncommon in open fractures.

Treatment

For skeletally mature patients, closed reduction and plaster cast stabilisation is

Forearm – radius and ulna fractures

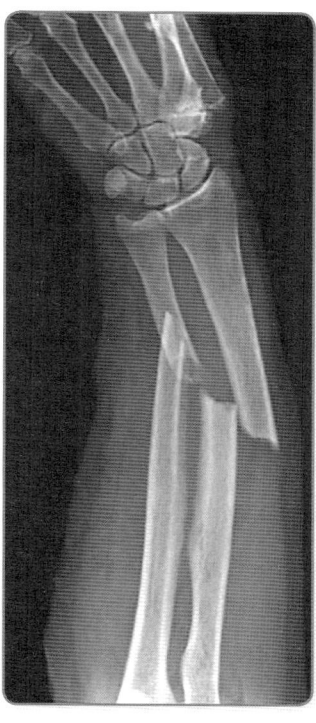

Figure 34.1 AP and lateral radiographs showing a both bone forearm fracture.

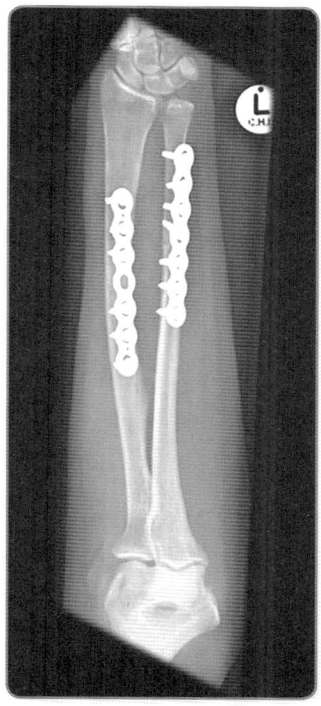

Figure 34.2 AP radiograph showing postoperative appearance of the fracture following open reduction and internal fixation with a compression plate.

almost universally unsuccessful. It may be attempted if the fracture is undisplaced, swelling minimal and the patient is prepared to accept a decreased range of movement. Loss of position in cast is all but inevitable and most surgeons would recommend early open reduction and internal fixation with either lag screw or dynamic plate compression (**Figure 34.2**). Bridging of comminuted fractures with locked plates may be required in multifragmentory fractures. If the construct is suitably stable early range of movement exercises may begin, if there is concern about stability then augmentation with a plaster splint is required. These fractures will take 8–12 weeks to heal in optimal conditions, in smokers, steroid users or in other compromised patients this may be significantly longer.

Intramedullary devices have been used to stabilise adult forearm fractures. The proposed benefit is of smaller incisions and less extensive dissection, however, the degree of fixation is compromised and as such this treatment is predominantly used in skeletally immature patients.

Open fractures should be treated with prompt antibiotics and temporary splintage with the limb straight. A thorough washout and debridement including inspection of the bone ends should be performed on the next available trauma list. If primary closure or immediate definitive cover is possible then the fracture may be internally fixed. If definitive coverage is to be delayed then external fixation should be employed either as a temporising measure or as definitive management.

Single bone forearm fractures are most commonly caused by raising the arm to protect the head, hence the term 'nightstick' injury. Isolated fracture of the radius is rare and in adults requires open reduction and internal fixation to counteract the rotational deforming forces applied to the bone (**Figures 34.3** and **34.4**). Isolated ulna fractures may be

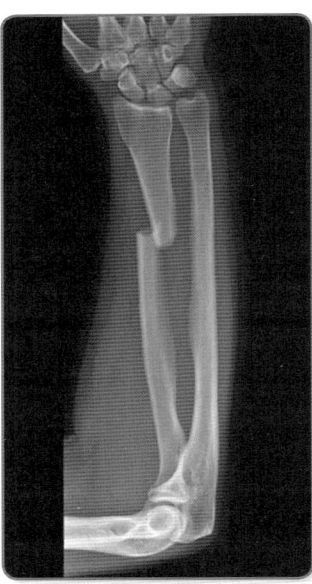

Figure 34.3 Isolated fracture of the radius caused by a kick from a horse.

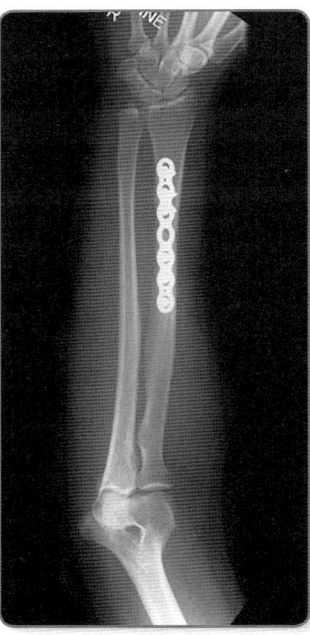

Figure 34.4 Isolated fracture of the radius caused by a kick from a horse-stabilised with a dynamic compression plate.

managed in a plaster splint if the alignment is acceptable, however, plate fixation may allow a faster return to function.

Complications
Early complications

- **Neurological injury** – this may occur at the time of injury or iatrogenically at the time of surgery. The posterior interosseus nerve is particularly at risk during exposure of the proximal radius
- **Vascular injury** – the dual blood supply of the hand from the radial and ulnar artery and an abundant collateral supply mean that direct arterial injury is rarely of significant consequence
- **Compartment syndrome** can occur in the forearm following fracture and surgery in any age group. The presence of an open injury does not exclude this condition. Be wary in particular of any patient who has had a difficult intramedullary nailing as significant trauma to the muscles can occur from multiple failed attempts to cross the fracture site

Late complications

- **Delayed union or nonunion** – patient factors such as smoking, steroid use and diabetes may delay union, as may local factors such as high-energy injury or open fracture. Mechanical factors such as implant selection and rigidity of fixation may contribute. Revision fixation with or without bone grafting may be required
- **Malunion** – as previously discussed the forearm relies on a complex anatomical relationship to allow movement. Small deformities can lead to significant disability. Furthermore, cross union may occur forming a synostosis between the two bones and a severe restriction in rotation. In the absence of synostosis corrective osteotomy may improve range of motion

Further reading

Burwell HN, Charnley AD. Treatment of forearm fractures in adults with particular reference to plate fixation. J Bone Joint Surg Br 1964; 46B:404–424.

Jones DB, Kakar S. Adult diaphyseal forearm fractures: intra-medullary nail versus plate fixation. J Hand Surg Am 2011; 36:1216–1219.

Smith DK, Cooney WP. External fixation of high-energy upper extremity injuries. J Orthop Trauma 1990; 4:7–18.

Related topics of interest

- Topic 33 Forearm – Galeazzi's and Monteggia's fractures
- Topic 53 Implants – plates
- Topic 73 Paediatric forearm fractures

35 Fracture healing

Key points
- Primary bone healing requires rigid fixation
- Secondary bone healing requires relative stability and results in progressive stiffening of callus prior to bony union

Primary bone healing

Primary bone healing requires absolute stability; a strain of <2%. The bone ends must also be closely apposed. There are two types: in contact healing, the bone ends are in contact and cutting cones cross between the two fragments in a process identical to the normal process of bony remodelling. In gap healing woven bone is laid down between the fracture ends transverse to the normal lamellae. Subsequently this two is remodelled. There is no callus formation.

Secondary bone healing

Secondary bone healing is, overall, a far more common mode of healing as, worldwide, very few fractures undergo rigid internal fixation. It is characterised by the production of callus. There are three main phases which overlap: inflammation, repair and remodelling.

The first stage involves a haematoma or inflammation. This peaks at 48 hours and resolves by 1 week. The injured tissues bleed, creating a haematoma. The haematoma forms a fibrin network, providing pathways for cell migration and, along with the damaged tissues and specifically platelets, releases cytokines. These stimulate cell migration, proliferation and differentiation. The chief cell types are neutrophils, macrophages and fibroblasts, and the chief factors released are IL-1, IL-6, BMPs, TNF-α, TGF-β, PDGF, FGF and IGF. The result is that granulation tissue replaces clots, and macrophages and osteoclasts begin to remove necrotic tissue, including ischaemia bone ends. The environment at this time is hypoxic and acidic, stimulating neutrophil and macrophage activity.

The second stage is repair or the formation of callus. This begins within the first few days before the inflammatory phase subsides. Callus stabilises the bony injury. There are two separate processes. Periosteal bony callus forms from pluripotent cells which differentiate directly into osteoblasts. It forms via intramembranous ossification; this phase normally only persists for the first 2 weeks postinjury. Fibrocartilaginous bridging callus (soft callus) forms in the periphery where there is lower oxygen tension. This undergoes endochondral ossification in a similar process to that observed in growth plates. Chondrocytes become hypertrophic then secrete proteoglycanases that degrade glycosoaminoglycans; high levels of which inhibit mineralisation. Chondrocytes and later osteoblasts secrete calcium phosphate complexes, further proteases and alkaline phosphatases which provide phosphate ions to precipitate with calcium. As the reparative phase continues the environment becomes first neutral and then alkaline promoting alkaline phosphatase activity and mineralisation of callus (medullary callus forms later and is important in delayed union if other mechanisms fail). If the fracture is unstable then type II collagen is formed first and later replaced by type I collagen.

Gradually, the calcified cartilage is reabsorbed. New vessels are formed, raising the oxygen tension locally. Osteoblasts follow the vessels laying down osteoid which then mineralises resulting in woven bone.

Differentiation of progenitor cells depends on local strain and oxygen tensions. If strain is very high, only granulation tissue can form. High strain promotes fibrous tissue, intermediate strain and low oxygen tension cartilage and low strain with high oxygen tension woven bone. Adequate blood supply is essential for fracture healing.

The final stage is remodelling which takes months to years. The process is the same as in primary bone healing. Cutting cones cross the woven bone. Osteoclasts reabsorb woven bone and osteoblasts lay down new lamellar bone. According to Wolff's law the bone resumes its normal configuration and shape; based on the stress to which it is exposed. The medullary cavity only reforms at completion of fracture healing.

Factors affecting bone healing

Local factors affecting fracture healing include the extent of soft tissue trauma: open fractures, associated neurovascular injury, soft tissue interposition and also bone loss, infection and neoplasia. The type of immobilisation will also affect bone healing.

Systemic factors affecting bone healing include smoking, nutrition especially protein intake and vitamin D levels, diabetes mellitus, age, steroids and head injury. A significant head injury stimulates abundant callus formation and bony union much before the expected time.

Young children heal much faster than adults. A general rule of thumb is 1 week to heal per year of age until age 6, after which it is 6 weeks, double if a lower limb fracture (and double again in smokers).

Immobilisation and bone healing

Cast treatment leads to secondary bone healing via either periosteal bridging callus or inter fragmentary enchondral ossification. Compression plates and other means of providing absolute stability should lead to primary bone healing. External fixators may give either healing as in casts or, if more rigid, primary bone healing. Intramedullary devices tend to give relative stability and so heal with secondary bone healing. Early on this is via either periosteal bridging callus and enchondral ossification; later through medullary callus and intramembranous ossification. It is important to respect the soft tissues. Although stabilisation methods improve position and therefore function of bony injuries the fracture generally heals despite the operation; not because of it.

Delayed or nonunion

Fracture nonunion is one that lacks potential to heal without further intervention. A minimum of double the expected healing time should have elapsed. The US FDA definition is 9 months elapsed time with no progress on serial radiographs over 3 months.

Check vitamin D levels and attempt to improve modifiable risk factors such as smoking.

If immobilisation is inadequate then this can lead to hypertrophic nonunion when blood supply is adequate. In this instance type II collagen predominates. If blood supply is inadequate then atrophic nonunion may result.

Further reading

Giannoudis PV, Einhorn TA, Marsh D. Fracture healing: the diamond concept. Injury 2007; 38:S3–S6.

Related topics of interest

- *Topic 9* Bone structure and physiology
- *Topic 67* Nonunion of fractures

36 Geriatric patients – perioperative management of hip fractures

Key points
- Hip fractures are associated with significant mortality and morbidity
- The National Hip Fracture Database aims to improve the quality and reduce national variability of care
- There is a best practice tariff attached to the management of patients admitted with hip fracture
- The perioperative management of hip fractures requires a multi-disciplinary approach
- Perioperative complications are common and without careful management there is an impact on length of stay, discharge destination, morbidity and mortality

Introduction

Hip fractures are common. Over 300,000 patients attend hospitals in the UK with fragility fractures and around a quarter of those have a fractured neck of femur. Fragility fractures are associated with a significant mortality and morbidity. The mortality at 30 days is 10% and this rises to 30% at 1 year. Hip fractures account for 4000 inpatient beds at any one time and the annual total cost to the NHS is over £2 billion pounds.

Evidence suggests that prompt, effective, multidisciplinary management can improve the quality of care and at the same time reduce costs. Accordingly, over the last 20 years, there has been an evolution of hip fracture care in countries such as the UK, making them leaders in the treatment of these injuries. What is written in this chapter reflects the standards of care delivered in the UK, standards that can be applied in any country or system.

Rigorous attention to formalised standards of perioperative care is required to achieve this.

The Blue Book and the National Hip Fracture Database

The Blue Book was published in 2007 by the British Orthopaedic Association in collaboration with the British Geriatrics Society and it summarised the evidence base for the perioperative management of hip fracture patients. Along with the National Hip Fracture Database (NHFD) it aimed to reduce the variation in the quality and cost-effectiveness of hip fracture care. The NHFD is a web-based, clinically-led audit of hip fracture care and secondary prevention. All 180 hospitals in England, Wales and Northern Ireland upload data on all their hip fracture admissions.

The Blue Book describes six standards of care and these reflect good practice at key stages of hip fracture care. The rationale for each standard is set out in *The Blue Book* and compliance is continuously monitored by participation in the NHFD.

1. All patients with hip fracture should be admitted to an acute orthopaedic ward within 4 hours of presentation.
2. All patients with hip fracture who are medically fit should have surgery within 48 hours of admission, and during normal working hours.
3. All patients with hip fracture should be assessed and cared for with a view to minimising their risk of developing a pressure ulcer.
4. All patients presenting with a fragility fracture should be managed on an orthopaedic ward with routine access to

acute orthogeriatric medical support from time of admission.
5. All patients presenting with fragility fracture should be assessed to determine their need for antiresorptive therapy to prevent future osteoporotic fractures.
6. All patients presenting with a fragility fracture following a fall should be offered multidisciplinary assessment and intervention to prevent future falls.

Best practice tariff

The best practice tariff (BPT) is a national tariff that offers a financial incentive to provide good quality cost-effective care. The BPT for fragility hip fractures was developed to encourage two key clinical characteristics of best practice: prompt surgery and appropriate involvement of geriatric medicine. There are currently seven criteria that need to be met for each patient for a hospital to earn the best practice tariff.

Best practice tariff criteria:
- The time to surgery is within 36 hours from arrival in an emergency department, or time of diagnosis as an inpatient, to the start of anaesthesia
- Admitted under the joint care of a consultant geriatrician and a consultant orthopaedic surgeon
- Admitted using an assessment protocol agreed by geriatric medicine, orthopaedic surgery and anaesthetist
- Assessed by a geriatrician in the preoperative period: within 72 hours of admission.
- Postoperative geriatrician-directed multi-professional rehabilitation team
- Fracture prevention assessments (falls and bone health)
- Two abbreviated mental tests scores to be performed. The first prior to surgery and the second postsurgery within the same spell

Preoperative care

Patients admitted with fragility fractures often have multiple co-morbidities and use numerous different medications. Therefore, as a high-risk group of patients, they should be assessed by an experienced anaesthetist and orthogeriatrician prior to surgery. Although assessment is a clinical priority it should not delay surgery. The evidence for improved outcomes with early surgery is inconsistent; however, there is evidence that it reduces length of stay, reduces the duration of pain and reduces the time spent heavily dependent.

Infection risk

The use of antibiotic prophylaxis significantly reduces the risk of superficial and deep wound infection following hip fracture repair. The development of a deep wound infection has a mortality of up to 50%.

Anaemia

Up to 40% of hip fracture patients have anaemia on admission; this is likely to be a reflection of their frailty and high co-morbid burden. Preoperative anaemia is an independent risk factor for death and readmission within 60 days. There is often a significant drop in haemaglobin following surgery, however higher postoperative haemoglobin measurements are associated with a shorter length of stay.

Postoperative care

Pain relief

Good postoperative analgesia is a vital part of management. Adequate pain relief encourages early mobilisation and reduces all the risks associated with prolonged bed rest. It also significantly decreases the risk of delirium and cardiovascular, respiratory and gastrointestinal morbidity. The use of peripheral nerve blocks reduce the opiate requirements, however evidence has not shown clear clinical benefits derived from this.

Fluid and electrolytes

A Cochrane review in 2016 concluded that there is no evidence that perioperative fluid volume optimisation strategies have an impact on outcomes for patients with a hip fracture. However problems with fluid and electrolyte balance are common in this group of patients. High-risk patients should be highlighted preoperatively and careful monitoring commenced following surgery.

Frail, elderly patients frequently develop a temporary hyponatraemia in the perioperative period. This occurs for a number of reasons, including:
- A delayed excretion to a water load (pre- intra- and postoperative intravenous fluids)
- A blunted renin response in the elderly. Renin is stimulated in response to hypotension, sympathetic stimulation and hyponatraemia and leads to increased water and sodium reabsorption. In the elderly this response is blunted leading to renal sodium loss in the perioperative period
- Syndrome of inappropriate antidiuretic hormone (SIADH). Common causes of SIADH include surgery, pain and opiates

Thromboprophylaxis

There is a high-risk of venous thrombo-embolism following hip fracture. There is evidence that both mechanical and pharmacological prophylaxis can reduce the risk (the use of both is what the current NICE guidance recommends, unless there are specific contraindications). Mechanical prophylaxis (intermittent pneumatic compression devices, antiembolism stockings or foot impulse devices) should continue until there is no significant reduction in mobility and pharmacological prophylaxis (fondaparinux, low molecular weight heparin or unfractionated heparin) should be continued for 28–35 days following surgery, depending on the agent used.

Delirium

Delirium is a complex neuropsychiatric syndrome with an acute onset and fluctuating course. It is common in all medical settings occurring in 15–20% of all general admissions to hospital, with a higher frequency in the elderly and those with pre-existing cognitive impairment. The risk is significantly higher in patients admitted with a hip fracture with 16–62% developing an acute state of confusion. It is associated with a prolonged length of stay, has a negative impact on the outcomes of rehabilitation, an increased number are discharged to placement and there is an increased mortality. Careful management and monitoring of pain control, oxygen saturations, blood pressure, signs of sepsis, bowel and bladder care, nutrition and medication will prevent some individuals developing delirium and will decrease the severity an episode of delirium.

Nutrition

A poor nutritional state is in itself a risk factor for hip fracture. Therefore, a significant proportion of hip fracture patients are malnourished prior to their fracture. In addition to this, hip fracture patients often receive only half their daily nutritional requirement while they are inpatients. It is therefore vital that there is a multi-disciplinary approach to maintaining good nutrition. Evidence suggests that although the use of oral supplement drinks does not have an impact on mortality it does lead to a decrease in long-term complications and reduces length of stay in rehabilitation. The use of nasogastric feeding in the severely malnourished may reduce length of stay in hospital.

Pressure care

Up to one-third of hip fracture patients will develop a pressure ulcer, many of which are preventable. There are a number of factors involved in the development of pressure ulcers, these include: time spent on the floor at home following the fall; time spent on a trolley in emergency department; the use of nonpressure relieving mattresses on the ward; prolonged theatre time; poor nutrition; anaemia and failure to mobilise following surgery.

Summary

The perioperative management of elderly patients with hip fracture needs a multidisciplinary approach and there are a number challenges specific to this condition. In the UK, the aim of the Blue Book, the NHFD, BOAST standards of care and NICE guidance is to highlight these challenges, encourage multidisciplinary service development and ultimately improve care for this cohort of patients. Countries around the world are copying this model.

Further reading

British Orthopaedic Association (BOA). Standards for trauma. BOAST 1 version 2. London: BOA, 2012.

Darowski A. The care of patients with fragility fracture. In: The Blue Book. London: British Orthopaedic Association, 2007.

Scottish Intercollegiate Guidelines Network (SIGN). Management of hip fracture in older people. Guideline 111. Edinburgh: SIGN, 2009.

Related topics of interest

- *Topic 69* Osteoporosis

37 Guidelines in trauma

Key points
- Guidelines do not substitute for clinical knowledge but should be taken into account, along with the patient's condition, when making decisions
- Guidelines are updated often; clinicians and surgeons should keep abreast of updates

Introduction

Clinicians should fully understand the guidelines which relate to their work and consider them carefully when managing patients. Guidelines do not replace clinical judgment, however, and patients should be involved in the decision-making process. It would be impossible to summarise the world's major evidence-based guidelines in a single chapter. Instead, this chapter outlines the key points of the UK guidelines most relevant to management of trauma patients, illustrating the breadth of topics on which guidance is especially helpful. Unless stated otherwise, the guidelines described here are for the treatment of all patients.

In orthopaedic trauma, UK guidelines are principally produced by two organisations: the National Institute for Care and Health Excellence (NICE) and British Orthopaedic Association (BOA). NICE guidelines are based on clinical evidence and take into account NHS funding constraints. NICE is accountable to the Department of Health, which selects topics for consideration and production of guidelines (accordingly, NHS England is legally obliged to provide funding for treatments recommended in NICE guidelines). The BOA's evidence-based guidelines supporting the management of injured patients are known known as the BOA Standards for Trauma (BOAST) guidelines.

Guidelines for surgical treatment

Transfusion in adults and children >1 year old (NICE, NG24, 2015)

Correction of coagulopathy
- Prothrombin complex should be used to reverse warfarin in trauma patients with severe bleeding or suspected intracerebral haemorrhage, or in those on warfarin who require emergency surgery, if there is significant bleeding risk
- Platelet transfusion should be considered if:
  - Platelets $<100 \times 10^9/L$ and severe bleeding/intracranial bleeding
  - Platelets $<50 \times 10^9/L$ in patients who are to undergo surgery (can use higher threshold if high blood loss expected)
  - Platelets $<30 \times 10^9/L$ and clinically significant bleeding

Minimise transfusion requirements
- Tranexamic acid should be offered to adults undergoing surgery with expected blood loss of >500 mL
- If very high blood loss is expected then intraoperative cell salvage should be considered
- Patients with iron deficiency anaemia should be offered iron supplementation pre- and postoperatively.

When transfusion is appropriate
- A threshold haemoglobin level for transfusion of 70 g/L is appropriate for healthy adults without ongoing bleeding. The target haemoglobin level post-transfusion in these patients is 70–90 g/L

- If there is no ongoing bleeding single unit transfusions should be considered. Reassess requirement after each unit
- Explain and provide written information for patients undergoing transfusion or their relatives, including the reasons for transfusion, risks, benefits and consequences of transfusion, giving the opportunity for questions

Fragility fracture of the hip in adults (BOAST 1, 2012)

- Fractures caused by other bone pathology or high-energy trauma do not fall under this guideline

Initial management

- Perform surgery either on the day of admission or the following day. Achieve this by early recognition and treatment of comorbidities, providing care on a dedicated orthopaedic or orthogeriatric ward with orthogeriatric input and scheduling surgery on a dedicated trauma list.
- Patients who cannot weight bear after a fall but have no fracture demonstrated on anteroposterior and lateral X-rays should be offered an MRI. If this is not possible within 24 hours then fine slice CT scan should be considered.

Surgical management

- Aim to allow full weight-bearing mobilisation postoperatively
- Displaced intracapsular fractures should be treated with hemi- or total joint arthroplasty, using a cemented femoral stem of a proven design. Total hip replacement should be offered to patients with displaced intracapsular fracture if the individual has no cognitive impairment and was able to walk outside independently, or with the use of a single stick prior to the injury, if they are medically fit for the procedure
- Extracapsular fractures falling into AO classes A1 and A2 should be treated using an extramedullary device such as the dynamic hip screw
- Subtrochanteric fractures should be fixed using an intramedullary nail

Postoperative management

- Postoperatively patients should be given the opportunity to mobilise at least daily and receive ongoing orthogeriatric input, with attention to falls prevention and bone health

Severe open lower limb fractures sustained by high-energy trauma (BOAST 4, 2009)

Initial management

- Neurovascular status should be assessed
- Intravenous coamoxiclav, cefuroxime or clindamycin is started within 3 hours of the injury and continued until wound closure or for 72 hours (whichever is sooner)
- Gross contamination is removed from the wound and it is photographed prior to dressing in saline soaked gauze
- The limb is splinted

Surgical management

- Immediate surgery is indicated for vascular compromise, compartment syndrome, polytrauma patients and if there is contamination with sewage, marine, agricultural matter
- Debridement and initial stabilisation should take place on a scheduled trauma list within 24 hours, with combined orthopaedic and plastic surgery input. Antibiotic bead pouch or a vacuum dressing should be used temporarily to cover the wound
- Definitive fixation and coverage of the wound should take place within 72 hours if possible, otherwise within 7 days

The management of traumatic spinal cord injury (BOAST 8, 2014)

- Patients with a spinal injury should have full examination of the peripheral nervous system, recorded on an American Spinal Injury Association chart available at www.asia-spinalinjury.org
- All units receiving trauma should have a linked Spinal Cord Injury Centre with

agreed common protocols for protecting the spine, anaesthesia, nursing, etc. When injuries are not covered by written protocols the on call consultant at the Spinal Cord Injury Centre should be informed within 4 hours of the injury and a management plan be formulated within 12 hours

Displaced supracondylar fracture of the distal humerus in children (BOAST 11, 2014)

Initial management
- On admission, full assessment of vascular status and each nerve should be recorded
- If there is threat to the skin or the perfusion of the hand then emergency surgery should be performed. Otherwise early surgery should take place, ideally on the day of admission, but avoiding overnight surgery

Surgical management
- Kirschner wires should be 2 mm in diameter where possible, and cross two cortices. Either divergent lateral or crossed wire configuration should be used, with efforts taken to avoid injury to the ulnar nerve recorded on the operation note

Postoperative management
- Postoperative monitoring for signs of compartment syndrome or vascular compromise should be performed until the risk has passed
- Fracture position should be checked on X-rays between 4–10 days, and wire removal undertaken at 3–4 weeks
- Monitoring for neurovascular compromise should continue until risk is passed
- A limb that is ischaemic after fracture reduction requires exploration by a surgeon who can perform reperfusion surgery if required. Expectant management is appropriate for a perfused limb without a radial pulse after the fracture has been reduced and also with nerve injuries associated with the initial fracture. Iatrogenic nerve injuries may require exploration

Peripheral nerve injury (BOAST 5, 2012)

Initial management
- The neurovascular status should be assessed and documented for all injuries, on presentation and after any intervention
- If a nerve injury is suspected the case should be discussed on an urgent basis, with a consultant who is skilled in managing nerve injuries. Any underlying unstable skeletal injury should be reduced and fixed on an urgent basis

Surgical management
- During surgery the nerve is usually explored (exceptions being axillary nerve injury following low energy shoulder trauma and lumbosacral plexus injury managed by sacroiliac screws). Intraoperative findings should be documented including the position of the nerve relative to any metalwork
- If a nerve is transected, repair should be performed on an urgent basis. If no surgeon who is experienced in nerve repair is available, the ends of the nerve should be gently tacked together using a fine-coloured suture

Arterial injuries associated with fractures and dislocations to the limbs (BOAST 6, 2014)

Initial management
- Limb injuries are assessed after immediately life-threatening injuries have been managed. Neurovascular status of the limbs should be recorded and active bleeding controlled with direct pressure or tourniquet

Surgical management
- Dislocations and grossly displaced fractures be reduced and splinted and neurovascular status reassessed
- If circulation is not restored with realigning fractures then exploration and reperfusion surgery should take place as

an emergency. Angiography should not be performed if it will significantly delay surgery
- A high index of suspicion for compartment syndrome should be held after reperfusion

Guidelines for fracture clinic services

Fracture clinic services (BOAST 7, 2014)

- Patients with acute orthopaedic trauma should be reviewed in consultant-led new fracture clinics, within 72 hours. Junior staff and extended scope practitioners should be supervised
- The management plan should be communicated to the patient and their general practitioner in writing. There should also be written information available to the patient covering common injuries, plaster cast and slings
- It should be possible to refer patients to physiotherapy, occupational therapy, falls prevention and fragility fracture services from clinic as appropriate
- Further imaging and operative intervention should be offered within a timescale that will not compromise outcome
- Rapid access back to clinic should be facilitated for patients with problems related to their initial injury

Fracture liaison services for patients age 50 years and over with fragility fracture (BOAST 9, 2014)

- All patients aged 50 years and over who present with a fragility fracture should enter a pathway to access a fracture liaison service should be offered written information about fragility fractures and bone health
- They should also receive a bone health assessment, including DEXA scanning where appropriate, within 3 months of the fracture

Falls in people aged >65 years: assessing risk and prevention (NICE, CG161, 2013)

Secondary prevention of falls

- Adults aged >65 years who present following a fall should be offered a risk assessment
- Risk factors should be mitigated where possible, e.g. by working on strength and balance, reviewing medications and making the home environment safer

Diagnosis and management of compartment syndrome of the limbs (BOAST 10 2014)

Assessment

- Compartment syndrome should be considered in all patients with significant limb injury and those who have undergone surgery that could lead to compartment syndrome
- Regional anaesthesia and patient controlled intravenous opiate analgesia can mask the diagnosis of compartment syndrome; the effect of such analgesia should be taken into account during assessment and the usage avoided in high-risk patients
- Where clinical signs are not diagnostic compartment pressure should be measured; Delta pressure (diastolic-compartment pressure) of <30 mmHg or absolute pressure of >40 mmHg are indications for decompression

Management

- Release of all circumferential dressings should be performed and the limb elevated to the level of the heart. If this does not relieve symptoms within 30 minutes surgery should be undertaken
- Fasciotomies should take place within 1 hour of the decision to operate with decompression of all affected compartments and excision of necrotic muscle tissue
- If diagnosis is made >12 hours after the onset of compartment syndrome nonoperative treatment may be appropriate; management decisions should be made by two consultants.

Child maltreatment: when to suspect maltreatment in under 16s (NICE, CG89, 2009)

Seeking information from multiple sources
- Listen to the history and seek to understand the explanation given by both the child and the parent, fully recording what is said. Discuss concerns with a senior or designated colleague for child protection, and gain collateral history from other healthcare professionals and agencies

Suspect abuse if physical injuries are not easily explained
- If the injury pattern or shape is not explained by the history
- If the location of the injury is not explained. For example, bruising on a non-bony body part or an abrasion in a place that is normally protected by clothing
- If injuries are incompatible with the developmental age of the child; including injuries to non-ambulant infants

Recognise signs of neglect
- Suspect neglect if the needs of a child appear not to be met, including personal hygiene and nutrition. This also includes appropriate supervision and accessing health services

Behavioural and emotional changes
- Maltreatment is possible if the emotional responses or behavior of a child are not appropriate for their age and situation. This also includes their interactions with parents and healthcare professionals

Summary

This is not a comprehensive list of UK guidelines. It is recommended that the full NICE online guidelines are consulted for more in-depth information on the above topics, and also for guidance on related topics such as acute kidney injury, head injury, delirium, surgical site infection and venous thromboembolism. NICE also produces evidence summaries, reviewing the evidence to support the off-label (unlicensed) use of various medications, e.g. the use of tranexamic acid in major trauma. These can be found online. At the time of writing, five further NICE guidelines relating to the management of major trauma, fractures and spinal injuries were in development.

Further reading

British Orthopaedic Association Standards for Trauma (BOAST). BOAST 7: Fracture Clinic Services. London: BOAST, 2013.
British Orthopaedic Association Standards for Trauma (BOAST). BOAST 9: Fracture Liaison Services. London: BOAST, 2014.
British Orthopaedic Association Standards for Trauma (BOAST). BOAST 10: Diagnosis and Management of Compartment Syndrome of the limbs. London: BOAST, 2014.
National Institute for Health and Care Excellence (NICE). Transfusion (CG 24). London: NICE, 2015.
National Institute for Health and Care Excellence (NICE). Falls in Older People: Assessing Risk and Prevention (CG 161). London: NICE, 2013.
National Institute for Health and Care Excellence (NICE). When to Suspect Child Maltreatment (CG 89). London: NICE, 2009.

Related topics of interest

- *Topic 62* Major trauma – Advanced Trauma and Life Support principles
- *Topic 100* Trauma outcome scores: using patient-reported outcome measures

38 Gunshot injuries

Key points
- Patients with gunshot injuries are managed in accordance with Advanced Trauma Life Support (ATLS) principles
- Carefully document distal neurovascular status
- Intra-articular or intracerebral fragments may require removal

Ballistics

Gunshot wounds are divided into:
- low velocity (<600 m/s muzzle velocity) and
- high velocity (>600 m/s).

Shotgun injuries are generally considered separately.

The passage of missiles through tissue results in cavitation. The permanent cavity is formed directly by the crushing and cutting effects of the passage of the presented portion of the missile through the tissue. When a bullet travels at high velocity a shockwave forms, resulting in the formation of a further temporary cavity due to transient lateral displacement of tissue. The permanent wound tract is compromised of the permanent central wound cavity in conjunction with a lateral zone of macroscopic tissue damage caused by radial tissue displacement from the temporary cavity. There is no evidence of further permanent damage outside the macroscopic area of tissue damage due to the formation of the temporary cavity.

Tissue damage

The wounding potential of a gunshot wound depends on the energy transfer to the tissues. This is a function of several factors which include the kinetic energy of the missile, the tissue density and the behaviour of the missile once it enters the tissues. In general penetrating missiles do more damage than perforating missiles. A missile that enters the leg and strikes the femur, fracturing it and not leaving the leg, thus transferring all the kinetic energy, will, overall, do more damage than one, travelling at the same speed, that travels through muscle only and exits the leg still possessing a proportion of its initial kinetic energy. Missiles do not necessarily follow predictable paths between entry and exit points as tissue density changes may result in a change of direction.

At short range, shotguns can produce a devastating amount of tissue damage; but this force is dissipated at longer ranges due to the spread of pellets. The wadding also enters the sound cavity at short range. This incites an intensive inflammatory reaction and should be removed.

Immediate management

The presence of a bullet wound should not detract from following the principles of ATLS management. The patient may have been exposed to multiple mechanisms of injury. Specific management depends on the area of injury. Give prophylactic antibiotics in accordance with local guidelines and ensure that tetanus status is up-to-date. Tourniquets may be required for initial control of catastrophic haemorrhage but worsen tissue damage and lead to further limb ischaemia. Apply the tourniquet as distally as is consistent with haemorrhage control. Prehospital tourniquets such as the Combat Application Tourniquet are less well tolerated than the standard pneumatic tourniquets available in theatre.

Nerve and vessel injury

There should be a high index of suspicion for nerve and vessel injury in a gunshot wound and distal neurovascular status should be carefully documented. Neuropraxia due to temporary cavitation is not uncommon. Missile injuries may result in pseudoaneurysm formation or arteriovenous fistula formation.

Spinal injuries

If a fragment has lodged in a vertebral body having passed through bowel this may be treated with antibiotics only. Cases with a progressive neurological deficit should be decompressed. Complete cord injury has a poor prognosis; cases involving the cauda equina alone may have a better outcome. If a projectile is retained in the spinal canal re-imaging should be considered prior to operation as there are reports of movement of fragments.

Operative management

Operative management depends on the nature of the injury. All wounds should be cleaned and debrided; delayed primary closure with a second look at 2–3 days postinjury is generally advocated.

In the presence of neurovascular injury or massive soft tissue destruction then external fixation is generally used to provide temporary stability prior to a more definitive procedure. Primary internal fixation may be appropriate in low velocity wounds without extensive tissue damage or vascular compromise. Those injuries may be treated as Gustillo–Anderson grade I open fractures although the entry and exit wounds should not be closed primarily. All high-velocity wounds associated with bony injury are, by definition, Grade III injuries due to the potentially contaminated nature the injury and the soft tissue damage associated.

Debridement

Wound extension should be by means of longitudinal incisions; where possible in the line of potential fasciotomies. Take a methodical approach to debridement either inside out or outside in removing all dead and devitalised tissue as leaving this increases the risk of deep infection – a feared complication of any open fracture – both through providing bacterial culture medium and by impairment of the host immune response. Bone fragments without adequate soft tissue attachments, that fail the 'tug test', should be removed; any resulting bony defect can be addressed at a later stage. Devitalised tissue can be recognised through the 4 Cs – colour, consistency, contractility and capillary bleeding. Foreign matter may also be drawn or propelled into the cavity and should of course be removed. The bullet tract does not need to be laid open.

Removal of fragments

Removal of fragments can be a satisfying procedure. However, the surgeon should be aware of the need to avoid additional tissue damage. Most retained fragments are well tolerated by the patient and do not need routine removal. However, both cerebrospinal fluid and synovial fluid are corrosive to bullet fragments and can result in synovitis or high lead levels if left in contact for extended periods of time; therefore, intra-articular fragments should be removed.

Further reading

Jordan DJ, Malahias M, Khan W, Hindocha S. The ortho-plastic approach to soft tissue management in trauma. Open Orthop J 2014; 8:399–408.

Stapley SA, Cannon LB. an overview of the pathophysiology of gunshot and blast injury with resuscitation guideline. Current Orthopaedics 2006; 20:322–332.

Sidhu GS, Ghag A, Prokuski V, Vaccaro AR, Radcliff KE. Civilian gunshot injuries of the spinal cord: a systematic review of the current literature. Clin Orthop Relat Res 2013; 471:3945–3955.

Related topics of interest

- *Topic 1* Amputations – mangled extremities and decision making
- *Topic 17* Damage control orthopaedics and trauma physiology
- *Topic 68* Open fractures

39 Hand and wrist – carpal dislocations

Key points
- Carpal dislocations are frequently missed – up to 25%
- Prognosis is dependent on early recognition and surgical treatment
- The defining feature is dislocation of the capitate head from the lunate concavity

Epidemiology
Difficult to establish incidence and prevalence, as this is a rare injury but perilunate injuries comprise 10% of wrist injuries.

Pathophysiology
Mayfield originally described the potential mechanism and the four stages of perilunate dislocation in 1980. The defining feature is dislocation of the capitate head from the lunate concavity. The most common mechanism for this injury is a fall onto the outstretched hand landing on the thenar eminence/radial side producing a supination moment in the wrist. The injury begins on the radial side of the wrist as it supinates progressing round the lunate to the ulnar side. In a fall landing on the hypothenar eminence first, such as with the hand behind you, the sequence is reversed due to the pronation forces on the wrist. The ligamentous and/or bony structures surrounding the lunate sequentially fail as the load and duration increases. The force can pass through bones and ligaments causing a perilunate fracture-dislocation, along the lines of the 'greater arc' or the injury can be purely ligamentous through the 'lesser arc' (**Figure 39.1**).

The most common pattern is a transscaphoid perilunate fracture dislocation (with a middle third scaphoid fracture) but trans-(radial) styloid, transcapitate, transhamate and transtriquetral injuries can also be seen. The structures that are

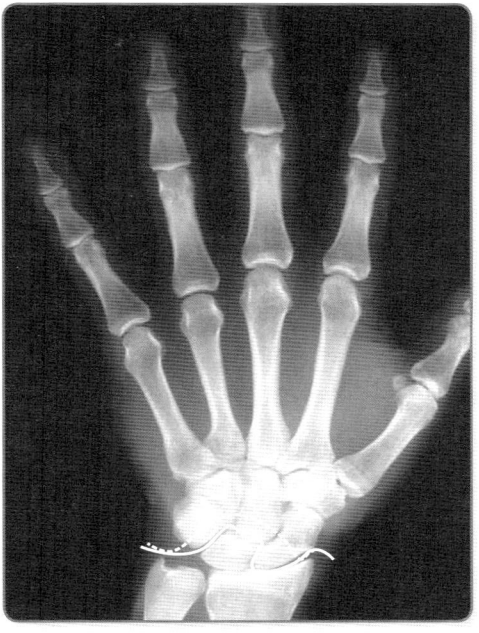

Figure 39.1 Greater (dotted line) and lesser arcs (smooth line).

sequentially injured in a typical supination injury are as follows: scaphoid bone or scapholunate (SL) and radioscapholunate ligaments (Mayfield stage 1), midcarpal disruption with radioscaphocapitate ligament rupture or capitate fracture (Mayfield stage 2), lunotriquetral (LT) ligament (Mayfield stage 3).

There are two main types of dislocation. They describe the direction of force generating the injury.
- The most common is a dorsal dislocation where an extended wrist forces the capitate and the entire distal row dorsally. The capitate dislocates from the lunate concavity and remains dorsal to the lunate or it can reduce into the lunate fossa thereby dislocating the lunate volarly through the space of Poirier. This is a potential weak spot in the volar capsular ligaments between the

proximal radiolunate ligaments and the distal arcuate ligament. This is a lunate dislocation or Mayfield stage 4
- If a volarly directed force is applied, the wrist flexes and the distal carpal row dislocates volarly. This injury is much less common. As the deforming force is removed the distal carpal row forces the lunate dorsally either into an extended position or the lunate can dislocate dorsally with the capitate coming to rest in the lunate fossa

The majority of patients have sustained high-energy injuries and a thorough ATLS search for other injuries must be performed. Up to 26% of patients will have other significant injuries and 11% will have ipsilateral upper limb injuries.

Axial dislocations are much less common. The force is directed through either the radial or ulnar side of the carpus, rupturing intercarpal ligaments in a longitudinal direction. Normally one or two metacarpals remain attached to the distal row carpal bones that are dislocated. This injury represents another form of high-energy injury and there is often associated soft tissue disruption. Beware of compartment syndrome in patients with axial dislocations.

Clinical features

These are devastating injuries and the history has a very significant role to play in diagnosing these injuries. Early identification and surgical management is one of the best prognostic indicators of future function. The assessing clinician must have a high index of suspicion as perilunate dislocations are often missed due to distractions of other more life-threatening injuries.

Swelling is usually pronounced. Tenderness is widespread but may be localised to an area just distal to Lister's tubercle, representing the radiocarpal joint. The capitate may be felt as a hard lump subcutaneously in this area or the lunate may be felt volarly as fullness in the carpal tunnel. The neurovascular status of the hand must be assessed and documented at regular intervals, as the median nerve is very vulnerable particularly if the lunate is dislocated volarly into the carpal tunnel.

Investigations

A perilunate dislocation is a surgical emergency and there is no role for nonoperative management of the ligament and bony injuries. Standard posteroanterior (PA), 45° pronated oblique and lateral radiographs are essential and should be obtained without delay. The PA radiograph can often be misinterpreted as normal as the displacement of the carpus is in the plane of the X-rays. There may be some overlap of the adjacent carpal bones such as the capitate and scaphoid. On a well-aligned PA radiograph this is always a significant finding. Gilula's lines are very useful in this regard and should be traced carefully (**Figure 39.2**).

The lateral radiograph is the most informative. Being familiar with some simple alignment angles on a lateral radiograph helps spot displacement of the carpal bones. Firstly identify the lunate. If the wrist is in neutral flexion/extension the concavity of the lunate should be pointing distally towards the metacarpals and most importantly should be full of capitate. The capitate should be aligned

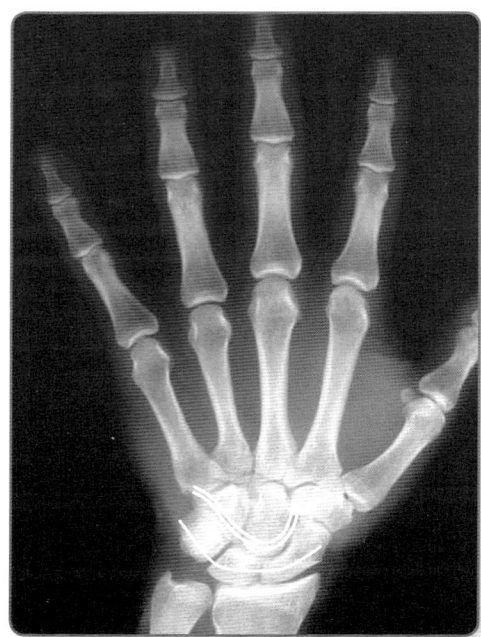

Figure 39.2 Gilula's lines.

(+/- 15°) with the lunate and the distal radius. The orientation of the scaphoid and the lunate is more difficult to plot on the lateral view. If you draw a line along the long axis of the scaphoid and another line perpendicular to the concavity of the lunate (like a mast in a boat), the angle should be between 30–60°. If it is more than 70° there has been a disruption of the SL ligament and perilunate disruption is likely. Excessive flexion of the scaphoid may be evident as a scaphoid ring sign where the distal scaphoid is so flexed that on a PA the distal half of the bone is seen end on with a circular outline of cortex looking like a circle or ring.

CT scan and MRI are usually unnecessary but may delineate any suspected fractures elsewhere in the hand.

Diagnosis

The diagnosis is made clinically and radiographically as above.

Treatment

As alluded to above, these injuries are a surgical emergency. Orthopaedic surgeons familiar with the treatment of perilunate dislocations should be responsible for attempting reduction in the emergency department. This can be performed under sedation, regional or general anaesthesia. If initial attempts are unsuccessful or if median nerve symptoms are present, the clinician should have a low threshold for transferring the patient to the operating theatre, with fluoroscopy available. A carpal tunnel decompression should be performed expediently if neurological compromise is evident or suspected, even if definitive fixation is not performed at this visit to theatre.

Traction should be applied for 5–10 minutes before reduction is attempted. If the carpus is dorsally dislocated, extend the wrist maintaining some traction, place a thumb over the volar aspect of the lunate to stabilise it and apply a volarly directed force on the dorsum of the wrist to engage the head of the capitate on the dorsal rim of the lunate. Further volar pressure on the lunate and traction of the hand should reduce the capitate back into the lunate concavity. Only then can the wrist be returned to neutral. True lunate dislocations are best-reduced open in theatre from the volar and dorsal sides.

These injuries are often highly unstable and gentle traction should be maintained until a plaster of Paris cast has been applied. The cast should ideally have plaster on the volar, radial and dorsal sides with anteroposterior moulding to prevent dislocation in the cast. All fingers and metacarpophalangeal joints should be left free and finger movements (into a full fist) encouraged, helping to reduce swelling. The hand should be elevated in a Bradford sling and neurovascular observations should be checked as soon as possible.

Traction views in theatre may give the clinician more information about the pattern of injury.

Options for definitive fixation include K-wire fixation of the carpus percutaneously or the ruptured ligaments can be repaired acutely as an open procedure. Percutaneous wires are still used to maintain the reduction for 6–9 weeks.

The key to a successful reduction and wiring is to reduce the lunate flexion/extension to neutral before stabilising the LT and SL joints.

Any concomitant scaphoid or other carpal fractures should be fixed at the time of definitive surgery.

Complications

Due to the high-energy involved in these injuries, complications are common:
- Immediate complications include median nerve neuropraxia and compartment syndrome
- Early complications include superficial and deep infection and adhesions causing stiffness (particularly if combined volar and dorsal approaches are performed)
- Late complications include early and rapidly progressive arthritic changes (although clinical and radiographic correlation is poor), chronic pain and instability requiring further surgery

Delay to diagnosis and poor quality initial reductions have been shown lead to worse outcomes.

Further reading

Jones DB Jr, Kakar S. Perilunate dislocations and fracture dislocations. J Hand Surg Am 2012; 37:2168–2173.

Melsom DS, Leslie IJ. Carpal dislocations. Current Orthop 2007; 21:288–297.

Vitale MA, Seetharaman M, Ruchelsman DE. Perilunate dislocations. J Hand Surg Am 2007; 40:358–362.

Related topics of interest

- *Topic 37* Guidelines in trauma
- *Topic 40* Hand and wrist – carpal fractures

Hand and wrist – carpal fractures

Key points

- Scaphoid fractures are common and account for up to 70% of all carpal fractures
- Scaphoid waist fractures can be part of a greater arc injury
- Beware of the high rate of associated scapholunate and lunotriquetral injuries

Epidemiology

Scaphoid fractures

The annual incidence of scaphoid fractures is 8 per 100000 for women and 38 per 10000 for men, although the variation in the literature is very large. 69% are caused by a fall on an outstretched hand (FOOSH).

Other carpal fractures

Triquetral fractures comprise up to 31% of all carpal fractures and are the second most common type of carpal fracture. Fractures have been described in all carpal bones. Hamate fractures comprise 7% or carpal fractures. Trapezium and pisiform fractures comprise 3% and 2% respectively. Lunate and capitate fractures comprise 1% each of all carpal fractures.

Pathophysiology

Scaphoid fractures

The scaphoid fracture is the most common and most difficult to treat. Its surface is mostly (80%) covered in cartilage and it is divided into three regions; proximal pole, distal pole and waist. It is the only carpal bone to span both proximal and distal carpal rows. Its blood supply is precarious and enters distally and dorsally on the ridge (dorsal carpal branch of radial artery) then travels intraosseously to the proximal pole. 20–30% of the bone is supplied by a volar artery entering in the distal pole (superficial palmar branch of the radial artery). There are many variations in arterial anatomy.

The trabeculae at the level of the waist are thin and sparsely distributed whereas the proximal pole is denser. The mechanism of injury is usually hyperextension with radial or ulnar deviation of the wrist causing the waist to impinge on the dorsal rim of the radius. As extension continues a fracture starts on the tensile (volar) side and propagates through to the dorsum. Proximal pole fractures are the result of dorsal subluxation in forced hyperextension.

No classification system predicts union well and all systems have poor inter- and intraobserver reliability. The descriptive classification of waist, distal and proximal poles as well as the degree of displacement is the most useful in describing the fracture. The greatest predictors of nonunion are >4 weeks from injury to immobilisation and a current history of smoking.

There is high percentage (up to 80%) of associated injuries to other carpal bones and ligaments in the wrist including the scapholunate and lunotriquetral intrinsic ligaments.

Nonunion

The natural history of scaphoid nonunion is for degenerative changes to progress from the radioscaphoid articulation (distally, stage I) to the scaphocapitate articulation (stage II) then to the lunocapitate articulation with panscaphoid arthritis [Stage III – scaphoid nonunion advanced collapse (SNAC)].

Triquetral fractures

The triquetral body can be injured by direct impaction of the ulnar styloid or hamate if an axial load is applied in ulnar deviation or as part of a perilunate fracture dislocation (greater arc injury). The other way is an avulsion of the dorsal intercarpal or radiocarpal ligament during a forced hyperflexion/radial deviation injury. This causes a flake of bone to be detached from the dorsal rim, visible on the oblique radiograph but belies a far greater injury to the ligamentous stability of the wrist.

Hamate fractures

Hamate fractures can occur to the hook or the body. The latter is more common and is associated with dorsal fracture dislocations of the 4th and 5th metacarpals. This occurs during an axial loading of the flexed carpometacarpal (CMC) joints. The lever arm dislocates the 4th and 5th CMC joints and shears a fragment from the dorsum of the hamate. Body fractures can also be part of a greater arc injury. The hook is invariably caused by a direct blow. Typically, this is caused during sports such as golf as the club strikes the palm but can occur as part of a FOOSH.

Trapezium fractures

These are similar in aetiology to triquetral fractures. Body fractures are caused by forced radial deviation (as opposed to ulnar deviation for triquetral fractures) compressing the trapezium between the thumb and the radial styloid causing vertical compression fractures. Avulsion of the transverse carpal ligament can be caused by a FOOSH causing a flake fracture to the ridge of the trapezium.

Pisiform fractures

The pisiform is a sesamoid bone attached to the flexor carpi ulnaris (FCU) tendon proximally and to the pisohamate, pisometacarpal, and pisotriquetral ligaments distally. Guyon's canal lies immediately radial to the pisiform. It articulates with the triquetrum only. The pisiform is most often injured by a FOOSH with either a stellate or transverse fracture. The former is caused by the direct blow and the latter by FCU causing an avulsion fracture.

Lunate fractures

The lunate has important ligaments attached volarly (long and short radiolunate and the strongest portion of the lunotriquetral ligaments) and dorsally (dorsal radiocarpal and the strongest portion of the scapholunate ligaments). Avulsion of these ligaments can cause rim fractures and should alert the clinician to a potentially unstable wrist. Body fractures occur by axial load.

Capitate fractures

The capitate is well protected and fractures are uncommon. They can occur transversely as part of a greater arc injury as well as forced hyperextension of the wrist. The capitate impacts on the dorsal rim of the radius, usually after the scaphoid has fractured, and a transverse fracture is created. The proximal fragment can rotate 180° end up with the articular surface pointing distally. The proximal fragment has no soft tissue attachments and is susceptible to avascular necrosis. 50% of all capitate fractures have associated injuries in the wrist such as part of a perilunate fracture dislocation.

Trapezoid fractures

Trapezoid fractures are extremely rare. The 2nd CMC joint is tightly bound with ligamentous attachments and the bone itself is locked in place by the capitate and trapezium. Fractures most often occur as part of a fracture dislocation of the 2nd CMC joint from an axial load. They are frequently associated with other injuries.

Clinical features

Scaphoid fractures

Clinical examination is difficult but several tests, when combined, have been shown to be superior to any single test. Anatomical snuffbox tenderness, with the wrist in ulnar deviation, has a sensitivity of 90% but specificity of 40%. Tenderness over the scaphoid tubercle, with the wrist extended, has a sensitivity of 87% and a better specificity of 57%. Absence of tenderness with these two manoeuvres makes a scaphoid fracture highly unlikely. Another examination is reproducing pain in the anatomical snuffbox with pronation of the wrist followed by ulnar deviation (52% positive predictive value, 100% negative predictive value), i.e. if the test is negative the patient does not have a scaphoid fracture.

Other carpal fractures

All the other carpal bone fractures will show localised swelling and the individual bones can be palpated. Tenderness can be elicited and the entire wrist including carpus and metacarpals as well as radius and ulna distally should be examined to rule out associated injuries. Few of these fractures have specific tests associated with them.

Hook of hamate fractures can be tested by resisted flexor digitorum profundus (FDP) flexion with the wrist in ulnar deviation. The hook acts as a pulley for the FDS tendons diverting the tendon from their central location in the palm to the border digit. Therefore, ulnar deviation and finger flexion forces the tendon in an ulnar direction against the hook, causing pain. The hook can be palpated at the intersection of two lines in the palm. The first line is drawn from the base of the ring finger directly to the wrist at the intersection of the ulnar 1/3rd and radial 2/3rd of the wrist crease. The second line is from the pisiform to the middle of the middle phalanx of the index finger. The intersection point is the location of the hook of hamate.

Investigations

Most carpal fractures can be identified using plain radiographs. Oblique radiographs can be helpful especially for dorsal hamate and triquetrum fractures.

A scaphoid series of radiographs should include posteroanterior, semipronated, lateral and Ziter's views (pronated ulnarly deviated view). Follow-up radiographs at 2 weeks for suspected scaphoid fractures are no longer indicated as they have been shown not to be of further diagnostic value. If a scaphoid fracture is suspected and initial radiographs are normal then either a CT scan or MRI should be requested. The national guidance (GEMNet 2013) suggests the gold standard is MRI but CT scan is an acceptable alternative if MRI access is limited. Both scans have similar sensitivities and specificities and the radiation dose for a wrist CT is 0.03 mSv, equivalent to 0.38 of the dose of a chest radiograph.

The hook of hamate can be visualised on a 'carpal tunnel view' with the wrist hyperextended and the beam tangential to the wrist. This can be painful in the acute setting.

Further imaging (CT or MRI) should be undertaken on most lunate, trapezium, capitate, hook of hamate and triquetrum body fractures.

Diagnosis

The diagnosis is made from a combination of history and clinical and radiographic assessment with further imaging as detailed above.

Treatment

Scaphoid fractures

Up to 95% of scaphoid fractures will unite in a cast in 6–8 weeks if treated nonoperatively. Operative management has the benefit of early mobilisation and return to work but results are equivalent at 1 year and operative management has associated surgical risks. Vascularised bone grafting is reserved for nonunions that fail to unite with standard grafting techniques.

The decision to operate or not depends on several factors:
- Degree of displacement; >1 mm displacement can lead to functional deficit
- Patients' wishes, comorbidities and concerns
- History of the injury; >4 weeks from injury to immobilisation increases risk of nonunion

Non-union

All but the most pain free patients, in exceptional circumstances, with scaphoid nonunion should be offered surgery in the form of open reduction and internal fixation (ORIF) with bone grafting.

Other carpal fractures

Minor avulsion fractures can be treated in cast for 4–6 weeks although rim avulsions of the lunate are treated with ORIF due to the potential sequelae of displacement. Body fractures are treated with ORIF unless undisplaced. Nonoperative management involves very close monitoring of displacement with radiographs and CT scans.

Complications

- Immediate complications of:
  - Fracture: dislocation or severe deformity can cause neurovascular injury
  - ORIF: neurovascular and tendon damage
- Early complications include:
  - Fracture: ongoing pain and instability
  - ORIF: infection, pain, hypertrophic scar
- Late complications include:
  - Fracture: nonunion and SNAC wrist, stiffness, need for fusion surgery.
  - ORIF: nonunion and SNAC wrist, stiffness, need for fusion surgery

Further reading

Geissler WB, Adams JE, Bindra RR, Lanzinger WD, Slutsky DJ. Scaphoid fractures: what's hot, what's not. J Bone Joint Surg AM 2012; 94:169–181.

Papp S. Carpal bone fractures. Orthop Clin N Am 2007; 38:251–260.

Shah MA, Viegas SF. Fractures of the carpal bones excluding the scaphoid. J Hand Surg Am 2002:3.

Related topics of interest

- *Topic 39* Hand and wrist – carpal dislocations
- *Topic 43* Hand and wrist – scaphoid fractures

41 Hand and wrist – metacarpal fractures

Key points
- Most metacarpal fractures are stable and can be treated nonoperatively
- Border digits are most often affected
- Correct splinting is essential

Epidemiology

Metacarpal fractures are common and account for up to 50% of all hand fractures. Men are up to 5.7 times more likely to sustain a metacarpal fracture than women and the peak incidence is in the age range 20–29 years. The mean annual incidence in one large study in the Netherlands was 1.6%. The mean annual incidence for men was 2.0% and for women was 1.0%. In the very young and those over 50 years the most common cause was an accidental fall and in those ages in between was a motor vehicle accident or an injury sustained during sport.

Pathophysiology

The vast majority of metacarpal fractures are to a single metacarpal and are stable. The thumb metacarpal is the most injured due to it having the least stability and no protection from adjacent bones. The border metacarpals are often affected due to the relatively strong attachments of the central two rays at each end and the protection that the border metacarpals afford them.

Thumb metacarpal fractures

Fractures can be extra- or intra-articular. The latter are either a Bennett's or Rolando type fracture. A Bennett's fracture describes a fracture line running through the articular surface leaving the volar ulnar corner in its anatomic position but the remaining articular surface and shaft dislocated radially and dorsally by the pull of abductor pollicis longus (APL). The fragment left behind has the strong anterior oblique ligament (beak ligament) still attached. A Rolando fracture describes a multifragmentary intra-articular fracture in a Y or T shaped configuration.

Extra-articular fractures tend to be at the meta-diaphyseal junction. The force of flexor pollicis longus (FPL) volarly pulls the distal fragment into flexion and APL maintains the proximal fragment in abduction.

Metacarpals 2–5

Fractures can occur at any point along the bone depending on the direction and magnitude of the injuring force. Axial loads can cause articular compression or shear injuries at either end, whereas axial load with a bending force can cause the familiar 5th metacarpal neck fracture – Boxer's fracture (**Figure 41.1**). At greater forces the bases of the 4th and 5th metacarpals dislocate dorsally with or without fractures to the metacarpals themselves (**Figures 41.2** and **41.3**) or the hamate (**Figures 41.4–41.6**). Further bending forces create diaphyseal fractures. Any rotational component to the force will cause spiral fractures and have the greatest risk of rotational malalignment.

More complex fracture patterns and multiple fractures indicate higher energy injuries and should alert the clinician to the possibility of other injuries and soft tissue compromise, including compartment syndrome.

It is helpful to be familiar with the shape of the bones and the differences in ligamentous anatomy across the metacarpals. The 2nd to 4th metacarpals have an apex-dorsal longitudinal bow (**Figures 41.7–41.9**) and together form the transverse arch of the palm. The heads of metacarpals 2–5 are trapezoidal and are elliptical in the sagittal plane. The true collateral ligaments originate in the depression on the sides of the dorsum of the head and insert into the volar radial and ulnar corner of the proximal phalanx. The accessory collateral ligaments insert from the true collateral ligament into the volar plate.

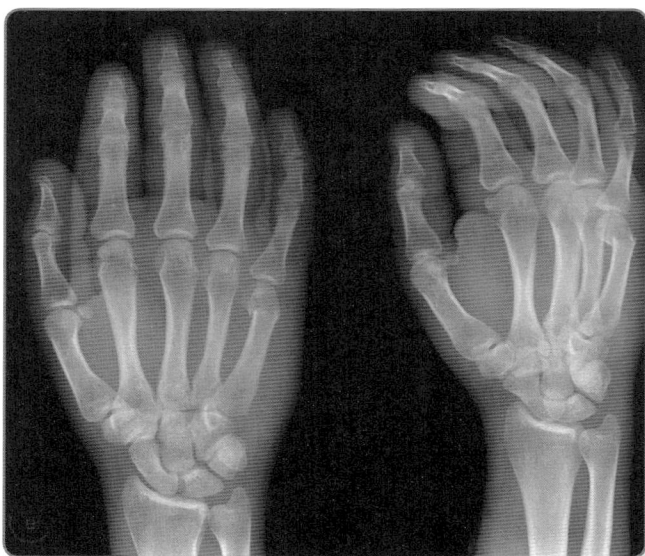

Figure 41.1 Boxer's fracture treated nonoperatively.

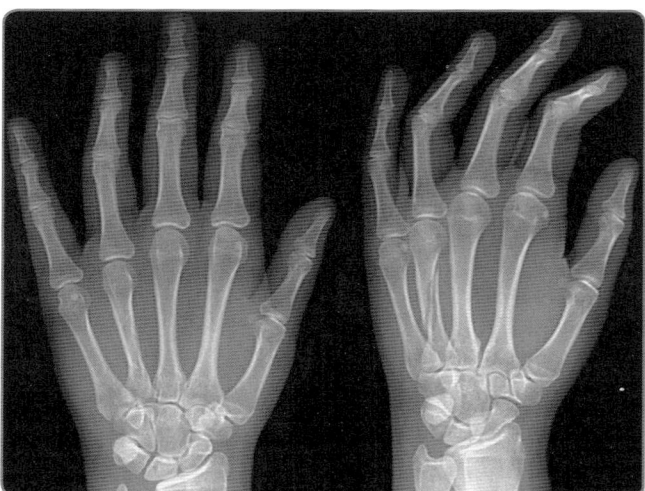

Figure 41.2 4th metacarpal fracture treated nonoperatively.

The true collaterals are tighter in flexion due the trapezoidal shape of the head and the accessory collaterals are tighter in extension when the true ligaments are looser.

The 2nd and 3rd metacarpal bases have tight ligamentous attachments across the carpometacarpal (CMC) joints and have very little movement. The 4th and 5th have sequentially looser CMC joint ligaments and therefore more range of motion. This is key to allowing the 4th and 5th heads to descend volarly when making a power grip. Malunion or dislocation at these joints causes significantly reduced power and early arthritis.

The dorsal capsules of the 2nd, 3rd and 5th CMC joints are reinforced by the insertions of extensor carpi radialis longus (ECRL), extensor carpi radialis brevis (ECRB) and

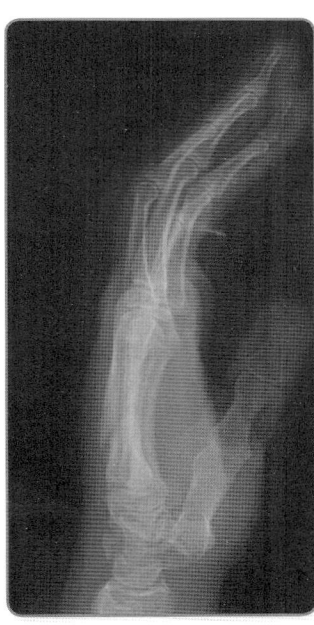

Figure 41.3 Metacarpal fracture.

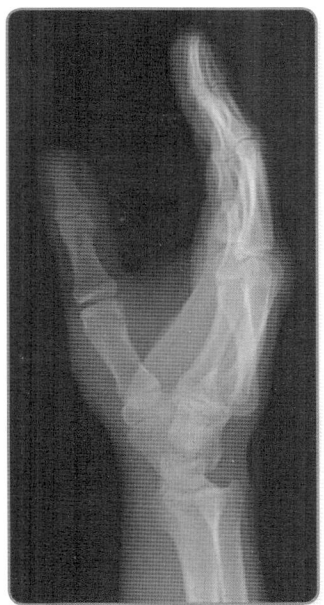

Figure 41.5 Dorsal dislocation of 5th metacarpophalangeal joint.

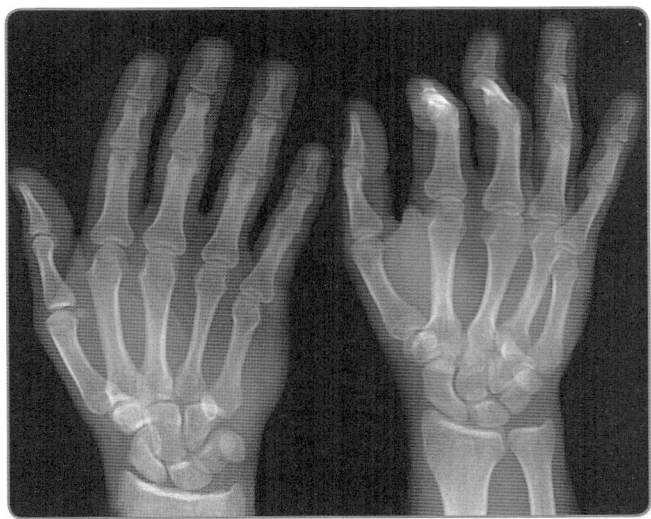

Figure 41.4 Dorsal dislocation of 5th metacarpophalangeal joint.

extensor carpi ulnaris (ECU) respectively. The latter acts as a deforming force when the base of the 5th metacarpal dislocates. The volar capsular ligaments of the 2nd CMC joint are reinforced by the flexor carpi radialis (FCR) insertion also.

The thumb and the 4th and 5th metacarpals can tolerate moderate degrees of angulation due to their increased range of motion at the CMC joint, but the 2nd and 3rd can tolerate very little. No metacarpal can tolerate much rotational deformity as it

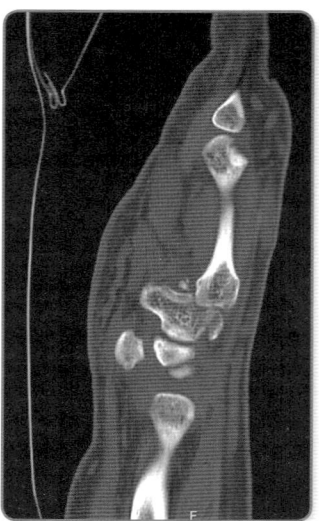

Figure 41.6 Sagittal CT slice showing 5th metacarpal dislocation and hamate fracture.

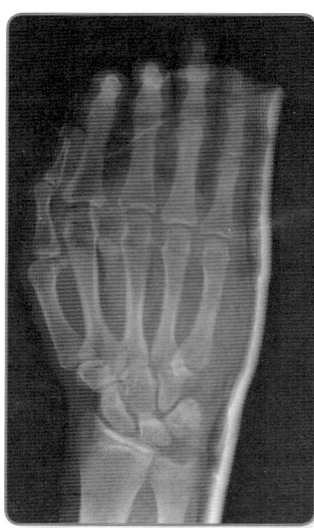

Figure 41.8 5th metacarpal shaft fracture – post manipulation under anaesthesia.

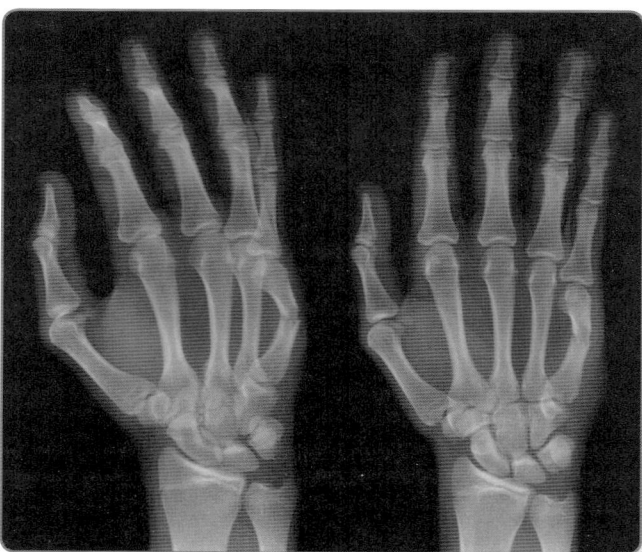

Figure 41.7 5th metacarpal shaft fracture treated with manipulation under anaesthesia (MUA) in the emergency department – pre-MUA.

affects the rotational profile of the digits and hence grip.

Clinical features

Injuries to the hand produce swelling and point tenderness. Palpation can be very precise as the anatomy is relatively superficial and bruising tends to be very localised. Swelling can be very pronounced, especially in higher energy injuries where compartment syndrome must always be considered. Compartment syndrome in the hand can be catastrophic if not detected early so vigilance is necessary.

Investigations

First line investigations are posteroanterior (PA), oblique and lateral radiographs.

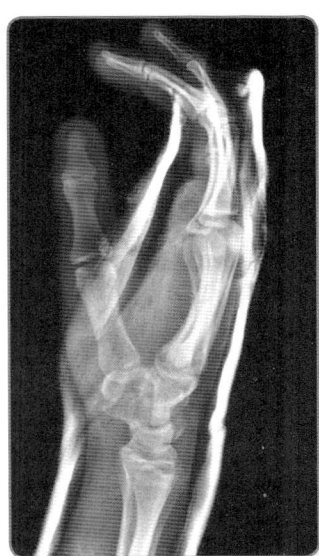

Figure 41.9
5th metacarpal shaft fracture – post manipulation under anaesthesia.

The oblique view is particularly helpful in metacarpal fractures as it is often difficult to separate out or trace each individual metacarpal on a lateral radiograph due to the overlap of four metacarpal shafts. This view is also helpful in diagnosing dorsal hamate fractures associated with subluxation of the bases of the 4th and 5th metacarpals and boxer's fractures of the metacarpal neck. Do not measure angulations of these latter fractures on an oblique radiograph however; use the lateral view.

Displacement of the bases of the metacarpals can be best seen on the lateral radiograph. All the metacarpal shafts should be parallel. Dorsal displacement of the base of the 4th and 5th is particularly visible on this view. Metacarpal shaft fractures often appear with a spike of bone protruding dorsal to the other shafts.

The PA view is often the clearest for diagnosing a fracture but rarely is helpful in assessing displacement as most displacement occurs in the sagittal plane for reasons discussed above.

Dedicated thumb PA and lateral views should be requested but the whole hand should be radiographed to rule out concomitant injuries.

Specialised views include the Brewerton's (with the dorsal side of the fingers flat on the X-ray plate, metacarpophalangeal (MCP) joint flexed to 65° and with the beam 15° in an ulnar to radial direction) and skyline views (fingers fully flexed and beam is angled tangential to the metacarpal head). They are particularly helpful to delineate the bony anatomy of the metacarpal heads in clenched fist injuries.

Diagnosis

The diagnosis should be suspected after a thorough history and sought for in the examination. The rotational profile of digits 2–5 is easier but patients are often too sore to move the fingers into a fist themselves. The clinician should assist with passive flexion of the fingers to check for rotational malalignment. A haematoma between the heads of the metacarpals can cause rotational defects and serial examinations should be performed and compared when the haematoma has dispersed at the one week appointment. Rotational malalignment often corrects itself when this has occurred.

Treatment

As with any fracture, initial management should consist of full ATLS precautions. Swollen hands should be elevated above the level of the heart as early as possible. Open fractures should be thoroughly cleaned in the emergency department.

Casting of metacarpal fractures (2–5) generally consists of a dorsal back-slab in emergency department in the position of safe immobilisation (POSI). This is a cast from forearm to fingertips with the wrist extended 30–40°, the MCP joints flexed to 70° and the fingers straight. It can exclude the index and middle fingers for ulnar sided injuries. This position ensures the ligaments of the respective joints are kept on stretch to help prevent future stiffness. Thumb metacarpal fractures are immobilised in a radially based cast including the wrist, CMC and MCP joints but not the interphalangeal joint.

Definitive treatment depends on the stability of the fracture. A fracture is considered functionally stable when it is possible to actively move the fractured digit by 50% of range of motion painlessly. Instability can be judged by the degree of initial displacement. A fracture is considered unstable if it cannot be reduced or maintained in an anatomic or near anatomic position when the hand is placed in the POSI.

Specialist hand therapists can then use thermoplastic splints to immobilise the fracture but not the surrounding joints. The vast majority of metacarpal shaft and neck fractures can be managed nonoperatively with a thermoplastic splint and early active movements. Operative intervention should be minimally invasive if possible, such as 'bouquet' antegrade intramedullary wiring or percutaneous wiring. Plates have higher rates of stiffness and complications and should be reserved for the most unstable fractures (Table 41.1).

Intra-articular fractures need anatomic reduction and internal fixation. Bennetts and Rolando fractures are highly unstable and usually displace even in the best-moulded thumb spica casts. Operative intervention with manipulation under anaesthesia (MUA) and wiring or open reduction and internal fixation with plates and screws is preferable.

Boxer's fractures and most single stable metacarpal fractures can be managed with no cast after the first week and with buddy strapping only. Encouraging full active motion can de-rotate rotational malalignment if instituted early enough due to the effect of the deep transverse metacarpal ligament. Boxer's fractures up to 70° and shortened, isolated metacarpal shaft fractures (2–5 only) can be managed in this way with little or no sequelae.

Table 41.1 Indications for surgical intervention to manage metacarpal fractures

Failure to achieve acceptable reduction
Open fractures
Collateral ligament injuries
Index metacarpal fracture
Rotational deformity
Multiple fractures of metacarpal
Intra-articular fractures
Polytrauma
Fracture with bone loss
Associated soft tissue injury (vessel, tendon, nerve, skin)

Complications

- Immediate complications include compartment syndrome and neurovascular injuries
- Early complications include pressure sores from poorly fitting splints or casts, malunion, rotational malalignment
- Late complications include stiffness, prominent metalwork such a plate, tendon attritional rupture and nonunion

Further reading

Khan A, Giddins G. The outcome of conservative treatment of spiral metacarpal fractures and the role of the deep transverse metacarpal ligaments in stabilizing these injuries. J Hand Surg Eur 2015; 40:59–62.

McNemar TB, Howell JW, Chang E. Management of metacarpal fractures. J Hand Therapy 2003; 16:143–151.

Orbay JL, Indriago I, Gonzalez E, Badia A, Khouri R. Percutaneous fixation of metacarpal fractures. Oper Tech Plast Reconstr Surg 2014; 9:138–142.

Related topics of interest

- *Topic 14* Compartment syndrome
- *Topic 40* Hand and wrist – carpal fractures
- *Topic 42* Hand and wrist – phalangeal fractures

42 Hand and wrist – phalangeal fractures

Key points
- Most phalangeal fractures are inherently stable and can be managed with simple splinting and early mobilisation
- Unstable fractures will often adopt a predictable pattern of deformity secondary to the intrinsic forces acting upon the digit
- Unstable fractures require surgical fixation however increased stability comes at a cost of increased surgical insult and consequently stiffness

Epidemiology

Fractures of the phalanges are the most common injuries to the human skeleton. They make up 10% of all fractures presenting to the emergency department. The distal phalanx is fractured most frequently, followed by the proximal and then the middle phalanx. The little finger and thumb are most frequently affected as they lie on the periphery of the hand and are therefore the least protected. The predominant mechanism of injury follows a trimodal distribution and is strongly associated with the age of the patient. The leading cause of phalangeal fractures in the under 30 age group is sporting injuries, in the 40–69 age group industrial machinery accidents and for over 69 age group, simple falls.

Principles

Most undisplaced fractures of the phalanges are inherently stable. That is to say they will not displace under normal physiological force. They may therefore be treated with buddy strapping and early mobilisation. In exceptionally painful injuries splinting with the metacapophalangeal (MCP) joints in 60° of flexion and the interphalangeal joints (IPJs) extended (Edinburgh position) may increase comfort. This position reduces, but does not exclude the risk of post immobilisation stiffness. Once the fracture is no longer painful than any form of splinting may be discarded. Full activities are usually resumed at 4–6 weeks.

In general, bony alignment is regarded as acceptable if there is less than 10° displacement in the anteroposterior (AP) and lateral X-rays, at least 50% opposition is present and no rotational deformity exists. Displacement exceeding these measures requires reduction and stabilisation. Rotational deformity is particularly poorly tolerated and may also not be apparent on the radiographs. Thorough clinical assessment is mandatory.

Almost all displaced fractures requiring reduction are unstable. They may still be managed nonoperatively if they have sufficient axial stability to resist the deforming force of the long flexors and extensors. Transverse and short oblique fractures that have been well reduced are usually sufficiently stable to control in an Edinburgh position splint. Splinting should not be continued for longer than 3 weeks, as this has been associated with increased stiffness and inferior function.

If reduction cannot be held in a plaster splint then surgical intervention is indicated. Open reduction and internal fixation with plates and screws can provide anatomic reduction and rigid internal fixation at the cost of significant soft tissue scarring from the surgical dissection. Fixation must be suitably stable that mobilisation exercises can begin immediately. Closed reduction and percutaneous pinning with K-wires is less of an insult to the soft tissues but at the cost of reduced stability.

Intra-articular fractures can lead to significant stiffness and loss of function. In general restoration of the articular surface is required. Specific intra-articular fracture will be discussed later in the chapter.

The pitfalls of managing phalangeal fractures have been succinctly captured by Alfred Swanson MD, 'Hand fractures may be complicated by deformity from no treatment, stiffness from over treatment and both deformity and stiffness from poor treatment'.

Clinical features

The injury must be appreciated within the context of the patient as a whole. Hand dominance, occupation and hobbies should be recorded. The precise mechanism of the injury can suggest the diagnosis and from this the fracture pattern may be predictable. The environment in which the injury occurred is important if there is a risk of wound contamination with marine or agricultural material. Fractures may occur following bites to the finger whether they are from humans or other animals. These are at particularly high risk of infection.

Phalangeal fractures classically present with pain, swelling, loss of mobility and deformity, however symptoms may be minor in the first instance and there may be more than one fracture in an injured hand. A thorough inspection of the entire hand and comparison to the contralateral side should be performed. Assessment for rotational deformity is essential as this is poorly tolerated and an indication for intervention. If flexion is possible then the fingers should converge on the scaphoid tubercle (**Figure 42.1**).

In the acutely fractured digit assessment may have to rely on the cascade of the fingernails. Neurovascular assessment is should be performed and documented. A thorough assessment of the condition of the soft tissues is required.

Investigations

Plain AP and lateral radiographs centred over the area of maximum tenderness are usually adequate to make the diagnosis, assess stability and alignment, and plan treatment in phalangeal fractures. The exception to this is proximal phalanx fractures where an oblique view may be required as the adjacent digits can obscure the view on the lateral projection.

Cross-sectional imaging is rarely required in the assessment of phalangeal fractures.

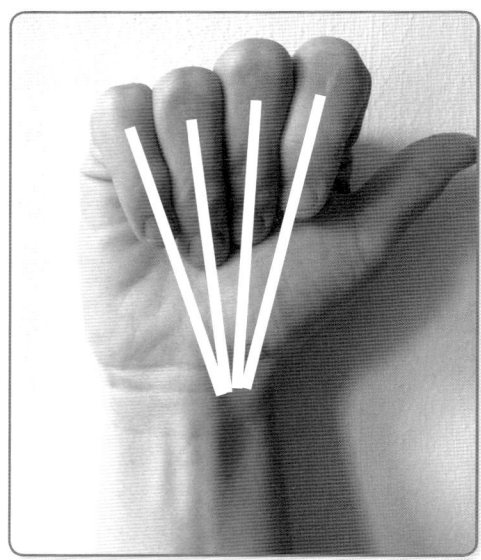

Figure 42.1 The fingers point towards the scaphoid tubercle in flexion. This alignment will be disrupted in the presence of rotational deformity.

Pathophysiology and specific fracture types

Distal phalanx fractures

Distal phalanx fractures are classified anatomically into tuft fractures, shaft fractures and intra-articular fractures.

Tuft fractures frequently occur as part of a crush injury and are often associated with a nail bed laceration. If the nail plate is intact a painful subungual haematoma may occur. This should be trephined to relieve the discomfort. Accurate repair of the surrounding soft tissues and a brief period (1–2 weeks) of splintage is usually sufficient treatment.

Shaft fractures are commonly transverse in nature. If undisplaced the surrounding soft tissue and nail plate will act as a splint however in open displaced fractures reduction and internal screw fixation may be required.

Intra-articular fractures occur due to avulsion of the tendinous insertions. Dorsal fractures occur secondary to the pull of the extensor tendon and volar fractures due the force of flexor digitorum profundus (FDP). If the joint is congruent then these fractures may be treated nonoperatively otherwise K-wire stabilisation of the distal interphalangeal joint (DIPJ) may be required.

Extra-articular proximal and middle phalanx fractures

Transverse fracture of the base of the proximal phalanx will adopt an apex volar deformity due to flexion of the proximal fragment by the interossei and extension of the dorsal fragment by the central slip of the extensor tendon (**Figure 42.2**).

These fractures are potentially unstable but can be reduced using a plaster or aluminium splint with the MCPJ flexed and the IPJs extended (the Edinburgh position). If these fractures cannot be controlled in a splint then percutaneous K-wires can be used to augment the reduction. The Eaton-Belsky method of passing the wire through the metacarpal head to stabilise proximal phalanx fractures is a simple and safe technique.

In transverse extra-articular fractures of the middle phalanx both volar and dorsal angulation can occur depending on the relationship between the fracture and the insertion of the FDS tendon. Fracture proximal to FDS leads to dorsal angulation whilst fracture distal to FDS produces a volar angulation deformity.

Spiral or oblique fractures of the proximal or middle phalanx are potentially unstable even if they are undisplaced at presentation. Multiple transverse K-wires or percutaneous screw fixation can be employed to stabilise the fracture.

Intra-articular fractures of the proximal and middle phalanx

Fractures involving the condyles of the proximal phalanx are unstable even if undisplaced at presentation (**Figure 42.3**).

If the decision is made to manage nonoperatively then vigilant clinical and radiographic follow-up is essential. Surgical stabilisation is therefore preferable (**Figure 42.4**). The decision to use K-wires or screws is made based on the size of the fragment.

T-shaped fracture affecting the base of the proximal phalanx is intra-articular and unstable. The AO principles should be applied as for any intra-articular fracture. Open anatomic reduction and rigid stabilisation is required.

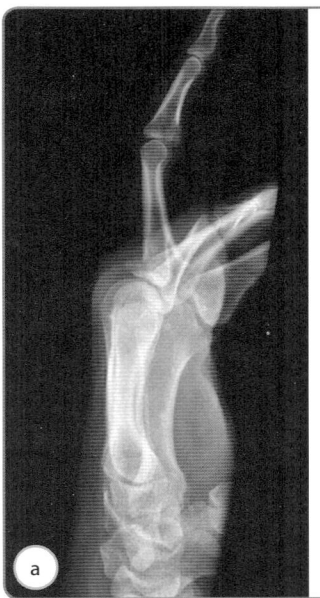
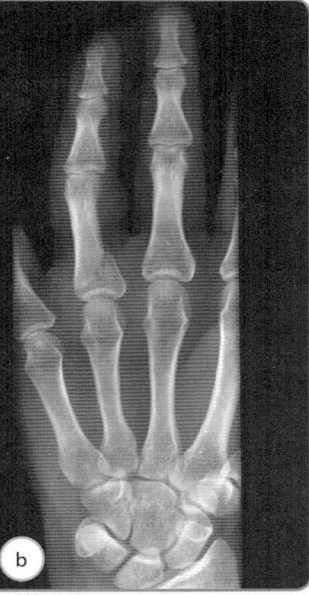

Figure 42.2 (a) Anteroposterior and (b) lateral radiographs showing the typical apex volar deformity occurring with a transverse fracture to the base of the proximal phalanx.

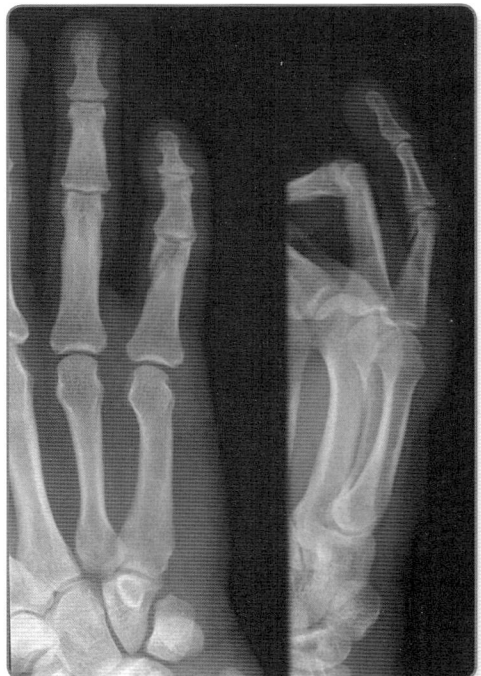

Figure 42.3 Radiograph showing a potentially unstable unicondylar fracture of the proximal phalanx.

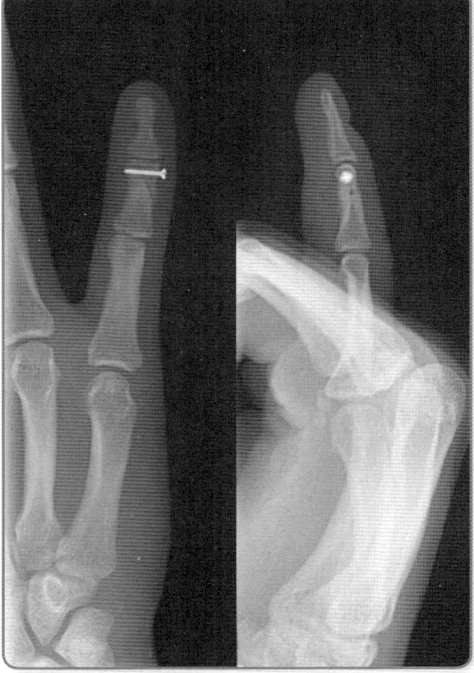

Figure 42.4 Radiograph showing screw fixation of an intra-articular fracture.

Axial load to the finger such as a cricket ball striking the fingertip can lead to a multi-fragmentary intra-articular fracture of the base of the middle phalanx. Open reductions with internal fixation and simple immobilisation have produced poor clinical outcomes. Therefore, these fractures are treated with dynamic external fixators and early motion. This takes advantage of the remodelling potential of the DIPJ and can lead to surprisingly good clinical outcomes.

Complications

Malunion
Angular and rotational deformity may occur compromising hand function. Malunion can be treated by corrective osteotomy, however, this may in turn lead to loss of range of movement.

Stiffness
It can lead to loss of extension and flexion. Loss of extension is better tolerated whilst loss of flexion can be severely disabling due to dysfunction of the common belly of FDP. This can leave the hand lacking dexterity and feeling weak. Stiffness may occur secondary to joint contracture and scarring or tendon adhesions. Equal passive and active range of movement is suggestive of joint contracture whilst an increased passive compared to active suggests tendon adhesions. I reality a combination of both pathologies usually co-exist. Treatment is with aggressive hand therapy and mobilisation with surgical release reserved for resistant cases. The results of surgery are unpredictable.

Nonunion
Only occurs in surgically treated fractures rigidly fixed in distraction. Revision fixation and bone grafting is required to achieve union.

Post-traumatic arthrosis
It should be treated as for primary hand osteoarthritis.

Further reading

Bulstrode C, Buckwater J, Carr A, et al. Oxford Textbook of Orthopaedics and Trauma. Oxford: Oxford University Press, 2002.

Green D, Hotchkiss R, Pederson C, et al. Green's Operative Hand Surgery, 4th edn. London: Churchill Livingstone, 1999.

Related topics of interest

- *Topic 41* Hand and wrist – metacarpal fractures
- *Topic 44* Hand and wrist – tendon ruptures
- *Topic 66* Nailbed injuries

43 Hand and wrist – scaphoid fractures

Key points

- The scaphoid plays a key role in the complex biomechanics of the carpus, unrecognised injury may therefore lead to rapid degenerative change and loss of function
- Fractures of the scaphoid may not be apparent on initial radiographs and as such may be overlooked or misdiagnosed. They are frequently the subject of medico-legal claims
- The blood supply to the proximal pole is predominantly retrograde and therefore avascular necrosis (AVN) is a recognised sequel of these fractures

Epidemiology

Fracture of the scaphoid is a common injury with an incidence of between 1.5 and 121 per 100,000 quoted in the literature. They make up 2.4% of all wrist fractures. There is a significant preponderance in males compared to females. The most frequent mechanism of injury is a fall from standing height on to an outstretched hand or a sporting injury. Male gender and sporting injury are strong predictors of true fracture.

Pathophysiology

The scaphoid is an irregular tubular S-shaped bone found on the radial side of the carpus. It is also known as the navicular of the wrist. It is the only bone to cross both rows of the carpus and as such has an essential role in co-ordinating the complex kinematics of wrist motion. 80% of the surface of the scaphoid is covered in articular cartilage and it articulates directly with the radius, capitate, lunate, trapezium and trapezoid. It is due to these complex biomechanical interactions that failure to immobilise scaphoid fractures may lead to excess strain across the fracture site and nonunion. Furthermore the blood supply to the proximal pole of the scaphoid runs in a retrograde fashion. The dorsal carpal branch of the radial artery enters the dorsum of the scaphoid just distal to the waist of the scaphoid and supplies the proximal 80% of the bone. It is for this reason that disruption to the waist or proximal pole of the scaphoid can lead to proximal AVN.

Clinical features

The clinical assessment of a potential scaphoid fracture begins with the clinician maintaining a high index of suspicion. Patient demographics and mechanism of injury may suggest the diagnosis. There may be a remarkable paucity of clinical signs on inspection although bruising, swelling and a fullness in the snuffbox may be apparent. The patient will complain of radial sided wrist pain and is likely to have a reduced range of movement of the thumb and wrist. Tenderness over the anatomical snuffbox and scaphoid tubercle are common clinical signs. Telescoping of the thumb will cause pain in scaphoid fractures. These clinical signs are highly sensitive but lack specificity individually; however, the presence of all three has been reported to have a specificity of 74% for fracture.

Investigations

Plain radiographs are the primary investigation of choice. Specific scaphoid views should be requested: a neutral posteroanterior (PA), a true lateral, a 45° oblique view and a scaphoid view with the wrist extended 30° and deviated 20° ulnarward (**Figure 43.1**). Routine PA and lateral views of the wrist are insufficient to diagnose or exclude scaphoid fracture. Even with standard four views 30–40% of scaphoid fractures are not seen at initial presentation. If there are positive clinical signs but negative radiology the wrist should be splinted and the imaging repeated at 10–14 days. By this stage resorption of bone surrounding hairline fractures may make the injury more apparent.

Hand and wrist – scaphoid fractures

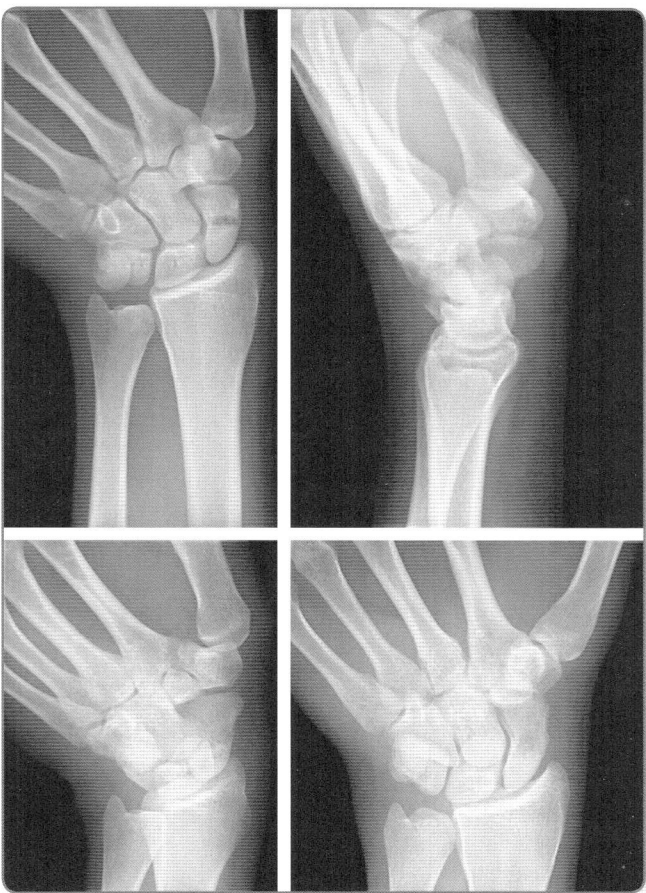

Figure 43.1 Plain radiographs showing standard four views required to assess a fracture of the scaphoid. A minimally displaced fracture through the waist is demonstrated.

Both CT scan and MRI have excellent sensitivity and specificity for diagnosing scaphoid fractures. MRI has the additional advantage of demonstrating soft tissue pathology accounting for the patient's symptoms in the absence of a fracture. However, acute access to cross-sectional imaging remains unavailable in many institutions.

Diagnosis

Initial diagnosis should be predominantly clinical. The assessing doctor should have decided whether to treat as a scaphoid fracture from the patient demographics, mechanism of injury and clinical examination. However as only 5–20% of patients attending the emergency department with a suspected scaphoid injury have a true fracture there is likely to be significant over diagnosis at first presentation. In the absence of radiological evidence at 10–14 days postinjury, if available, cross-sectional imaging should be employed to prevent unnecessary treatment.

Classification

The Herbert classification of scaphoid fractures may be used. Type A is stable, type B unstable; Type C includes delayed union whilst type D is for established Nonunion. **Table 43.1** demonstrates the full classification including subtypes.

Treatment

The AVN in scaphoid tubercle fractures (Herbert A1) has not been described and nonunion is rarely symptomatic. These fractures may therefore be treated symptomatically with immobilisation by plaster or removable wrist splint.

Undisplaced (Herbert A2) fractures can be treated with immobilisation in plaster cast for 6–8 weeks. Above and below elbow plasters with and without thumb involvement have been shown to be equally effective with comparable rates of nonunion, however, patients better tolerate below elbow casts with the thumb left free. Undisplaced fractures can be treated by percutaneous screw stabilisation. No cast is required. This has been shown to allow more rapid return to work and sporting performance at the cost of increased risk of intraoperative complication. An improved rate of union although anticipated has not been demonstrated in the literature.

Unstable fractures (Herbert B) require reduction and stabilisation. If reduction can be achieved closed then percutaneous screw stabilisation may be performed (**Figure 43.2**). For open reduction of a proximal pole fragment a dorsal approach is utilised while a volar approach is employed for displaced waist fractures.

Complications

Nonunion occurs in up to 10% of scaphoid waist fractures and 80% of proximal pole fractures. This figure increases with degree of displacement and delay in appropriate care. Nonunion disrupts the kinematics of the wrist leading to a predictable pattern of degenerative change known as a scaphoid nonunion advanced collapse wrist. This a disabling and difficult to treat condition that can severely compromise a patient's quality of life and ability to work. Open reduction and internal fixation with bone grafting should be performed prior to the development of secondary arthrosis.

Table 43.1 Herbert classification of scaphoid fractures.

A	Acute stable	A1	Tubercle
		A2	Nondisplaced crack at waist
B	Acute unstable	B1	Oblique distal third
		B2	Displaced waist
		B3	Proximal pole
		B4	Fracture dislocation
		B5	Comminuted
C	Delayed union		
D	Established nonunion	D1	Fibrous
		D2	Sclerotic

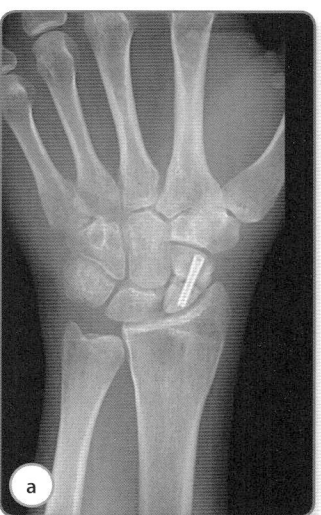
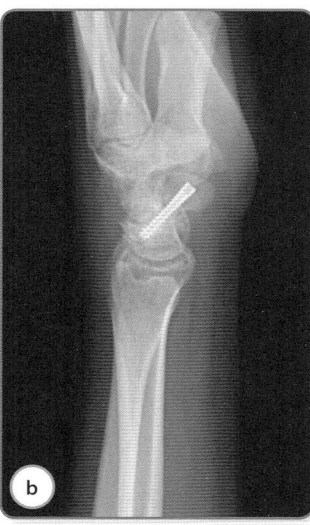

Figure 43.2 (a) Lateral and (b) anteroposterior radiograph showing a scaphoid waist fracture stabilised with a variable pitch screw.

Malunion of displaced scaphoid fractures disrupts the kinematics of wrist movement. Whilst mild deformity is well tolerated wrist instability pain and degeneration can occur in severe malunion.

The AVN occurs in up to 30% of proximal pole fractures. The pathological change begins immediately but may not become radiologically or clinically apparent for the first 1–2 months. Left untreated rapid degenerative change occurs in the wrist. Scaphoid excision and four-corner fusion may be required as a salvage procedure in untreated scaphoid AVN.

Further reading

Buijze GA, Doornberg JN, Ham JS, et al. Surgical compared with conservative treatment for acute nondisplaced or minimally displaced scaphoid fractures: a systematic review and meta-analysis of randomized controlled trials. J Bone Joint Surg 2010; 92:1534–1544.

Dias JJ, Singh, HP. Displaced fracture of the waist of the scaphoid. J Bone Joint Surg Br 2011; 93:1433–1439.

Duckworth AD, Ring D, McQueen MM. Assessment of the suspected fracture of the scaphoid. J Bone Joint Surg Br 2011; 93:713–719.

Related topics of interest

- Topic 39 Hand and wrist – carpal dislocations
- Topic 40 Hand and wrist – carpal fractures
- Topic 67 Nonunion of fractures

44 Hand and wrist – tendon ruptures

Key points
- With tendon ruptures in the wrist and hand, early and accurate diagnosis is key and timely but not emergent repair essential
- Early active movements improve results so repair well and refer to hand therapy early
- Repair under local anaesthetic with adrenaline, if possible, to test repair intraoperatively

Epidemiology

The incidence of extensor tendon injuries in the hand is 18/100,000 per year and mallet injuries alone are 9.9/100,000 per year. The incidence of flexor tendon injuries is lower; 4.83/100,000 per year. The ratio of men to women is 8:2 and injuries are most common in the 3rd and 4th decade of life.

Pathophysiology

Anatomy

The extensor tendons to the hand and wrist are innervated by the radial nerve (ECRL, ECRB) and its continuation, the posterior interosseous nerve (in order of branches: EDC, ECU, EDM, EPL, EPB, EIP). There is a large amount of variation in branching of the radial nerve and the configuration of tendons supplying the hand.

The ulnar and median nerves supply the intrinsic muscles, which add to the extensor apparatus via the lateral bands. The intrinsics are the principal extensors of the interphalangeal joints (IPJs) and secondary flexors of the metacapophalangeal joints (MCPJs). The central extrinsic tendons are the principal extensors of the MCPJs and secondary extensors of the IPJs. There is a loose connective tissue attachment of the extrinsic tendons to the proximal phalanx adding some power to extension of the fingers.

If the fingers were flexed by just using the flexor tendons, they would flex from the tips first as this is where flexor digitorum profundus (FDP) inserts, then the proximal interphalangeal joint (PIPJ) due to the FDS tendon insertion. There is no flexor tendon insertion to the proximal phalanges of the fingers. In order to flex the MCPJ, PIPJ and distal interphalangeal joint (DIPJ) smoothly and synergistically the lateral bands (mostly from the lumbrical muscles, via the FDP tendons in the palm) add an extension force to the PIPJ and DIPJ as the tendon retracts. This allows preferential flexion of the MCPJ and then flexion of the more distal joints when the lumbrical tendon loses its tension as the MCPJ flexes. This enables the hand to close around larger objects in particular but also allows it to position the fingers in space with far greater accuracy. It is because of this complex interaction of all three nerves and both the flexor and extensor apparatus that repair of tendons in the hand and wrist is an exacting technical exercise.

The flexor tendons are supplied by the median nerve apart from FCU and the ulnar half of FDP. They enter the carpal tunnel with the median nerve and fan out in the palm beneath the palmar fascia to enter the fingers and thumb via the A1 pulleys. The FCU inserts into the pisiform as a sesamoid bone and continues to attach to the base of the 5th metacarpal and the hook of the hamate. The ulnar nerve lies beneath the tendon in the forearm.

Extensor zones of injury

I-IX (zone IX is the muscle itself, see **Figure 44.1**). Odd numbered zones lie over the joints.

Extensor tendons can be injured at any level by a laceration and also by closed means in zone I, III, V and VII. Most lacerations can be primarily repaired. In zones II and IV the tendon is often lacerated <50% due to the shape of the bones and in these circumstances nonoperative management can be instituted if the patient can still actively extend the finger.

A mallet injury is an example of an avulsion of the extensor tendon in zone I usually caused by resisted finger flexion. The extensor tendon attempts in vain to overcome the flexion force applied to the DIPJ and the tendon is pulled from the distal phalanx causing the characteristic flexed DIPJ.

Volar PIPJ dislocations can cause closed zone III injuries where the central slip is avulsed from its insertion. Both these injuries are challenging to diagnose initially and a high index of suspicion should be encouraged due to the long-term sequelae of not instituting treatment early. Empirical splinting should be employed if suspicion is aroused during history and examination to avoid a mallet deformity causing a swan-neck deformity and a central slip injury causing a boutonniere deformity. These are both much more difficult to treat than the original injury.

Zone V injuries are frequently caused by bites or impact with the human mouth – the 'fight bite'. They are open joint injuries until proven otherwise and require urgent washout and debridement in theatre under regional or general anaesthesia. Flexing the MCPJ will deliver the laceration into the wound exposing the rent in the extensor hood or sagittal bands and down through the capsule. Not performing this manoeuvre intraoperatively can lead to the false impression the laceration does not go into the joint. The articular cartilage is not infrequently damaged and foreign bodies such as teeth should be removed! A thorough washout must be performed, the extensor tendon repaired and the wound left to granulate unless it is pristine. Tendon repair should not be attempted until infection is controlled.

Closed injuries in zone V can be caused by degenerative or traumatic means. The former is common in rheumatoid arthritis and the latter during pugilist sports. The sagittal band ruptures causing the central tendon to sublux ulnarly and volarly. The MCPJ cannot be extended actively but the patient can maintain MCPJ extension if the joint is passively extended.

Closed injuries in zone VII usually involve iatrogenic injury by protruding screws after fixation of the distal radius volarly or attritional injury from dorsal fixation. An EPL rupture can occur after undisplaced distal radius fracture.

Flexor zones of injury (Figure 44.2)

Zone I lies distal to the insertion of FDS. Zone II lies between zone I and the proximal end of the A1 pulley. Zone III lies between Zone II and the transverse carpal ligament (the carpal tunnel). Zone IV lies beneath the carpal tunnel. Zone V lies proximal to the carpal tunnel. The thumb zones are: zone I distal to the oblique pulley, zone II lies between zone I and the proximal end of the A1 pulley and zone III corresponds to the same zone in the palm, proximal to the A1 pulley.

Avulsion of the FDP tendon in zone 1 – the 'rugger jersey finger' – is caused by a forced extension of the DIPJ while the FDP contracts eccentrically. The tendon can avulse all the way back to the palm. These are frequently missed or treated as mallet injuries due to the

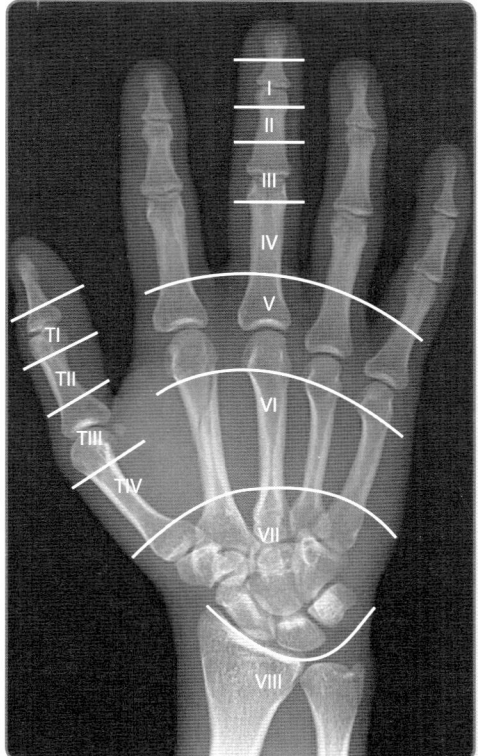

Figure 44.1 Extensor tendon zones of injury in the hand.

Topic 44

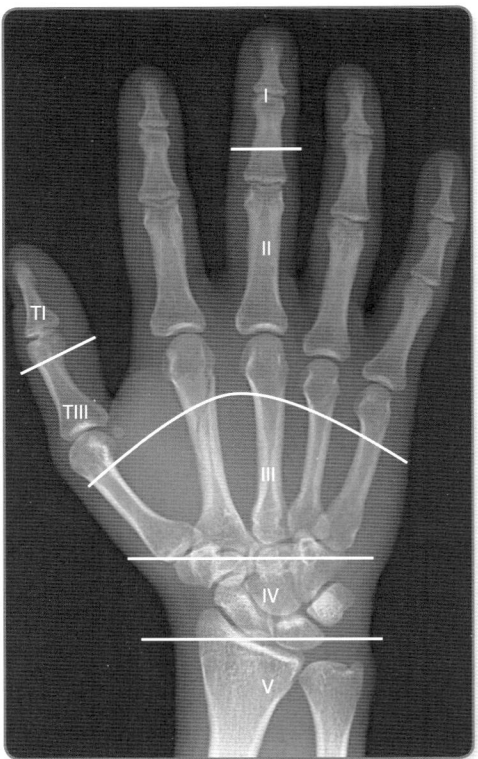

Figure 44.2 Flexor tendon zones of injury in the hand.

bruising. They require surgical reattachment. A similar injury occurs in the thumb with avulsion of FPL.

There are frequently associated injuries to neurovascular structures in the fingers, palm and wrist when a tendon is lacerated. These must be investigated preoperatively and repaired during surgery.

Clinical features

Open extensor tendon injuries are usually not difficult to identify clinically. The tendon is superficial and easily viewed in the base of a wound and resisted extension is either painful or absent. Pain on testing a tendon usually indicated damage but not the extent of injury to the tendon. Determining the extent of injury often requires local anaesthesia but this will facilitate thorough irrigation also. If pain prevents a definitive diagnosis, local anaesthetic can be used as a ring block and the examination repeated. This is a most useful test.

Closed injuries are more difficult diagnoses to make but using local anaesthetic, again, can help.

Open flexor tendon injuries often have associated injuries and the neurovascular status of the digits should be documented clearly in the notes before any local anaesthetic is used. Wounds should be thoroughly washed out with copious saline or under a running tap. Resisted flexion of each joint should be tested and a ring block used if pain prevents this. The digit may rest in a characteristic extended posture when a fist is made.

Investigations

Routine radiographs should be obtained in all tendon injuries as it has a profound effect on the diagnosis, healing and the requirements during surgery. Many mallet injuries and FDP avulsions have bony flakes or fragments of articular surface associated with them, which can easily be seen on radiographs.

Diagnosis

The diagnosis is usually made after a thorough history and examination. Specialist imaging techniques are rarely required but simple exploration in the emergency department under local anaesthetic can be most helpful.

Treatment

Extensor tendons

The extensor tendon is both thinner and flatter more distally and repair can be very difficult. More proximal to zone V the tendon can be repaired using familiar methods used in flexor tendon repairs. A guide for recommended types of repair at each zone is given in **Table 44.1**. Care must be taken in zone III & IV not to over-tension the repair and defunction the lateral bands.

Mallet injury: if joint is congruous; extension splinting for 8 weeks for soft-tissue injury and 6 weeks for bony injury. If joint not congruous; consider operative management with reduction of joint and K-wiring in extension. This is followed by active exercises and night splinting for 4–6 weeks.

Early active rehabilitation, such as the Norwich regime, for extensor tendon injury in zones III-VIII is now widely practiced. Exceptions include patients likely to be or unable to be compliant such as small children or those with multiple fractures in the hand. This active mobilisation prevents adhesions, which potentially may prevent full active flexion of the digits. Loss of flexion is far more disabling than loss of extension.

Flexor tendons

Flexor injuries are frequently open injuries and should be treated with copious washout under local anaesthesia if necessary to prevent flexor sheath infection.

The principles of repair of a flexor tendon is to achieve a meticulous repair with the ability to perform early active mobilisation to prevent adhesions. A non-absorbable braided (e.g. Ti-cron, Covidien) or monofilament suture (e.g. Prolene, Ethicon) should be used with diameter 3/0 and the peripheral suture being 5/0 or 6/0. A plethora of suture techniques are available but a locking suture technique, such as the Adelaide modification of the Savage repair has been shown to have superior gapping strength. The A2 and A4 pulleys should be protected at all times to confer biomechanical advantage to the tendon and prevent bowstringing. Flexor tendons should be repaired with a minimum of 4 strands crossing the tendon ends and a peripheral suture such as the Silfverskiöld technique should be employed. This can add up to 40% to the strength of the repair and aids gliding of the tendon.

Table 44.1 Extensor tendon zones and suitable type of repair

Zone I	Running 5/0 Prolene and transarticular K-wire for 6 weeks
Zone II	Running 5/0 Prolene and oversewn with Silfverskiöld repair (dorsum only)
Zone III–V	4/0 Prolene modified Kessler and oversewn with 5/0 Silfverskiöld repair (dorsum only)
Zone VI–VII	4/0 Prolene modified Kessler and oversewn with 5/0 Silfverskiöld repair (circumferential)

Rupture rates remain stubbornly between 5–10% but appear to be less when using 'wide awake hand surgery' techniques with intraoperative active movements. This utilises lignocaine with adrenaline and dispenses with the tourniquet. Patients actively flex their repaired tendon so the repair can be checked and adjusted as required.

Active mobilisation should begin within the first 4 days and many centres use the Belfast regime where a dorsal splint is applied with the wrist in 20–30° of flexion and MCPJs at 50–70° of flexion. The splint is worn constantly for 6 weeks and specialised hand therapists supervise the exercises. Excellent results can be obtained in 4 out of 5 patients but patients who rupture fair less well ultimately after revision repair or reconstruction.

Complications

- Immediate complications: damage to other neurovascular structures from the injury
- Early complications include infection, stiffness, rupture of repair, adhesions
- Late complications include stiffness, reduced grip strength, need for tenolysis (after 6 months)

Further reading

Langley C, Hobby J. Focus on: flexor tendon repair. J Bone Joint Surg Br 2009; 22:1-3.

Milner C, Russell P. Focus on: extensor tendon injury. J Bone Joint Surg Br 2011.

Related topics of interest

- *Topic 14* Compartment syndrome
- *Topic 40* Hand and wrist – carpal fractures

45 Head injury

Key points

- A low threshold for CT scan should be held for intoxicated patients with signs of head injury as they are at risk of intracranial bleeding and clinical examination can be difficult
- The cervical spine should be protected in all patients with blunt head injury until it can be proven to be clear of injury
- Urgent neurosurgical advice should be sought for patients with traumatic brain injury and care should be taken to avoid secondary brain injury

Introduction

Head injuries encompass trauma to the scalp, skull, dura, brain and to the blood vessels which supply these structures. A traumatic brain injury is a head injury which alters the level of consciousness. The severity is graded by the worst Glasgow Coma Score (GCS) score which occurs within the first 48 hours: 8 or less indicates a severe head injury, 9–12 is moderate and 13 or above is mild. Most head injuries are mild but around 0.2–0.3% of population in Europe and the United States will require admission to hospital each year.

Primary brain injury is due to haemorrhagic contusions, vessel disruption and nerve fibre disruption. Injuries can be considered as either focal or diffuse, although the two types often co-exist, particularly in more severe trauma. The primary brain injury also initiates neurochemical cascades which lead to cell death. These cascades are amplified by secondary insults to the brain. The primary brain injury cannot be treated, so the objective when managing patients with a head injury is to prevent secondary brain injury and further complications.

Assessment

Initial management of patients should be in line with Advanced Trauma Life Support (ATLS) guidelines. Mechanism of injury is an important indicator of the energy imparted, and may also raise concerns about abuse or intimate partner violence. Further assessment of patients with a brain injury should also include an accurate assessment of GCS. In the history, it is important to consider whether there could have been a medical reason for the accident (e.g. an arrhythmia or seizure) and also to record the duration of any loss of consciousness, retrograde or anterograde amnesia.

The presence of vomiting, a scalp haematoma or laceration should raise the suspicion of a skull vault fracture; depressed fractures should be palpated for due to the high incidence of associated underlying brain injury. Bilateral periorbital bruising and subconjunctival haemorrhage are seen when blood tracks from the back of the orbital cavity and are signs of a base of skull fracture. Other signs include leak of cerebrospinal fluid (CSF) from the nose or ear, blood leaking from the middle ear and, after 24–48 hours, the presence of mastoid bruising (Battle's sign).

Localising signs such as unilateral limb weakness should raise the suspicion of a space occupying lesion. Swelling or haematoma above the tentorium cerebellum can lead to with compression of the oculomotor nerve causing an ipsilateral dilated pupil with reduced response to light.

Investigation

CT scanning is the investigation of choice, as it is quick to obtain and sensitive for diagnosis of skull fractures, foreign body and space-occupying haematomas. 10% of patients with a severe head injury also have a spinal injury; the cervical spine should be imaged along with the head CT and the whole spine protected until it can be safely cleared. A low threshold should be adopted for scanning intoxicated patients as risks of head injury are increased accurate assessment is difficult. The National Institute for Health and Care Excellence (NICE) recommendations are outlined in **Table 45.1**.

Table 45.1 NICE guidelines for a CT scan in adults with a head injury	
Scan required within 1 hour of identifying one or more of the following:	Scan required within 8 hours of identifying one or more of the following:
• GCS score <13 upon initial assessment • GCS score <15 2 hours after initial assessment • Post-traumatic seizure • Focal neurological abnormality • Suspected open/depressed/base of skull fracture • Vomiting more than once	• Age >65 years • Coagulopathy/anticoagulant medication • High energy mechanism of injury • Retrograde amnesia for >30 minutes

MRI is more sensitive than CT scanning at detecting small areas of haemorrhage deep within the brain. However, most of the time this level of detail is not required for decision making in the early phases.

Since CT scanning has become so widely available, skull X-rays are mainly used for identifying facial fractures.

Skull fractures

Skull fractures may be linear or depressed, closed or open. A skull fracture increases the risk of intracranial haemorrhage, especially if the fracture line crosses one of the venous sinuses or the middle meningeal artery branches. Depressed fractures can directly cause a mass effect and also increase the risk of post-traumatic epilepsy. Most undisplaced skull fractures can be managed nonoperatively. Indications for surgery include fractures with depression of >1 cm and those with significant intracranial bleeding.

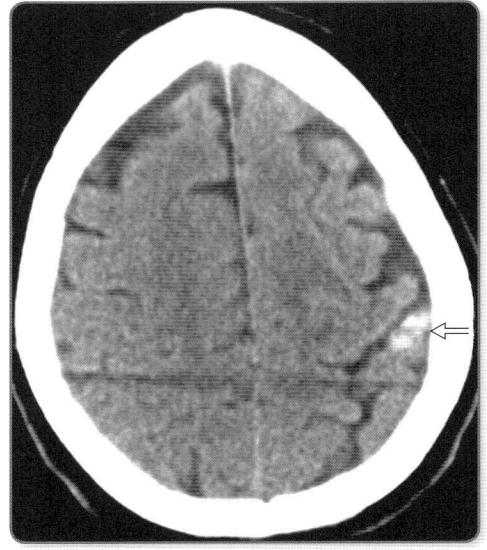

Figure 45.1 Haemorrhagic contusions with no significant mass effect.

Focal brain injury

Contusions occur when the brain impacts against the inside of the skull, as a result of sudden acceleration or deceleration. They may be seen either beneath the point of impact or on the opposite side of the brain (contre-coup) injury. The frontal and temporal lobes are frequently involved as head injuries are frequently caused by impact from the front. Bleeding may be seen on CT scan (**Figure 45.1**) but often the full extent of the contusion is not apparent on the initial scan. Bleeding and swelling associated with the contusions can lead to a reduction in level of consciousness.

Parenchymal injuries are caused by shearing forces within the brain, injury occurs by laceration of the small blood vessels.

Intracranial haematoma

Subarachnoid, subdural and extradural bleeding may be seen in isolation or in combination. **Figure 45.2** shows the relevant anatomy and dural layers.

Subarachnoid bleeding is most commonly caused by trauma, but it can also occur spontaneously from a ruptured aneurysm. Decompression can be performed if there is compromise due to a high intracranial

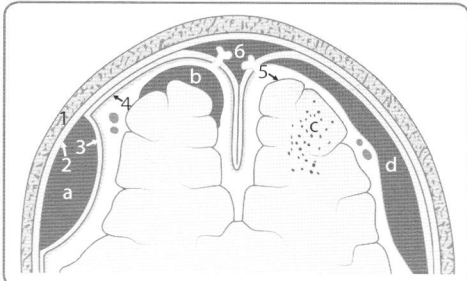

Figure 45.2 Anatomy relating to head injury. 1, skull; 2, periosteum; 3, dura mater; 4, arachnoid mater; 5, pia mater; 6, venous sinus. Extradural haematoma (a) is due to bleeding between the periosteum of the skull and the dura mater. Traumatic subarachnoid haemorrhage (b) refers to bleeding between the pia mater and the arachnoid mater; (c) shows parenchymal bleeding. A subdural haematoma (d) occurs when blood accumulates between the arachnoid mater and the dura mater.

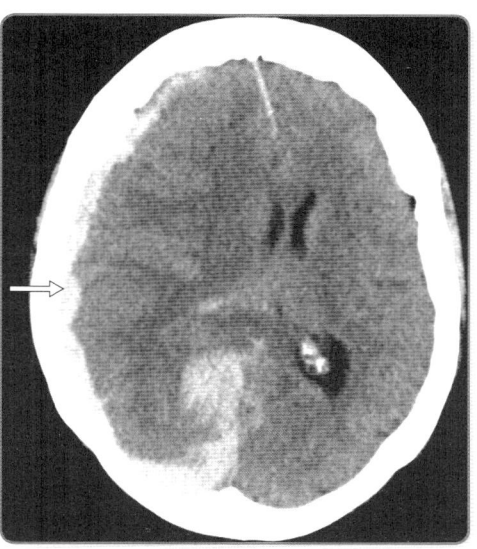

Figure 45.3 Subdural haematoma around the right cerebra hemisphere and in the interhemispheric fissure, with midline shift and partial effacement of the right lateral ventricle.

pressure which cannot be controlled by medical management.

A subdural haematoma is shown in **Figure 45.3**. The commonest causes of a subdural haematoma are tears to either a bridging vein which crosses the subdural space or a cortical vessel which runs across the surface of the brain. Subdural haematomas do not cross the midline, but can cross suture lines in the skull. Surgical evacuation of the haematoma should be considered in haematomas with a depth of >10 mm and those with >5 mm of midline shift.

Extradural (also known as epidural) bleeding is most often caused by a fracture that injures the middle meningeal artery or its branches although bleeding from a venous sinus will also lead to an extradural haematoma. They are less common in infants and the elderly as in these patients the dura is tightly adherent to the skull. Extradural haematomas rarely cross suture lines but may cross the midline (unlike subdural haematomas).

Most extradural haematomas are high-energy injuries and the patient is unconscious from the time of the impact. However in some patients there is a lucid interval of between 10 minutes and 8 hours as the haematoma collects. Surgery to relieve the pressure of the haematoma and to control the bleeding is indicated in patients with loss of consciousness, a large haematoma, or midline shift of 5 mm.

Generalised brain injury

Diffuse axonal injuries are due to high-energy trauma. There is shearing injury to the nerve fibres, particularly around the midline and the deep lobar white matter. Early CT scanning may show some associated haemorrhage but MRI is more sensitive.

Secondary brain injury

Secondary brain injury refers to brain damage caused after the initial trauma. Such damage can be minimised, by the following means:
- Maintaining tissue oxygenation. The blood pressure should be maintained at a normal level for the patient (often a mean arterial pressure of 90 is aimed for) with oxygen saturations of over 90%. The intracranial pressure should be controlled to give

a cerebral perfusion pressure (mean arterial blood pressure minus intracranial pressure) of at least 60 mmHg
- Normal electrolyte and metabolic status; in particular normoglycaemia should be maintained
- Prevention of seizures and pyrexia as these are associated with increase in the brain's metabolic requirements
- Prevention and treatment of coagulopathy to prevent secondary haemorrhage

Intracranial pressure and mass effects

The brain normally occupies 80% of the intracranial volume, blood around 10% and CSF around 10% and normal supine intracranial pressure is between 10 and 15 mmHg. The Monro–Kellie doctrine is based on the cranial cavity being rigid, and its contents being incompressible. **Figure 45.4** shows the relationship between intracranial volume and pressure.

Displacement of the brain can be caused by intracranial bleeding or oedema, giving rise to 'mass effects' such as midline shift or herniation. CT features depend on the location and size of the mass lesion. Herniation of the cingulated gyrus through the falx cerebri can obstruct CSF flow through the lateral ventricle, resulting in hydrocephalus. Herniation of the base of the temporal lobe through the tentorium cerebellum compresses the midbrain. Ultimately, with increasing mass effect, herniation of the cerebellar tonsils through the foramen magnum or 'coning' occurs.

Outcome and complications

Factors which affect outcome after traumatic brain injury include initial GCS, co-morbidities and concomitant injuries. Age is a strong independent determinant; elderly people who are comatose following head injury rarely have a good outcome and management decisions should take this into account.

Common complications include chest and urinary infection and venous thromboembolic disease. Seizures may occur at any time from immediately after the injury to some years later. Most patients who have a seizure within minutes of the trauma will not go on to have further seizures but some people who develop later onset epilepsy will require long-term treatment with phenytoin or carbamazepine. The CSF leak develops in 10% of patients who have a base of skull fracture. Most patients who have a dural tear present with rhinorrhoea or otorrhoea, within the first 48 hours of trauma although CSF rhinorrhoea can present months later. Air is seen on CT scan in a third of cases (**Figure 45.5**) and rarely the neurosurgical emergency of 'acute tension pneumoencephalus' can

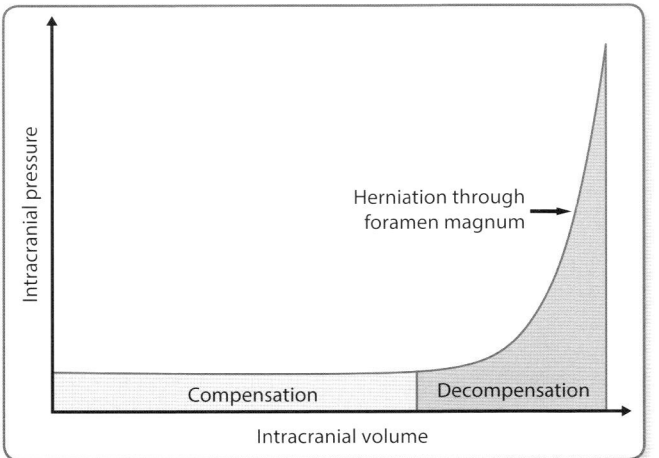

Figure 45.4 Initially swelling of the brain or haematoma formation can be compensated for by increased venous return, displacement of CSF to the spine and reuptake of CSF by the arachnoid villi. Once compensatory mechanisms have been exhausted small increases in volume lead to greater rises in intracranial pressure.

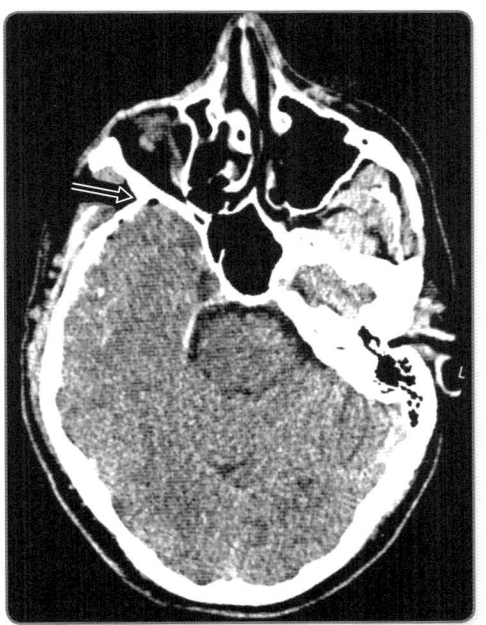

Figure 45.5 Presence of air bubbles within the cranium indicates a dural injury. CSF leakage may be observed and there is a risk of infection.

occur, if the dural tear communicates with the nasal cavity. The CSF rhinorrhoea can be differentiated from normal nasal discharge by glucose testing; normal CSF contains about 1/3 of the blood glucose level, whereas normal nasal discharge does not contain glucose. Dural tears can be complicated by meningitis or abscesses, therefore antibiotic prophylaxis should be considered. Treatment is initially nonoperative but fistulas which do not quickly resolve may need surgical repair. Syndrome of inappropriate antidiuretic hormone (SIADH) is the most common endocrine system problem that occurs following head injury. Low serum sodium is seen in conjunction with high urinary sodium.

Further reading

Corps KN, Roth TL, McGavern DB. Inflammation and neuroprotection in traumatic brain injury. JAMA Neurol 2015; 72:355–362.

Hutchinson PJ, Kolias AG, Timofeev IS, et al. Trial of decompressive craniectomy for traumatic intracranial hypertension. N Engl J Med 2016; 375:1119–1130.

Raj R, Mikkonen ED, Siironen J, et al. Alcohol and mortality after moderate to severe traumatic brain injury: a meta-analysis of observational studies. J Neurosurg 2016; 124:1684–1692.

Related topics of interest

- Topic 17 Damage control orthopaedics and trauma physiology
- Topic 62 Major trauma – Advanced Trauma and Life Support principles

46 Humeral fractures – distal

Key points
- Fractures of the distal humerus are relatively uncommon
- They can present very challenging injuries to manage
- Preoperative planning is essential
- Care must be taken to protect neurovascular structures

Epidemiology

Fractures of the distal humerus are relatively uncommon. They can occur as an isolated fracture to the distal humerus or as part of a more complex elbow injury. Single column fractures are rare, representing only 3% of all distal humerus fractures, and within this lateral column fractures are more common than medial. Bicolumn fractures contribute up to 70% of all distal humerus fractures.

As with many fractures, distal humerus fractures mainly occur in two population groups: younger men in high-energy trauma or elderly women with osteoporotic bone. Both of these cohorts can present very challenging injuries to manage, as there is often significant articular comminution and multiplanar fracture patterns.

Pathophysiology

The mechanism of injury for distal humerus fractures is usually either a direct below to the elbow or a fall on outstretched arm with the elbow in full extension. The force of the injury is transmitted along the ulna, causing it to drive into the distal humerus resulting in a fracture. The position of the elbow, direction of force and its magnitude will determine the fracture configuration. Higher energy injuries or poorer quality bone results in more comminuted fractures with more extensive metaphyseal involvement.

There is an associated risk of both neurological and vascular injury. The ulnar nerve is situated in the cubital tunnel next to the medial condyle; the median nerve lies with the brachial artery anteriorly; the radial nerve lies between brachialis and brachioradialis, just proximal to the elbow, and crosses anterior to the lateral condyle before dividing into the superficial radial nerve and posterior interosseous nerve. (**Figure 46.1**). The anatomical location of the nerves means they are vulnerable to injury from fracture fragments in displaced injuries.

Clinical features

The elbow is likely to be very painful, bruised and swollen and there may be clinical deformity. There may also be a feeling of instability. The forearm and wrist should be examined for any associated bony injury distally or clinical signs of compartment syndrome. A missed compartment syndrome can lead to Volkmann contracture. The soft tissues should be inspected for any evidence of an open injury. A formal assessment of the range of movement will be painful and unlikely to contribute to the diagnostic process.

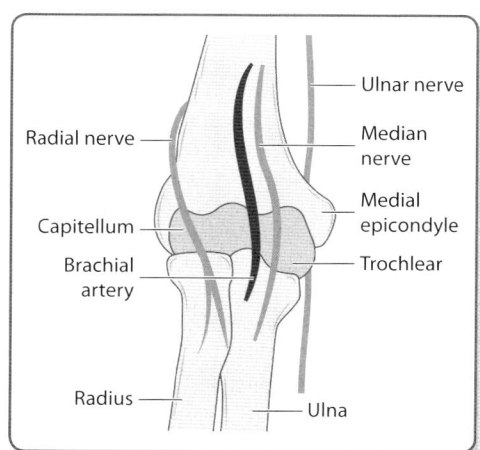

Figure 46.1 Neurovascular structures around the elbow.

Humeral fractures – distal

The neurological and vascular status of the limb can be compromised. A detailed neurovascular examination should be performed and documented. This should be repeated after application of plaster cast, as movement of the fracture or excessive flexion at the elbow can cause subsequent neurovascular compromise.

Investigations

Plain anteroposterior (AP) and lateral radiographs of the elbow are essential (**Figure 46.2**) and further AP and lateral radiographs of the forearm and wrist are recommended. Radiographs of the elbow should be repeated following application of a plaster cast.

Classification systems for these injuries are based on plain radiographs alone. However, current practice would suggest that CT imaging with 3D reconstructions should be performed routinely, particularly for complex fractures with articular involvement. CT imaging is valuable to analyse the fracture configuration to optimise pre-operative planning through consideration of the surgical approach, the articular reconstruction or any additional kit requirements.

Classification

There are many different classifications used for distal humerus fractures.

- The Milch classification: This addresses isolated unicondylar fractures (see **Figure 46.3**). This classification describes type I and type II fractures for either the lateral or medial condyle. The important feature is that in type I fractures the integrity of the relationship between the humerus and forearm is preserved, and therefore the elbow is stable. However, in type II injuries the fracture crosses the capitello-trochlear groove, disrupting the elbow joint making it an unstable injury.
- The Mehne and Matta classification: This was designed for preoperative planning for two column injuries. It describes the fracture pattern according to the shape of the fracture lines (see **Figure 46.4**).
- The Jupiter classification and the AO/OTA classification are both extensive detailed classification systems that can also be used categorise fracture pattern.

Treatment

The aim of management of these injuries is to restore normal joint anatomy and to regain elbow range of movement.

Nonoperative management

As stated earlier, stable unicondylar injuries are rare, so the indications for nonoperative management are few. Nondisplaced Milch type 1 fractures can be immobilised in an

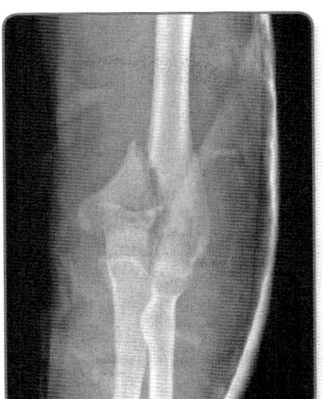

Figure 46.2 AP radiograph of a Milch type II medial condyle fracture.

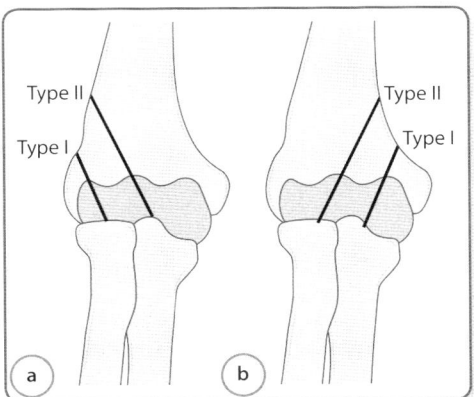

Figure 46.3 Milch classification of distal humerus fractures. (a) Lateral condyle fractures. (b) Medial condyle fractures.

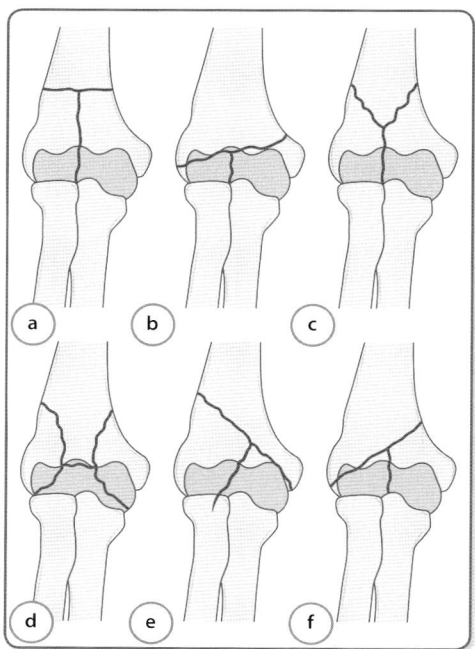

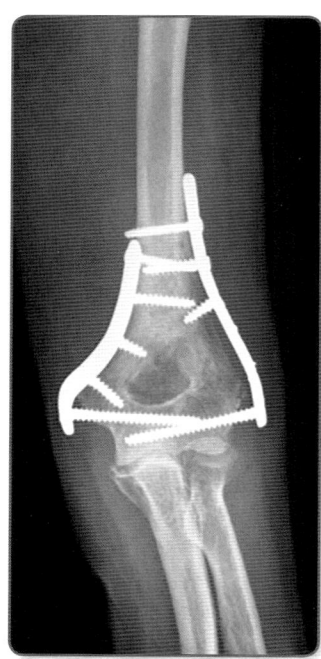

Figure 46.5 AP radiograph postoperative open reduction and internal fixation.

Figure 46.4 Mehne and Matta classification of distal humerus fractures. (a) High T. (b) Low T. (c) Y. (d) H. (e) Lateral lambda. (f) Medial lambda.

above elbow plaster. For medial condyle fractures, the forearm should be positioned in pronation; for lateral condyle fractures the forearm should be in supination. The other indications for nonoperative management are patients with bicolumn injuries who are not medically fit to be a surgical candidate. In these cases, the 'bag of bones' approach can be adopted using a collar and cuff or hinged brace, promoting early range of movement to limit stiffness. A functional range of movement to facilitate self-care, i.e. feeding and personal hygiene is the goal in these cases.

Operative management

- Closed reduction and percutaneous fixation – this can be used for displaced Milch type 1 fractures. Supracondylar fractures in adults do not have the same tough periosteum to reinforce K-wire fixation as they do in children; therefore, it is not usually a stable enough fixation construct to manage adult supracondylar type fractures.
- Open reduction internal fixation – this is the mainstay of operative treatment to achieve a stable fixation to allow early gentle range of movement. The principles of fixation are to reconstruct the articular surface and then attach the articular unit to the humeral shaft with bicolumn plate fixation. Anatomical contoured plates with locking screw options are often used (see **Figure 46.5**). A good exposure to the joint is necessary and olecranon osteotomy is sometimes required to visualise the joint surface. Ulnar nerve transposition should be considered to protect the nerve from compression from the plate.
- Total elbow arthroplasty – this is an option for elderly patients with bicolumn injuries or significant comminution with poor quality bone, in cases when the elbow is not reconstructible.

Complications

Early complications
- Nerve injury is the most commonly reported postoperative complication, surgeons must be meticulous to protect the neurovascular structures
- Vascular injury

Late complications
- Stiffness is the main problem as most patients are unlikely to regain full extension after a significant injury, although enabling an early range of movement with targeted physiotherapy has been shown to be beneficial
- Malunion can occur if there is collapse of the medial or lateral column causing cubitus valgus and cubitus varus respectively
- Heterotopic ossification

Further reading

Court-Brown C, Heckman JD, McKee M, et al. Rockwood and Green's Fractures in Adults, 8th Ed. Philadelphia, PA: Lippincott Williams and Wilkins; 2014.

Jupiter JB. Internal fixation for fracture about the elbow. Op Tech Orthop 1994; 4:34.

Jupiter JB, Mehne DK. Fractures of the distal humerus. Orthopaedics 1992; 15:825–833.

Related topics of interest

- *Topic 18* Elbow – dislocations and associated fractures
- *Topic 47* Humeral fractures – proximal
- *Topic 75* Paediatric humeral condylar fractures

47 Humeral fractures – proximal

Key points
- The majority of proximal humerus fractures can be managed nonoperatively
- Early physiotherapy input is essential

Epidemiology

Fractures of the proximal humerus represent approximately 5% of all fractures. They mainly occur in two differing populations: low-energy injuries in elderly osteoporotic patients and high-energy injuries in younger patients. Proximal humerus fractures most often occur in falls from a standing height onto an outstretched arm. Due to the association with osteoporosis, these fractures are more common in females at a ratio of 2:1 and the incidence is increasing with an ageing population.

Fractures of the proximal humerus can be associated with dislocation of the humeral head and can be complicated by the presence of a neurovascular injury, particularly in higher energy injuries.

Pathophysiology

Proximal humerus fractures occur in large variety of fracture patterns (**Figure 47.1**). The fracture pattern often dictates subsequent management and outcome; therefore, it is essential to understand the fracture configuration. Furthermore, there may be a pre-existing pathology in the shoulder, such as a rotator cuff tear, which may impact on decision making in the management of the fracture.

Clinical features

The patient presents with swelling and pain in the shoulder. There is often significant bruising extended down the arm, to the elbow and across the chest. The neurological and vascular status of the limb should be

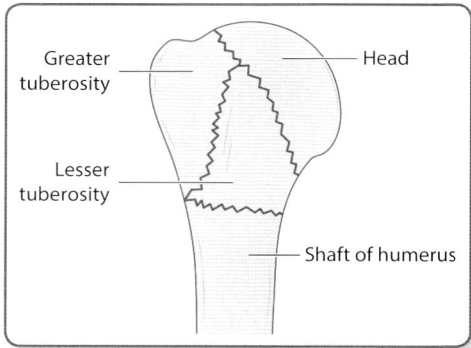

Figure 47.1 Fracture segments of the proximal humerus.

thoroughly examined and documented. The most commonly affected nerve is the axillary nerve. Compromise of the axillary nerve will result in altered sensation over the regimental patch, however, motor function can be difficult to ascertain due to pain on moving the arm although it should be possible to see or feel the fibres of the deltoid muscle contracting.

The axillary vessels may also be damaged causing impaired blood flow or pseudoaneurysm. Any suspicion of injury should prompt further imaging such as Doppler studies or CT angiography and the involvement of the vascular team.

Proximal humerus injuries can also present as open injuries, these may only be small breaches in the skin due to sharp bone spikes in fragile soft tissues so careful examination is required to identify these. In addition, the whole patient should be examined for any concurrent injury.

Investigations

Plain radiographs including anteroposterior (AP), scapular Y lateral and axillary views are recommended. CT scans are useful to more clearly delineate the fracture configuration, particularly for comminuted and intra-articular fractures, to guide both management and preoperative planning. Assessing the muscle bulk in the supraspinatus and subscapular fossae on CT scan can help formulate an impression as to whether or not there has been a pre-existing rotator cuff tear, as the presence of a tear will result in atrophy of the muscles. However, MRI is the investigation of choice for a more detailed assessment of the soft tissues.

Classification

The Neer classification is the most commonly used classification for proximal humerus fractures (**Figure 47.2**). It is based on the anatomy of 4 constituents of the proximal humerus: the greater tuberosity, lesser tuberosity, humeral head and humeral shaft. The Neer classification considers a fragment displaced if there is >45° of angulation or the fragment has displaced >1 cm. It is important to understand there may be up to 4 fracture lines yet this would still be classified as a one-part fracture if none of these fragments are displaced by >45° or >1 cm.

The AO/OTA classification provides a detailed system for categorising proximal humerus fractures. This system has three main categories: extra-articular unifocal, extra-articular bifocal and intra-articular fractures. The AO/OTA system also includes fracture dislocations.

Treatment

The function of the upper limb is to place the hand in space in order to perform tasks. This requires a pain free, functional range of movement at the shoulder. This is the aim for management of proximal humerus fractures,

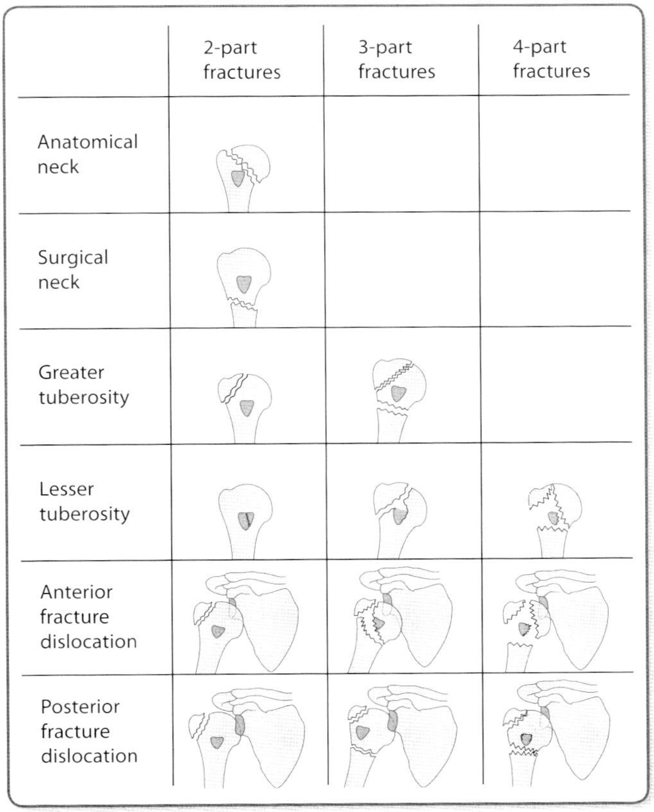

Figure 47.2 Neer classification of proximal humerus fractures.

whilst also minimising complications such as nonunion, malunion and avascular necrosis. Early physiotherapy is essential to promote early movement and rehabilitation can last up to 18 months.

Nonoperative management

The majority of proximal humerus fractures can be managed nonoperatively. This includes one and two-part fractures, multifragmentary fractures if they are minimally displaced, and also displaced fractures in a population who are not medically fit for surgery. Collar and cuff immobilisation allows ligamentotaxis to help maintain good alignment. Early physiotherapy input is essential to minimise stiffness in the shoulder, elbow and wrist, which can occur from prolonged immobilisation in a sling.

Operative management

There is a variety or surgical interventions available according to the fracture configuration and the patient's fitness for surgery.

- Open reduction internal fixation (ORIF) – can be used for 2-, 3- or 4-part fractures, especially in younger patients. There has been a move towards anatomically contoured plates with locking options for osteoporotic bone (**Figure 47.3**)
- Intraoperative imaging must be scrutinised to prevent screw penetration into the joint
- Intramedullary nail – is a useful option in segmental fractures and for pathological fractures, the entry point of the nail can cause damage to the rotator cuff so care must be taken
- Hemiarthroplasty – for use in severely comminuted fractures or articular fractures in the elderly. Reduction of the tuberosities is essential to achieving rotator cuff function
- Total shoulder arthroplasty – for use with concurrent glenohumeral osteoarthritis with an intact rotator cuff
- Reverse geometry shoulder replacement – for use in elderly patients with poor rotator cuff function, either due to nonrepairable tuberosities or due to pre-existing pathology (**Figure 47.4**)

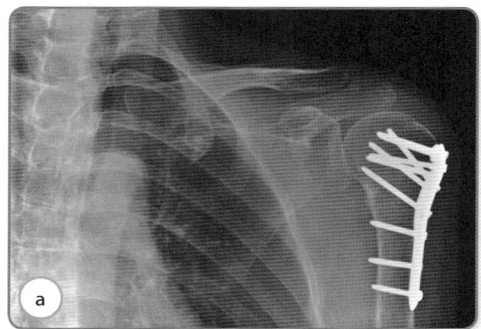
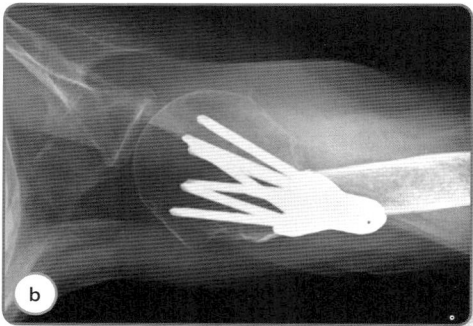

Figure 47.3 ORIF following proximal humeral fracture: anterior (a) and posterior (b) views.

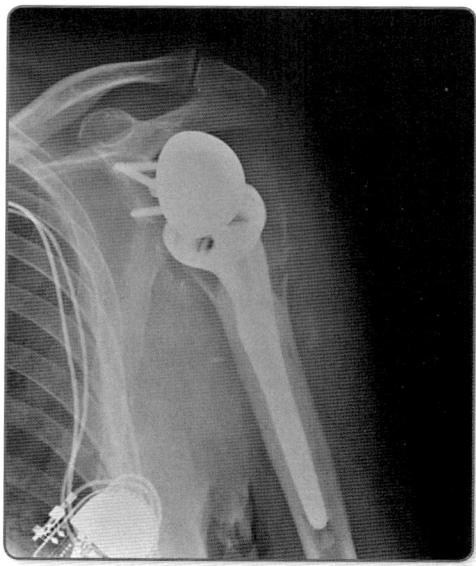

Figure 47.4 Postoperative anteroposterior radiograph – reverse shoulder arthroplasty.

Humeral fractures – proximal

Complications

Immediate complications
- Neurological or vascular injury (see previously)

Early complications
- Stiffness and adhesive capsulitis
- Postoperative infection

Late complications
- Avascular necrosis occurs due to loss of blood supply to the humeral head and may necessitate replacement arthroplasty
- Malunion is often well tolerated as there is an innate ability for the shoulder joint to compensate due to its natural capacity for a wide a range of movement. In symptomatic malunions, treatment is corrective osteotomy or arthroplasty
- Nonunion can be managed operatively or nonoperatively. In the elderly, arthroplasty is the mainstay of treatment
- Implant failure; the use of replacement arthroplasty in shoulders for trauma is increasing, but the implant survivorship in these cases is as of yet not known

Further reading

Boyle MJ, Youn SM, Frampton CM, Ball CM. Functional outcomes of reverse shoulder arthroplasty compared with hemiarthroplasty for acute proximal humeral fractures. J Shoulder Elbow Surg 2013; 22:32–37.

Kontakis G, Koutras C, Tosounidis T, Giannoudis P. Early management of proximal humeral fractures with hemiarthroplasty: A systematic review. J Bone Joint Surg Br 2008; 90:1407–1413.

Neer CS. Displaced proximal humeral fractures part II. Treatment of three-part and four-part displacement. J Bone Joint Surg Am 1970; 52:1090–1103.

Related topics of interest

- *Topic 46* Humeral fractures – distal
- *Topic 89* Shoulder dislocations
- *Topic 84* Principles of nonoperative management of fractures

48 Imaging – description and interpretation

Key points

- Accurate description is essential for communication
- Clinical context is key to guiding interpretation
- Seeking an expert opinion from a radiologist is invaluable

Introduction

In orthopaedics, the history and examination of a patient is often supplemented with further imaging. There is a wide range of imaging modalities available, as discussed later, but the basic concepts for describing all imaging remains constant. An accurate description is essential for clear communication and correctly interpreting the image is essential in generating a diagnosis and formulating a management plan.

Fracture terminology

There are many different terms used to describe imaging as listed below. The description should always relate to the position of the distal part of the fracture in relation to the proximal part.

Describing the fracture location:
- Identify the bone
- Proximal, middle or distal third
- Intra-articular or extra-articular

Describing the fracture displacement (Figure 48.1):
- Translation – the shift of the fragment as a percentage, 100% translated is 'off-ended'
- Angulation – varus/valgus and anterior/posterior or radial/ulnar and volar/dorsal in the forearm and hand. This relates to the distal fracture fragment in relation to the proximal part. Describing which direction the apex of the fracture is pointing is helpful too
- Length – shortening or distraction
- Rotation – a twist on the longitudinal axis
- Impaction – compression of the bone
- Avulsion – a fragment of bone that has been pulled off by its soft tissue attachments

Describing the fracture type (Figure 48.2):
- Transverse
- Oblique
- Spiral
- Comminuted

Paediatric terminology:
- Greenstick – an incomplete fracture involving the tension side of the bone
- Torus – an incomplete fracture involving the compression side of the bone

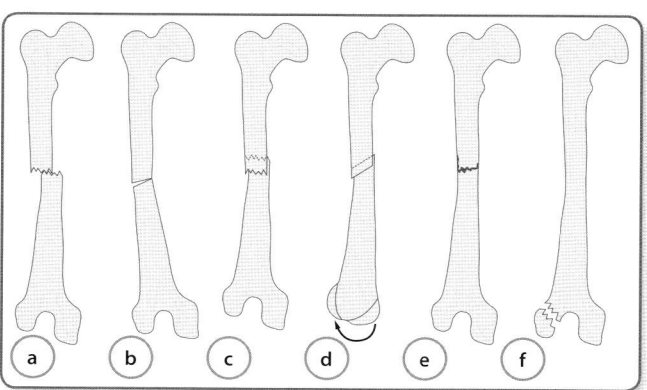

Figure 48.1 Types of fracture displacement. (a) Translation. (b) Angulation. (c) Shortening. (d) Rotation. (e) Impaction. (f) Avulsion.

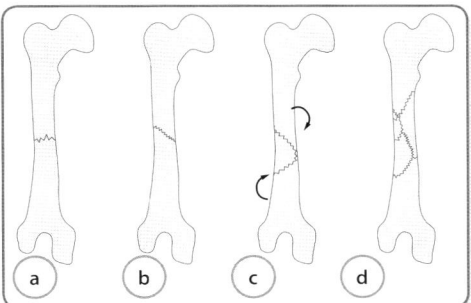

Figure 48.2 Types of fracture. (a) Transverse. (b) Oblique. (c) Spiral. (d) Comminuted.

Describing joint congruity:
- Dislocation – loss of congruity between two joint surfaces
- Subluxation – partial or incomplete dislocation

Describing the plane:
It is important to note on 3D imaging such as MRI and CT scanning, the plane of the imaging should be identified: axial, sagittal and coronal.

Interpretation

When interpreting any form of imaging it is important to be aware of the clinical context: the age of the patient, the mechanism of injury, relevant medical history and examination findings.

It also needs to be established whether or not the imaging is appropriate to answer the clinical question and there are several components that determine this. Firstly, is this the correct imaging modality? Secondly, is it an adequate study? For example, for a plain radiograph there must be orthogonal views (two perpendicular), the joints above and below should be imaged and the radiograph should have adequate exposure and penetration to enable interpretation.

Moving on to analysing and interpreting the image, it is useful to have a systematic approach to ensure nothing is missed. Moving from superficial to deeper structures may be a useful technique.

- Soft tissue – is there any obvious skin or soft tissue loss? Are there any foreign bodies? Is there any soft tissue swelling? Is there any gas evident that may suggest an open injury?
- Bones – is there any cortical irregularity or discontinuity? Are there any bony lesions? Is there any callus present?
- Joints – are there signs of a joint effusion, e.g. elevated fat pads around the elbow? Is there a lipohaemarthrosis? Are there any signs of degenerative disease?

Additional factors that may aid interpretation are whether or not there has been previous imaging, or if the contralateral side has been imaged. This can be very useful for comparison or to see a change over time. In difficult cases, or with more complex imaging modalities, seeking an opinion from a musculoskeletal radiologist is extremely useful.

Further reading

Greenspan A, Beltran J. Orthopaedic imaging: a practical approach. 6th Ed. Philadelphia, PA: Lippincott Williams and Wilkins; 2014.

Raby N, Berman L, Morley S, de Lacey G. Accident and emergency radiology: a survival guide. 3rd Ed. Philadelphia, PA: Saunders Ltd, 2014.

Related topics of interest

- *Topic 11* Classification of fractures
- *Topic 49* Imaging modalities
- *Topic 77* Paediatric physeal fractures

49 Imaging modalities

Key points
- Exposure to ionising radiation for patients and surgeons should be minimised
- Ultrasound and MRI provide the best imaging of soft tissues

Ionising radiation and radiographs

Radiographs are produced using X-rays. X-rays are ionising radiation and therefore may damage cells either by direct interaction with DNA or through free radical production. Different tissues absorb different amounts; the remainder strike a receiver, originally photographic film; now more commonly a fluorescing substance coupled with an electronic receiver producing an image.

All radiation exposure must be justified, optimised (kept as low as reasonably achievable) and limited – the exposure of individuals should be kept below annual dose limits – 20 mSv for the occupationally exposed and 1 mSv for a member of the public.

The voltage controls the number of X-rays produced and their energy; increasing the current increases the number of X-rays only. An X-ray machine contains an aluminium filter to remove low energy rays that would be absorbed by the body and increase dose without contributing to the effect of imaging. X-rays obey the inverse square law where doses fall in inverse proportion to the square of the distance to the receiver – double the distance gives a quarter of the dose.

To minimise the dose when using fluoroscopy maximise your distance from the fluoroscope, decrease number and duration of exposures – avoid real time screening, position the patient as close as possible to the detector reducing dose and scatter. Use PPE including thyroid shields. Do not use the detector as an operating table – not only does this increase dose but if pierced may result in an explosion.

Computed tomography scans

CT scans also use ionising radiation. The source and receiver rotate around the patient and a computerised algorithm reconstructs this data into a three-dimensional (3D) image. Densities are reported in Hounsfield units which are calibrated from the density of pure water – 1000 and air – 0. Different windows can be applied to the scan emphasising tissues of different densities. Images are displayed in slices which represent the average density over that thickness. Modern scanners acquire data as they move in a spiral around the patient rather than a step-wise movement of the patient for discreet slices. They also tend to have multiple detectors resulting in faster scan acquisition and reduced artefact. The data received can be reformatted to give coronal or sagital images or 3D reconstructions.

Contrast may be given with CT scans to highlight vascular anatomy. This is generally iodine based. It can cause renal failure, generally in those with pre-existing renal impairment.

The main disadvantage of CT scanning is the associated radiation dose. A CT head gives a 2-mSv dose equivalent to 100 chest X-rays. A CT abdomen and pelvis is 10 mSv. Thinner slices increase the dose.

Nuclear medicine

Nuclear medicine involves the administration of an intravenous radioactive agent. This is taken up by different areas and the decay begins. The resulting γ-radiation is detected by a γ-camera which works in a similar manner to an X-ray detector. The metastable isotope of Technetium (Tc99m) is most commonly used. The 6-hour half-life allows reasonable imaging times and reduces the dose required. It may be labelled with other compounds to control where it is taken up. Bone scans use Tc99m labelled methyl diphosphinate which is taken up by osteoblasts and will therefore show areas of increased bone turnover such as fractures or tumours. However, if there is osteoclastic activity only, such as in myeloma, or if the spread of disease is such that there are no discrete tumours; then bone scans may give a false negative. Bone scans are also used for investigation of painful prosthetic joints with increased signal suggestive of loosening but although this is a sensitive investigation it is not specific and will not discriminate between infection or aseptic loosening.

Single-positron emission photon computerised tomography rotates the camera around the patient to form images that represent a slice of tissue in a similar manner to CT scans allowing 3D localisation of a tumour although the images generated are not as good as a CT scan with more noise and poorer resolution.

Positron emission tomography scans use 18 F labelled deoxyglucose to highlight areas of increased metabolic activity. This can be combined with CT.

Ultrasound imaging

Ultrasound uses sound waves rather than ionising radiation. These are produced by a transducer which uses the piezoelectric effect: application of an electric current to a material deforms it and this mechanical deformation produces ultrasound waves. When the waves pass between tissues of different densities a proportion, depending on the difference between densities, is reflected back. This is picked up by the detector, again via the piezoelectric effect and converted into the picture. Doppler ultrasonography detects the frequency shift from flowing fluid and can therefore demonstrate flow in vessels.

Fine density differences within a tissue type also give a signal; the resolution can be much better than CT or MRI. During a musculoskeletal scan the structure of interest can be moved allowing a dynamic picture to be developed. Ultrasound can also be used in real time to guide needle placement for injections, aspirations or biopsy.

A coupling gel is necessary to avoid the abrupt changes in density between room air and skin. Bowel gas also obscures imaging of underlying structures. Cortical bone or other calcified structures strongly reflect back the signal leading to acoustic shadowing – nothing behind the structure can be seen – or reverberation – a series of echogenic lines on the interface. In the obese patient or if deeper imaging is required then a lower frequency probe is used; but this reduces resolution. There is a learning curve and review of saved images imparts less information than is gained at the time of the examination.

Magnetic resonance imaging

MRI does not involve ionising radiation as it is based on the absorption and emission of energy by atoms in an external magnetic field. Scanning is principally based on the behaviour of hydrogen atoms although gadolinium, a paramagnetic element may be used as a contrast agent as its nucleus also has an odd number of proton and neutrons. The atoms are placed in a high magnetic field, generally of between 1.5–3 Tesla and due to unbalanced spin act almost as tiny magnets and become aligned. They are then subjected to radiofrequency pulses that flip them at right angles to the magnetic field. As they flip back they emit a further pulse that is detected by the voltage receiver coils. Again computer algorithms are used to derive a 3-D picture from the received signal.

Hydrogen ions that are bonded in fat have different behaviour to ones in water. The main elements are described as T1 and T2. T1 measures the exponential growth or gain of magnetism (of alignment) by the tissue. T2 measures exponential decay or for how long the tissues remain magnetically aligned. Fat has short T1 and T2, liquids have long T1 and T2. Other tissues are intermediate depending on the fat/water mix.

Different sequences are acquired by varying TR – the time to pulse repetition – and TE – the time to echo or to reform and receive the pulse. Short TR and TE emphasise T1, fat and fluid are bright. Increasing TE and TR increases T2; water is brighter, fat dark, and pathology, or at least oedema, shows up better.

As the signal characteristics for each sequence vary; each separate sequence is acquired separately. Data cannot be reformatted or post processed. Multiple sequences require more time.

Other common sequences are proton density (PD) – a mix of T1 and T2, good for looking at menisci. Short tau inversion ratio (STIR) has both a long TE and TR, therefore, decreases fat signal intensity and makes fluid more visible. This is useful for, as an example, demonstrating ongoing oedema in vertebral fractures. T2* alters the flip angle to 16–80°. This increases signal from fluid but also increases artefact. This is useful in looking for haemorrhage. Fast spin/turbo – T2 and PD together – faster acquisition time but decreased sensitivity this sequence also reduces artefact from metal.

MRI does not involve ionising radiation but the safety of the scan in the first trimester is not yet established. In addition, the strong magnetic field can have unfortunate effects on ferromagnetic objects including oxygen cylinders, trolleys, wheelchairs; also hearing aids, jewellery, watches, glasses and credit cards.

Some modern pacemakers, cochlear implants, aneurysm clips and intravascular coils, filters and stents are MRI compatible but most are not. Implantable cardioverter defibrillators (ICDs), neurostimulators, insulin pumps, Swan-Ganz catheters are not. Metallic orbital foreign bodies are a contraindication. Orthopaedic implants are not contraindicated. They may degrade images and should be mentioned in the request so appropriate sequences can be planned. Surgical staples are compatible as are intrauterine contraceptive devices (IUCDs), halo vests and most heart valves and penile implants although again this must be checked.

Some patients cannot tolerate the tight confines of the scanner, some morbidly obese patients will not fit. Open magnet scanners are available but operate at lower magnetic field strength and give poorer quality images. They are not widely available.

Further reading

Dewey P, George S, Gray A. Ionising radiation and orthopaedics. Current Orthop 2005; 19:1–12.

McKie S, Brittenden J. Basic science: magnetic resonance imaging. Current Orthop 2005; 19:13–19.

Related topics of interest

- *Topic 1* Amputations – mangled extremities and decision making
- *Topic 11* Classification of fractures
- *Topic 48* Imaging – description and interpretation

50 Implants – circular external fixators

Key points
- Circular external fixator is based on the mechanical principles of beam loading
- Limb reconstruction units provide specialist care

History of the circular external fixator

The circular external fixator was developed in the 1950s by the orthopaedic surgeon Gavriil Abramovich Ilizarov to treat nonunions, and he discovered distraction osteogenesis by chance.

Since that time there have been different evolutions of circular external fixator frames. Dr Charles Taylor from the USA developed the Taylor Spatial Frame, which is based on a hexapod system but designed to be easier to use and more accurate, and and its use was expanded in the field of deformity correction. Computer software has subsequently been developed to assist in the fine-tuning of frames in deformity correction.

The use of circular external fixators requires sub-specialist expertise and an infrastructure to facilitate specialist patient care, from surgeons and nurses, as an inpatient and outpatient. Due to this, the use of circular frames is mainly based in specialised limb reconstruction units.

Pathophysiology

Distraction osteogenesis is based on the principle of tension–stress, in which new bone is formed in response to an increase in tension.

Callus forms at the site of injury, or in a planned osteotomy, tension is applied through the wires of the frame causing a controlled distraction force. The distraction continues at a rate of 1 mm a day, as 0.25 mm increments four times a day. This stimulates callus to form in a column to fill the defect and subsequently ossify to consolidate the bony column.

Indications

These include:
- Treatment of nonunion
- Limb lengthening
- Bone transport
- Deformity correction
- Management of fractures, open and closed

Construction

Circular external fixators consist of a series of rings, interconnected by struts. A combination of half pins, olive wires and fine wires are then positioned through the bone and connected to the rings. A foot plate can also be added to enable weight bearing.

Altering the following factors can increase the stability of the frame:

- Increasing the number of rings
- Decreasing the diameter of the rings
- Moving the rings closer around the defect or site of injury
- Increasing the number, and the diameter of wires
- Increasing the tension on the wires
- Placing the wires in an orthogonal configuration

Case examples

Bone transport: The patient was involved in a road traffic accident sustaining an open tibial fracture. A circular frame was used for bone transportation to fill the bony defect (**Figures 50.1–50.3**).

Topic 50

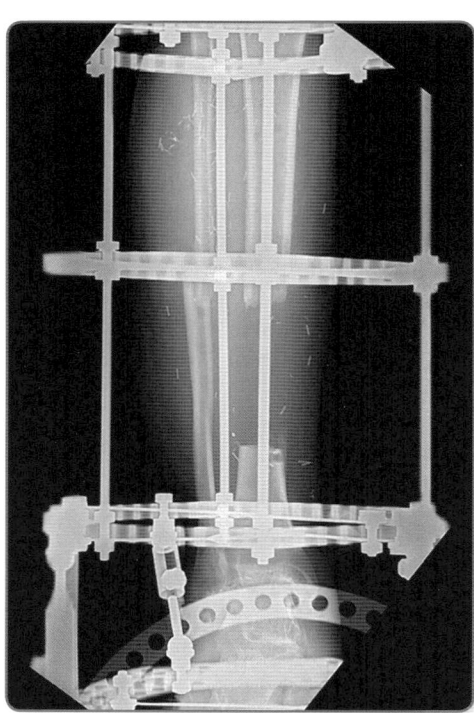

Figure 50.1 Bony defect.

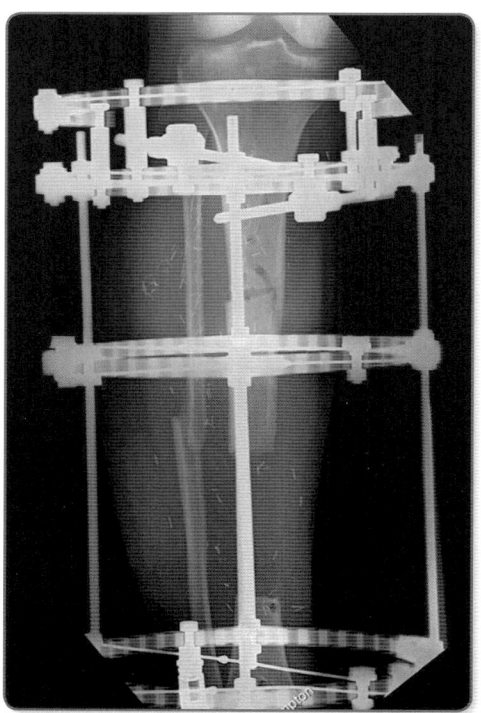

Figure 50.2 Proximal osteotomy and bone transport.

Implants – circular external fixators

Deformity correction: The patient presented with an impending stress fracture due to varus malunion from a previous fracture (**Figures 50.4–50.6**).

Complications

- Pin site infection is a common complication and can usually be managed with oral antibiotics
- Periprosthetic fracture may necessitate revision surgery
- Patient compliance can be an issue as the circular frames have a significant bio-psycho-social impact, therefore, patient selection and counselling is important

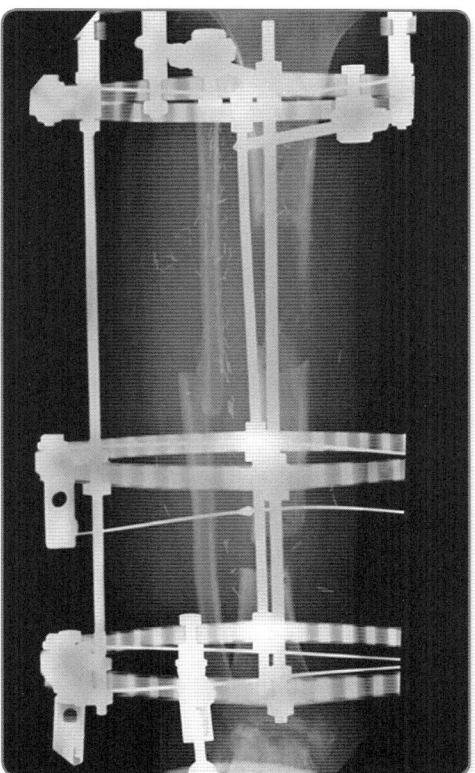

Figure 50.3 Bone transport continues. Note the proximal ossification filling in the defect.

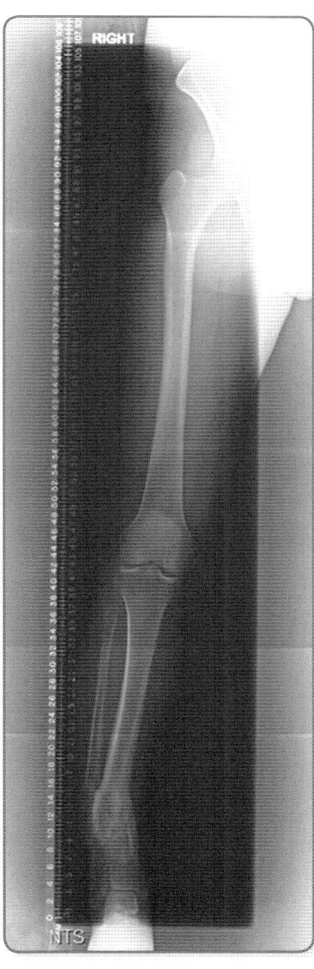

Figure 50.4 Varus malunion of a tibial fracture.

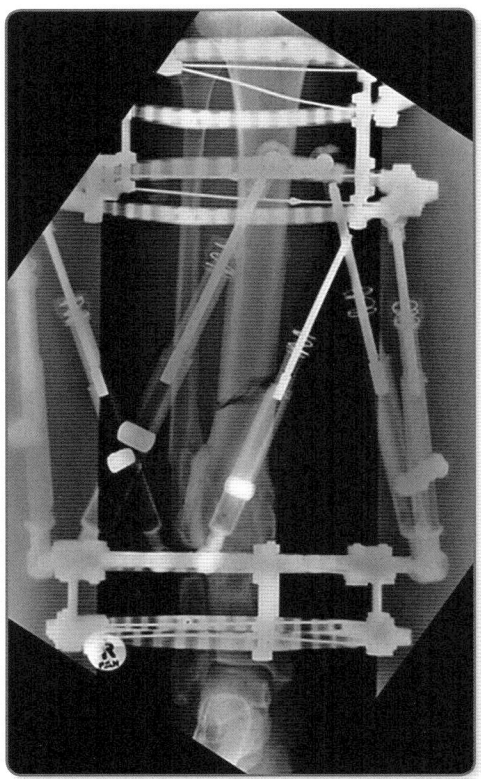

Figure 50.5 Application of circular frame and osteotomy.

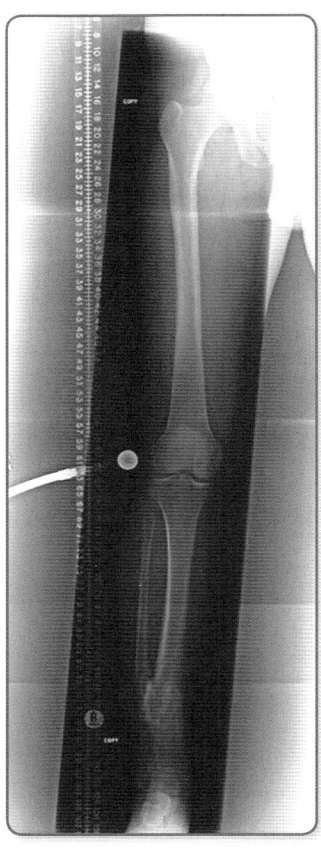

Figure 50.6 Long leg alignment views following removal of the frame.

Further reading

Horas K, Schnettler R, Maier G, Schneider G, Horas U. The role of soft tissue traction forces in bone segment transport for callus distraction. Strategies Trauma Limb Reconstr 2015; 10:21–26.

Ilizarov S, Rozbruch R. Limb lengthening and reconstruction surgery, 1st ed. Boca Raton, FL: CRC Press; 2006.

Solomin L. The Basic Principles of External Skeletal Fixation using the Ilizarov device. Berlin: Springer; 2008.

Related topics of interest

- *Topic 8* Bone loss – options for reconstruction
- *Topic 51* Implants – monolateral external fixators
- *Topic 67* Nonunion of fractures

51 Implants – monolateral external fixators

Key points
- External fixators allow rapid stabilisation of injuries
- They can be used with a compromised soft tissue envelope
- External fixation can provide either temporary or definitive management strategies

Introduction
External fixators allow relatively basic and rapid stabilisation of fractures. This can be temporary, as part of a damage control protocol or soft tissue stabilisation, or definitively taking the fracture all the way to union. They can be used in compromised soft tissues to obtain fracture fixation with percutaneous pin placement.

Advantages of external fixation
- Rapid application
- Minimal disruption to the soft tissue envelope
- Minimal disruption to bone vascularity
- Management of open fractures
- Staged management of closed fractures (tibial pilon, plateau, etc.)
- Allows other surgical specialties (vascular, plastics) to work on the limb with skeletal control
- Potentially adjustable without further surgery

External fixator structure (Figures 51.1 and 51.2)
A. **Pin** – drilled into the bone and allows the fixator to be coupled to the bone
B. **Clamp** – attaches the bone pin to the bar or the other bar to another bar
C. **Bars or rods** – attaches bone pins to each other and hence joins bone segments together via a frame construct
D. **Clamp** – bar-to-bar connection

Bone pins
- Increasing the diameter of the bone pin subsequently increases the frame stability. However, the pin size shouldn't exceed 30% of the bone diameter as has been related to an increased fracture risk
- The pins are radially preloaded with the pin being slightly larger than the pilot hole
- Two pins are required in each segment to provide rotational control
- The thread length should exceed the diameter of the bone diameter. To maximise pull-out strength all threads should be in contact with the bone
- Self-drilling, self-tapping pins lead to increased rates of thermal necrosis and have been related to pin loosening. Therefore, it is recommended that bones should be predrilled and tapped, especially if the fixator is to be retained for any significant period of time
- Some pins are coated, with for example hydroxyapatite, to reduce likelihood of loosening
- Pin location should be away from the zone of injury and if possible away from any

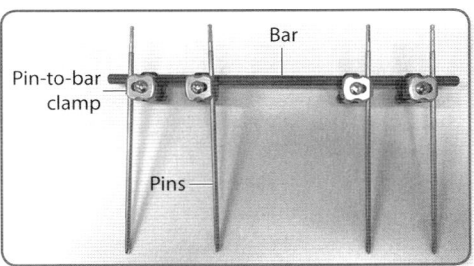

Figure 51.1 Basic monolateral fixator components.

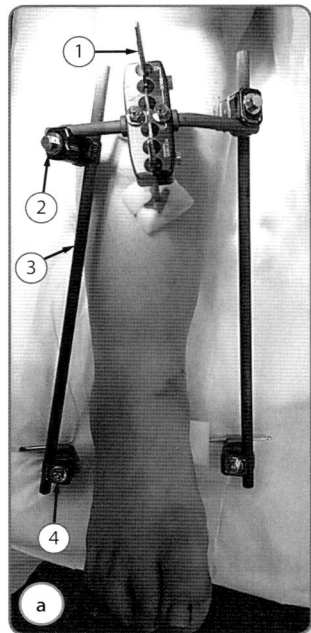

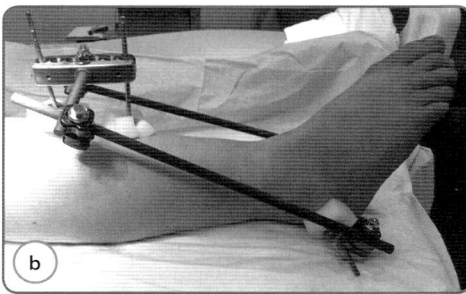

Figure 51.2 A standard A-frame construct for a distal tibial fracture. (a) Lateral and (b) anterior views. ① Pins. ② Bar-to-bar clamp. ③ Bar. ④ Pin-to-bar clamp.

and relaxing skin incisions minimise disruption. Pre-drilling and cooling reduces thermal necrosis. Postoperative pin site care should be meticulous

Bars

- Are composed of stainless steel or carbon fibre
- They connect bone pins and thereby connect bone fragments
- The bars connect directly to bone pins or to other bars via clamps

Clamps

- Used to connect pins to bars or bars to bars
- Are multiaxial allowing connections in any direction
- Often hand tightened initially prior to definitive tightening

Biomechanical properties

- Allowing fracture ends to come into contact is the most important factor for stability of fixation with external fixation

Other factors that enhance stability (rigidity) include (**Figure 51.3**):

- Larger diameter pins (second most important factor)
- Increased number of pins
- Increased spread of pins
- Reduced working length
- Minimised distance between the bar and bone
- Increased number of bars
- Increased number planes of construct (rods in different planes)
- Second rod in the same plane – increases bending resistance
- Increased spacing between pins (near-far construct)

Frame design

- Standard monolateral: Creates a stable construct for usually diaphyseal fractures. This obtains a stable reduction and allows mobilisation of adjacent joints.
- Joint spanning: Usually for periarticular fractures or dislocations as either temporary or definitive fixation methods. External fixation spans the affected joint immobilising

future incision sites planned for definitive fixation but as close to fracture site as possible. It is therefore a good tactics to contact the definitive surgeon, if not performing external fixation, to discuss optimal placement
- The working length is the distance across fracture site between closest bone pins
- When constructing an external fixator, the bone frame interface in important. Therefore, meticulous care in pin insertion is paramount. Soft tissue protection

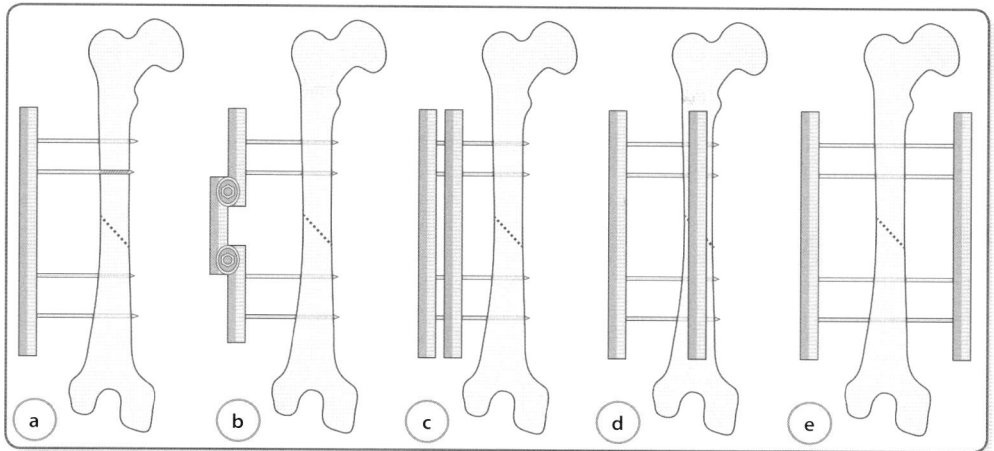

Figure 51.3 Different external fixation constructions with differing stabilities. (a) Unilateral, uniplanar fixator, (b) unilateral, uniplanar modular fixator, (c) unilateral, uniplanar double bar fixator, (d) unilateral, multiplanar fixator, (e) bilateral fixator.

it temporarily. Often (for the distal tibia) in a Delta or 'A' frame configuration.

Damage control

Damage control aims to achieve rapid control of life-threatening injuries to stabilise the trauma patient. Long bone injuries are easily and rapidly stabilised with the application of an external fixator. This then allows for optimisation of the patient, without the 'second hit' of definitive surgery. The limb fracture is then treated with a staged management protocol. The staged approach has in itself been shown to produce beneficial results with reduced infection rates in high-energy fracture patterns associated with soft tissue compromise.

Further reading

Egol KA, Tejwani NC, Capla Elm Wolinsky PL, Koval KJ. Staged management of high-energy proximal tibial fractures (OTA types 41): the results of a prospective, standardised protocol. J Orthop Trauma 2005; 19:448–455.

Miller M, Tompson S, Hart J. Review of Orthopaedics, 6th edn. Philadelphia, PA: Saunders, 2012.
Ruedi T, Buckley R, Moran C. AO Principles of Fracture Management, 2nd ed. Stuttgart, Germany: Thieme, 2007.

Related topics of interest

- Topic 17 Damage control orthopaedics and trauma physiology
- Topic 50 Implants – circular external fixators
- Topic 56 Initial management of fractures

52 Implants – nails

Key points
- Intramedullary nails provide on-axis (or close to on-axis) fracture fixation
- Intramedullary nails can be both load sharing and load bearing
- Intramedullary nails allow for relative stability and secondary bone healing
- Modern nails are cannulated to facilitate their passage over a guidewire

Biomechanical principles

Intramedullary nails are designed to withstand bending and torsional forces and allow the bone to share the axial load.
- The strength of the nail is dependent on its design. Therefore, the nail strength is affected by changes in nail diameter, wall thickness and the material used
- Torsional rigidity represents the amount of torque required to produce torsional deformation. It is the measure of resistance of a specific material to torsional forces. This is calculated by the shear modulus and polar moment of inertia of a material. Therefore, the torsional rigidity is proportional to the fourth power of the radius (r^4). Thus, an intramedullary nail with twice the thickness shows 2^4 (16) times the rigidity. In practice, we can influence torsional rigidity, by reaming, allowing for the passage of a larger diameter nail. Torsional rigidity is decreased by slotting of the nail
- Bending rigidity represents the amount of force required to produce a bending deformation. This is dependent on the material properties (Young's modulus) and its distribution across the material (second moment area). Bending rigidity of intramedullary nails is related to the fourth power of the radius (r^4)

Intramedullary nails (**Figure 52.1**) are better at resisting bending forces than torsional forces.

To increase the strength of a nail it should be:
- Unslotted
- Solid

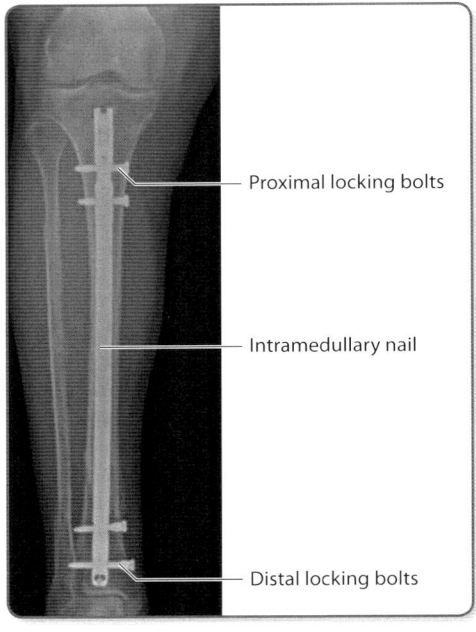

Figure 52.1 Intramedullary nail.

- Increase wall thickness (if cannulated)
- Increase nail diameter

Reaming
- Reaming increases the intramedullary canal diameter by using a side cutting reamer. This allows the torsional resistance to be increased by:
  - Increasing the contact area between the nail and the cortex
  - Passage of a larger diameter nail, with increased rigidity and strength
- Reaming results in an increased intramedullary pressure. This was a considerable worry, historically and thought to contribute to embolisation. More recent studies have shown that high intramedullary pressures are most prominently seen at the breaching of the medullary canal rather than during incremental reaming, and thus occur similarly in undreamed nailing.

- Reaming compromises the endosteal blood supply of that bone. There is a reactive increase in periosteal blood flow and change from centrifugal to centripedal blood flow within the bone. The endosteal circulation is thought to return after 6–12 weeks
- Risks of reaming include thermal necrosis, marrow embolisation

Slotted nails

- The slotting of nails was invented to allow flexibility within the construct to adjust for bone shape and anatomy, and particularly to allow ease of insertion
- Using slotted nails reduces the bending stiffness and torsional stiffness of the nail Therefore, larger diameter nails are needed to create the same stiffness as an unslotted nail
- Modern anatomical nails with bends or double bends negate the need for the increased flexibility gained with the slotted design

Interlocking

It is recommended that all nails are locked. Locking screws provide axial and rotational stability to the intramedullary nail. Locking screws are often the weakest part of the fixation and care must be paid to the size of locking options with incremental nail sizes.
Locking options are either:
- Dynamic – for axially and rotationally stable fractures
- Static – for axially and rotationally unstable fractures
- Secondary dynamisation – some axial shortening is allowed and subsequent compression when using dynamic locking options
- Active compression may be possible through the nail

Working length

This represents the distance across the fracture site between the points where the bone and nail are coupled. In a multi-fragmentary fracture pattern this may represent the distance between locking screws. In contrast a transverse fracture pattern with significant bone/nail contact at the isthmus significantly reduces the working length, stiffening the fixation construct.

The bending stiffness is the inverse to the working length squared. The rotational stiffness is inversely proportional to the working length.

Further reading

Miller M, Tompson S, Hart J. Review of Orthopaedics, 6th ed. Philadelphia, PA: Saunders, 2012.
Pape HC, Giannoudis P. The biological and physiological effects of intramedullary reaming. J Bone Joint Surg Br 2007; 89:142–146.

Ruedi T, Buckley R, Moran C. AO Principles of Fracture Management, 2nd edn. Stuttgart: Thieme, 2007.

Related topics of interest

- *Topic 51* Implants – monolateral external fixators
- *Topic 53* Implants – plates
- *Topic 54* Implants – screws

53 Implants – plates

Key points
- Plates are generally load-bearing devices, unless there is anatomic reduction and compression of the fracture
- Plate fixation can allow absolute or relative fixation techniques
- Numerous designs and applications to aid fracture fixation

Biomechanical principles
- The strength of a plate varies with the material used and its moment of inertia
- The bending stiffness of a plate is proportional to the third power of the thickness (t^3). Therefore, doubling the thickness increases the bending stiffness eight-fold (2^3)
- Plates are load-bearing devices when bridging fractures or with any residual fracture gap. Therefore, these are most effective when placed on the tension side of the bone during fixation

Plate design
- **⅓ tubular:** Plates that have a constant curvature of ⅓ of a circumference of a cylinder. Most modern versions of this plate are actually ¼ tubular. These plates are malleable having a low rigidity being only 1 mm thick. They are therefore easily contoured and often conform to the shape of the bone on compression
- **Dynamic compression plate (DCP):** These plates are of uniform thickness throughout their length. They contain oval screw holes to allow eccentric screw placement to generate compression
- **Low contact dynamic compression plate (LC-DCP):** These plates are of variable thickness and display a reduced plate footprint via scallops on their undersurface. This minimises periosteal compression on the underlying bone surface. They were designed to combat bone loss underlying the plate seen in early plating systems
- **Locking plates:** The threads on the screw head interlock with corresponding screw holes on the plate. This creates a fixed angle system with an increased resistance to pullout forces. Locking screws create no compression between the screw thread and the screw head. This minimises any compression on periosteum and plate can stand proud of bone surface. Locking principles make this technology suitable for minimally invasive techniques as plates require less contouring
- **Locking compression plate (LCP):** These are the modern incarnation of the DCP and LC-DCP, with combination holes for both nonlocked and locked screws, and scallops to reduce their footprint. These plates allow a combination of lag/compression principles with the benefit of locking technology
- **Precontoured (periarticular) anatomical plates:** These are contoured site-specific plates often with locking screw clusters in the metaphyseal region. They are good for periarticular locations

Plate mode
The way a plate is applied – the mode in which it is used – can affect the mechanical function. Therefore, plates of the same design and material can be used to obtain different functions and influence bone healing.
1. Methods to achieve absolute stability and primary bone healing:
   - **Neutralisation:** The plate acts to protect an interfragmentary lag screw from rotational forces. The process requires a plate to be applied to the bone to supplement or in conjunction with a lag screw
   - **Buttress:** The plate is used to push and reduce a fragment subject to shearing forces against an intact column of bone. The description originates from the similarities to a flying buttress in a cathedral or church supporting the roof and upper wall
   - **Compression (Figure 53.1):** The plate provides interfragmentary compression

Implants – plates

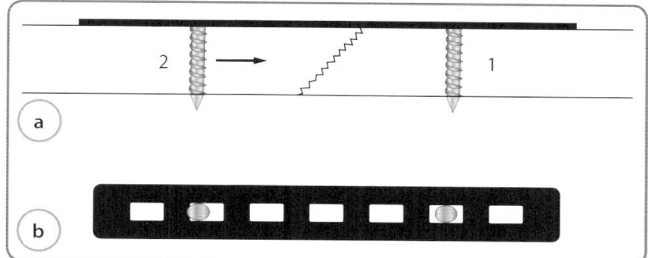

Figure 53.1 Compression plating. (a) Side view. (b) Top view.

by use of the dynamic sliding hole. This is not as efficient as a lag screw at generating compressive forces across a fracture gap. The system works best in short oblique or transverse fracture patterns. Compression can also be gained with the use of adjuncts such as a plate tensioning system. Compression plates can also be used in combination with lag screw fixation. Maximal stability can be gained when a lag screw is used through the plate. The best construct is to apply the plate first with compression and then to lag through the plate

- **Tension band plates:** The plate is applied on the convex surface of the bone which is subject to a tensile force. The plate resists this force, and allows for generation of compressive forces at the fracture gap

- Pre-bending the plate (in a concave fashion) prevents gapping at the far cortex in this scenario and generates further compressive force across the fracture

2. *Method to achieve relative stability and secondary bone healing:*
- **Bridge plating:** Provides relative stability and results in callus formation. This technique spans fracture site using the plate to achieve reduction with alignment, stability and length. This process is good for extra-articular, multifragmentary fracture patterns where absolute reduction would be hard to achieve. Bridging allows minimal disturbance of the fracture site and surrounding soft tissue envelope. This endeavours to preserve blood supply and the bone healing material within the zone of injury

Further reading

Miller M, Tompson S, Hart J. Review of Orthopaedics, 6th edn. Philadelphia, PA: Saunders, 2012.

Ruedi T, Buckley R, Moran C. AO Principles of Fracture Management, 2nd edn. Stuttgart: Thieme, 2007.

Stannard JP, Schmidt AH. Surgical Treatment of Orthopaedic Trauma. Stuttgart: Thieme, 2011.

Related topics of interest

- *Topic 50* Implants – circular external fixators
- *Topic 51* Implants – monolateral external fixators
- *Topic 52* Implants – nails
- *Topic 54* Implants – screws

54 Implants – screws

Key points

- A screw converts a rotational torque force into longitudinal translation
- Biomechanical properties and structure are related to function
- Variety of different functions to aid orthopaedic fixation

Characteristics of a screw

The structural characteristics of a screw determine its biomechanical properties (Figure 54.1).
- **Pitch** – the distance between screw threads
- **Lead** – the distance advanced in one complete 360° revolution. With a single thread the pitch and lead are interchangeable
- **Root diameter** – the inner diameter from the root of the threads. This is also known as the core diameter. This is proportional to the tensile strength of the screw
- **Outer diameter** – the outer diameter from the crest of the threads. This is related to the holding power (pull-out strength) of the screw
- **Screw working length** – length of bone traversed by the screw

Structure of a screw

- **Core:**
  - Internal diameter of the screw
  - Is proportional to the tensile force of the screw
  - The size of drill bit required is equivalent to the core diameter of the screw
- **Thread:**
  - Thread diameter is the distance between opposite thread crests
  - Thread depth is the distance between the crest and the core (trough)
  - Pitch is the distance between adjacent thread crests
  - The thread depth is proportional to pull out strength of the screw
  - The tap size is equivalent to the thread diameter of the screw
  - Thread profile – can be V-shaped, buttress, reverse buttress
  - Double thread – the lead is double the pitch, which allows faster tightening of the screw
- **Head:**
  - Prevents screw subsidence into bone
  - Generates compression
  - Shaped to allow force transmission to bone, which can be improved by washers. The head shape is generally congruent with plate holes to allow optimal force distribution. This can be mimicked on bone surfaces with the use of the countersink to increase the contact surface area
  - Screwdriver interface is generally screw specific, e.g. hexagonal, star, square
- **Tip:**
  - Can be blunt/conical
  - Self-tapping – tapping creates a channel for the thread to pass and increases the hold of the screw within the bone. A self-tapping screw has a fluted tip, which cuts a channel for the screw thread. These screws are slightly longer than a conventional screw to allow for the tap. If the screw has to be replaced

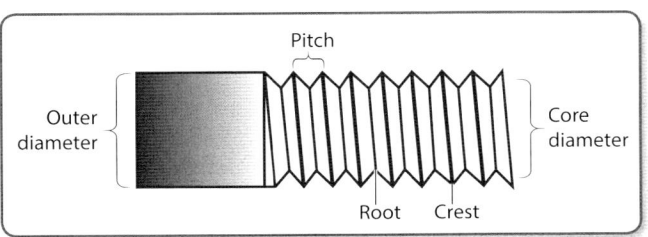

Figure 54.1 Structural characteristics of a screw.

and is inserted in a slightly altered path then this can destroy thread tap and lead to suboptimal bone hold. In thinner bone, self-tapping screws have been found to have an improved hold
- Self-tapping/self-drilling – no need for a separate drill or tap. However, these screws have a significantly longer tip before the thread commence and often protrude through the bone surface

The design features to maximise the pull-out strength of a screw include:
- Larger outer diameter
- Small root diameter
- Fine pitch
- Buttress thread profile
- Good bone quality
- Tapping prior to insertion

Types of screw

- **Cortical:** These screws have a smaller pitch and an increased number of threads. They are generally used in cortical bone with good bone quality. They have a reduced thread diameter to core diameter (reduced thread depth)
- **Cancellous:** These screws have a greater pitch and an increased depth of threads. This increases the bone contact area and subsequently increases the pull-out strength in poorer quality bone. These screws display a greater thread diameter to core diameter than cortical screws
- **Non-locking:** A compression force is generated from the thread against a smooth screw head. The head has no thread and creates a frictional force between itself and a bone surface or plate
- **Locking:** A separate thread located on the head, 'locks' into a specific plate hole with a reciprocal thread. Locking screws generate no friction and thus no compression but together with a locked plate act as rigid internal scaffold devices.

The locking mechanism generates a greater pull-out force than conventional non-locked designs
- **Cannulated:** This system allows the passage of a screw over a wire, as the screw has a hollow core. This enables more accurate screw placement. These screws are often used in isolation rather than with a plate, e.g. as malleolar screws. The cannulation potentially alters the core diameter, thread depth and tensile strength. For a screw of the same diameter, a cannulated screw is weaker
- **Partially threaded:** Generates compression towards the head of the screw. An example of their use is in malleolar fractures
- **Headless:** The head of these screws is buried within bone or cartilage. These screws are often used in intra-articular fracture fixation to minimise articular cartilage disruption. The screws have a differential thread pitch, with a different thread pitch at each end of the screw. Therefore, as the distal screw advances more with each turn it generates interfragmentary compression. This was first developed for the scaphoid (Herbert screw)

Functions of a screw

- **Lag screw** – generates interfragmentary compression. The Lag principle states that the screw thread must engage the far cortex, not the near cortex. This generates compression between the screw head and the distal thread-bone interface
- **Positional screw** – holds bone fragments in appropriate position, e.g. a syndesmosis screw
- **Reduction screw** – allows manipulation of fracture fragments via compressive forces
- **Poller screw** – guides the passage of an intramedullary nail

Further reading

DeCoster TA, Heetderks DB, Downey DJ, Ferrles JS, Jones W. Optimising the bone screw pull-out force. J Orthop Trauma 1990; 2:169–174.

Miller M, Tompson S, Hart J. Review of Orthopaedics, 6th edn. Philadelphia, PA: Saunders; 2012.

Roberts TT, Prumm CM, Papallodis DN, Uhl RL, Wagner TA. History of the orthopaedic screw. Orthopaedics 2013; 36:12–14.

Related topics of interest

- *Topic 50* Implants – circular external fixators
- *Topic 52* Implants – nails
- *Topic 53* Implants – plates

55 Infection

Key points

- Early administration of antibiotics and wound debridement is mandatory in the treatment of open fractures
- Osteomyelitis is a complex condition requiring multidisciplinary management
- Tetanus still exists, e.g. 7 cases were reported in the UK in 2014
- Orthopaedic surgeons are at severe risk of occupational exposure to blood-borne pathogens

Susceptibility to infection depends upon:
- Patient (host) factors – comorbidities, immune status and nutritional status
- Pathogen factors –– virulence of the micro-organisms, resistance to antimicrobial therapies, biofilm formation
- Wound factors – location and degree of necrotic or devitalised tissue, initial contamination
- Surgeon factors – adequacy of debridement in open fractures, tissue handling, tourniquet time, wound closure/coverage

Antibiotics in the management of acute fractures

All open fractures are contaminated. Increased infection rates are reported in severe open fractures, those with extensive contamination, associated vascular injuries, and in elderly patients, and those with certain comorbidities (i.e. diabetes mellitus). The use of prophylactic intravenous antibiotics has been shown to reduce the infection rate in elective clean orthopaedic cases and open fractures. The addition of antibiotics to the irrigation solution has become common in an attempt to further decrease the rate of postoperative infection. However, the efficacy of using antibiotics in irrigation fluid has not been proven.

Treatment of closed fractures

To maximise the beneficial effect of prophylactic antibiotics while minimising adverse effects, the correct antimicrobial must be selected, the drug must be administered just before incision and prior to tourniquet inflation, and duration of administration should not exceed 24 hours. Most hospitals have their own policy depending on local antibiotic stewardship rules.

Treatment of open fractures

Primary surgical treatment
This comprises wound excision, debridement and lavage, fracture stabilisation (temporary or definitive) and covering the wound.

Antibiotic administration
The literature supports early administration of antibiotics as the single most important factor influencing the rate of infection. Antibiotics should be given within 3 hours of injury. The British Orthopaedic Association Standards for Trauma (BOAST) state that in the management of open fractures:
- Co-amoxiclav (1.2 g) or cefuroxime (1.5 g) are given 8-hourly and are continued until wound debridement. Clindamycin 600 mg, 6 hourly is given instead if penicillin allergy is suspected
- Co-amoxiclav (1.2 g) and gentamicin (1.5 mg/kg) are administered at wound excision and continued for 72 hours or until definitive wound closure, whichever takes place first
- Heavily contaminated wounds and farm wounds require the use of cephalosporin, aminoglycosides, and high-dose penicillin
- Fresh water wounds require the use of fluoroquinolones (ciprofloxacin, levofloxacin) or 3rd- or 4th-generation cephalosporin (ceftazidime)
- Salt water wounds require the use of doxycycline and ceftazidime or a fluoroquinolone

Acute infection

Early infection after an open fracture or open reduction with internal fixation of a closed fracture is commonly due to *Staphylococcus aureus*, *Staphylococcus epidermidis*,

Pseudomonas aeruginosa, or gram-negative bacilli. An early biopsy and culture, with adjustment of antibiotic treatment according to culture results, is ideal. If the infection extends to the bone, then removal of all necrotic bone is mandated.

Implant removal is controversial. Consider initial removal, removal after fracture union, implant exchange or conversion to external fixation. However, in all cases stability of the fracture is required and thus it is often impossible to avoid use of hardware of some sort.

Osteomyelitis

Osteomyelitis is an infection of the bone and marrow. It can present acutely or chronically. Chronic osteomyelitis can develop as a result of a neglected or misdiagnosed infection. In the presence of infection, devitalised bone fragments become sequestra and granulation tissue is transformed into a layer of dense fibrous tissue, forming a membrane. This membrane acts as a barrier around the sequestra isolating the host from the infected area. Periosteal new bone formation around the periphery of the infected area produces an involucrum which increases the isolation of the host from the infection.

It is imperative that this complex condition is managed in an appropriate unit with the necessary multidisciplinary expertise. This includes orthopaedic and plastic surgeons, microbiologists, specialist nurses and therapists.

Diagnosis

Osteomyelitis is diagnosed primarily by thorough history and clinical examination, and plain radiographs (**Figures 55.1** and **55.2**). Pain, systemic malaise, local erythema and discharge may all be signs of osteomyelitis. Laboratory analysis including erythrocyte sedimentation rate, C-reactive protein and differential white cell count are not particularly useful other than to monitor trends in response to treatment. Plain radiographs may show lucency and localised bone resorption, or implant loosening. Further imaging studies such as CT, MRI, bone scans and SPECT may be useful. Biopsy may be necessary in both diagnosing and identifying the causative organism.

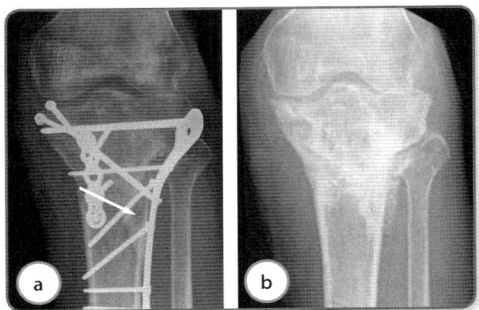

Figure 55.1 (a) Osteomyelitis (arrow) of proximal tibia following internal fixation demonstrating osteolysis under the lateral plate. (b) Postoperative image after hardware removal, debridément and local antibiotic impregnated calcium sulphate graft application.

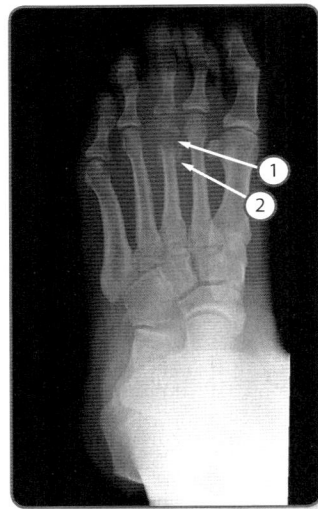

Figure 55.2 Anteroposterior radiograph showing osteomyelitis: infection of the 3rd metatarsal in a patient with diabetic foot. Lysis ① is a consequence of bony destruction. New subperiosteal bone has formed involucrum ②.

Classification

Osteomyelitis can be classified as:
- Paediatric or adult, according to age at the onset of the infection
- Haematogenous or exogenous, distinguishing on the basis of the pathogenesis;
- Acute or chronic, distinguishing the infection on the basis of whether it requires pre-existing osteonecrosis

The staging system developed by Cierny and Mader in 1985 is currently the most widely used for the classification of osteomyelitis. This classifies on the basis of anatomic area of bone involved and the inmunocompetence of the host. **Table 55.1** demonstrates staging for chronic adult osteomyelitis.

Treatment

Whenever possible, host comorbidities are addressed before initiating surgical management. If the patient is well, antibiotics should not be commenced until multiple samples and biopsies have been taken. Empirical antibiotic therapy is utilised initially and adjusted based on culture results.

There are several important steps in the management of osteomyelitis:
- Debridement of all dead, devitalised, necrotic and nonviable tissue
- Sampling/identification of organisms
- Dead space management/eradication
- Skeletal stabilisation
- Appropriate antibiotics
- Definitive soft tissue and skeletal reconstruction

Tetanus

Tetanus is an acute disease caused by the action of tetanus toxin, released following infection by the bacterium *Clostridium tetani*. It is characterised by generalised rigidity and spasms of skeletal muscles. The muscle stiffness usually involves the jaw and neck and then becomes generalised. The bacteria grow anaerobically at the site of the injury and have an incubation period of between 4 and 21 days (most commonly about 10 days).

Prophylaxis

Tetanus-prone wounds include those that require surgical intervention that is delayed for more than 6 hours, wounds that show a significant degree of devitalised tissue or a puncture-type injury, particularly where there has been contact with soil or manure, projectile injuries, frostbites and those containing foreign bodies. **Table 55.2** demonstrates the appropriate prophylaxis depending on the patient's immunisation status.

Treatment

A diagnosis of acute tetanus infection requires urgent medical attention. Primarily the aim is to control muscle spasms with diazepam or equivalent. Initial antibiotic therapy includes penicillin G or doxycycline; alternative therapy includes metronidazole.

Gas gangrene

Gas gangrene is a bacterial infection caused by *Clostridium perfringens*, *Clostridium septicum* and other histotoxic *Clostridium* species. Spore-forming rods produce

Table 55.1 Cierny–Mader staging system for chronic adult osteomyelitis

Lesion type

Stage 1 (medullary): infection within the medullary cavity, usually without involvement of the epiphyseal area.

Stage 2 (superficial): involves the outer cortical area, the subcutaneous tissue and the skin. The infection resides within an isolated area consisting of cortical sequestra and granulation tissue

Stage 3 (localised): involves full thickness of cortex and the adjacent medullary canal

Stage 4 (diffuse): involves the cortex and the medullary cavity as well, leading to an extensive of devitalisation of a bone segment

Host category

Type A normal

Type B (L/S) compromised by local and systemic conditions

Type C (L/S) severely compromised by local and systemic conditions

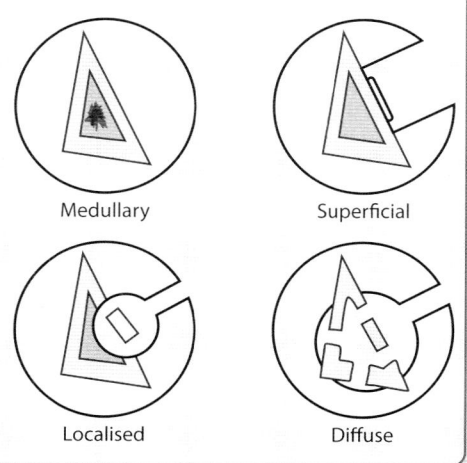

Table 55.2 Guidelines for tetanus prophylaxis

Wound	Immune history	Prophylaxis
Tetanus prone	Unknown or <3 immunisations	Tetanus, diphtheria toxoids Tetanus immune globulin (human)
	Immunisation complete	Tetanus toxoid if: • No booster immunisation within past 5 years • Severe wound or >24 hours old
Nontetanus prone	Unknown or <3 immunisations	Tetanus toxoid

exotoxins that cause fat and muscle necrosis and thrombosis of local vessels. These micro-organisms are typically to be found in grossly contaminated wounds, traumatic wounds, in farmyard related injuries, in wounds contaminated by bowel content and in patients with diabetes mellitus.

The incubation period is <24 hours, and symptoms include severe pain, oedema (distant from the wound), foul-smelling, serosanguineous discharge, high fever, chills, tachycardia and confusion. It is typical to find widespread gas in the soft tissues on plain radiographs.

The mortality of gas gangrene is 100% if the treatment is delayed. Overall, the mortality is 25%.

Treatment is based on surgical debridement, fasciotomies, hyperbaric oxygen (the data for this are inconclusive), and early administration of the antibiotics penicillin G and clindamycin. A cephalosporin and an aminoglycoside are added to cover other organisms.

Necrotising fasciitis

Necrotising fasciitis (NF) is an uncommon soft-tissue infection, with rapidly spreading inflammation and extensive necrosis of the skin, subcutaneous tissue, and superficial fascia. It is most commonly a polymicrobial infection, with group A β-haemolytic streptococci being most commonly involved. Early stages of the disease are often misdiagnosed as cellulitis or abscess because of the absence of specific clinical features.

Red flags for NF include recent surgery, pain-out-of-proportion, diarrhoea, hypotension, altered mental status, erythema progressing along the limb, fluctuance, haemorrhagic bullae and skin necrosis. The mortality of NF and limb loss incidence is 15–29% and 20.3–26% respectively.

Treatment is based on emergent aggressive debridement of all involved tissues and immediate empirical antibiotics covering aerobic, anaerobic, gram positive and gram negative bacteria, and adjusting antibiotic treatment once the microorganism has been defined.

Occupational hazards

Orthopaedic surgeons are at risk of occupational exposure to blood-borne pathogens. The surgeon must follow basic infection control strategies that can significantly reduce the risk of pathogen transmission such as the use of gowns, gloves, masks, eye protection, face shields, hands-free technique, blunted surgical needles and most of all, safe etiquette.

Human immunodeficiency virus (HIV)

The average risk of transmission of HIV to a healthcare worker after percutaneous exposure to HIV-infected blood has been estimated as 0.3%. This risk increases if the exposure involves a large amount of blood. The risk of seroconversion from mucous membrane exposure is 0.09%.

The risk of transmission from blood transfusion is 1/500,000 per unit transfused, and the risk of transmission from frozen bone allograft is <1 per million.

Donor screening is the most important factor in preventing viral transmission. If the

HIV status of the donor is unknown, consent must be provided for testing, performed by a doctor but never by the doctor that has been exposed.

Post exposure prophylaxis is administered in case of percutaneous injury or contact of mucous membrane/broken skin with blood, tissue, or potentially infectious body fluids. Cerebrospinal, synovial, pleural, peritoneal, pericardial, and amniotic fluids are considered potentially infectious.

Hepatitis B

Among the blood-borne viruses, hepatitis B virus it is the most highly communicable. Following needlestick injury, 37–62% will eventually seroconvert and 22–31% will develop clinical hepatitis B infection. After blood exposure such as a sharps injury in a previously unimmunised individual, the combination of vaccination and passive immunotherapy with hepatitis B immune globulin has been recommended. The hepatitis B vaccine consists of recombinant hepatitis B surface antigen and it is highly recommended for all healthcare workers with potential blood-borne exposure.

Hepatitis C

Healthcare workers with blood exposure are at risk for infection with hepatitis C virus (HCV) although, relative to hepatitis B virus (HBV), the risk is much lower. The risk of transmission from needlestick injury is 0.5–1.8%. No vaccine or immunoglobulin has proven useful and prevention is based on prevention of sharps injuries.

Further reading

British Orthopaedic Association (BOA) and British Association of Plastic, Reconstructive and Aesthetic Surgeons (BAPRAS). BOAST 4: The management of severe open lower limb fractures. London: BOA and BAPRAS, 2009.

Public Health England. Immunisation against infectious disease (The Green Book). London: Public Health England, 2014.

Related topics of interest

- *Topic 56* Initial management of fractures
- *Topic 68* Open fractures
- *Topic 85* Principles of operative management of fractures

56 Initial management of fractures

Key points

- In the initial management of a fracture thorough neurovascular examination of the limb should be undertaken, including an assessment for compartment syndrome
- The limb should be inspected for open injuries or significant soft tissue damage
- Two orthogonal radiograph views (AP and lateral) of the fracture should be obtained
- The patient should be given analgesia prior to any manipulation and splintage

Definition

A fracture is a break in the continuity of the bone (**Figure 56.1**). They are typically caused by the application of high energy to the bone – greater than normal physiological loading. However, fractures can also be the result of normal physiological stresses applied to weakened bone as seen in osteoporosis, malignancy, rickets and osteogenesis imperfecta.

Pathophysiology

Fractures are painful. The disruption of the periosteum activates nociceptors, whilst the localised inflammatory response and muscle spasms of surrounding muscle attachments exacerbate this. Patients are reluctant to move the affected limb and hold it in a position that guards it from further trauma. They are often unable to tolerate the external pressure over the fracture site.

Clinical assessment

The affected limb is typically swollen and possibly deformed. Neurologic and vascular examination of the affected limb is mandatory. Distal pulses, capillary refill time (CRT) and peripheral nerves traversing around the fracture site should all be assessed.

A careful inspection of the surrounding skin and soft tissue envelope should be undertaken and prompt identification of an open injury made. In closed injuries, the limb should be examined for fracture blisters and closed degloving.

The compartments of the affected limb should be examined for any evidence of compartment syndrome. The incidence is greatest in diaphyseal tibial shaft fractures, followed by forearm fractures. Open fractures may also be complicated by compartment syndrome.

These assessments must be documented in the notes, and repeat assessments (especially for compartment syndrome) must be made where necessary.

Investigations

Plain radiographs should be obtained with a minimum of two orthogonal views (AP and lateral) in which the fracture is centered. The joints proximal and distal to the fracture should be examined and further imaging obtained if clinically indicated.

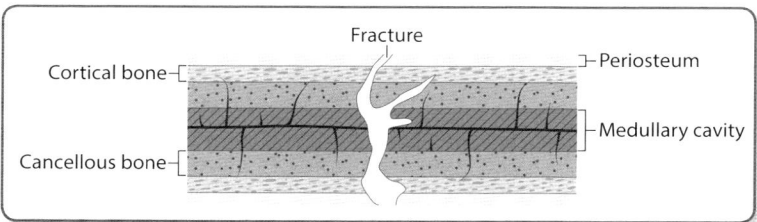

Figure 56.1 Anatomy of a fractured bone.

CT scans offer further information to aid the surgeon in preoperative planning. They are useful in assessing intra-articular fractures, grossly comminuted fractures, and fractures where the fracture pattern is not wholly obvious on plain radiographs.

CT angiograms can be used to assess for occult vascular injuries in open fractures as an additional tool to the clinical examination. These can detect vascular lesions that may have otherwise been missed.

Classifications

There are numerous classifications and eponyms for fractures. Fracture classification should be broken down in the first instance to basic principles. A distinction should be made between intra-articular and extra-articular fractures, since this also dictates principles for fracture management.

Common fracture patterns include transverse (horizontal fracture), oblique (angulated fracture), and spiral. The pattern produced is a consequence of the type of stress applied to the bone.

The fracture deformity should then be described in terms of any shortening, translation, angulation, rotation and number of parts. Classically, the deformity is described in terms of the position of the distal fragment in relation to the proximal fragment. Fractures with more than two parts are described as comminuted; these are associated with higher energy.

In addition, the AO-OTA alphanumeric classification system can be used to describe fractures. This though is mainly used for research and communication.

Treatment

Principles of fracture management are dictated by the location of the fracture and the patient's requirements. According to AO principles, intra-articular fractures should be managed with anatomical reduction and rigid internal fixation. In comparison, extra-articular fractures may be managed with relative stability techniques.

Initially, all fractures regardless of their definitive management are treated in a temporary splint to stabilise and protect the fracture, and allow for soft tissue oedema. This may occur after a manipulation.

Nonoperative/noninvasive

Minimally displaced fractures, regardless of whether or not they involve the articular surface, may be treated nonoperatively in a cast or splint. Depending on the location of the fracture it may be protected with a period of nonweight-bearing before progressing to full weight-bearing. The functional demands of the patient, their comorbidities, and wishes, should be taken in to account.

Some fractures to be managed with manipulation and casting require an anaesthetic for reduction of the fracture. This is therefore considered noninvasive rather than nonoperative.

Operative

Fractures can be stabilised operatively by either internal fixation or external fixation. External fixation is used as a means of damage control surgery in polytrauma patients; offers stability to soft tissues in high-energy fractures; and can be used in the presence of infection.

Extra-articular fractures will heal with relative stability – this can be achieved with definitive external fixation, intramedullary nailing or plate fixation.

Intra-articular fractures require anatomical reduction and rigid internal fixation with compression to permit a return to early range of movement and primary bone healing. This may be achieved through the use of screw fixation often along with plates to support the articular block's reduction to the diaphysis.

Complications

Immediate

- Vascular injury – this is due to either the force causing the initial fracture, or the sharp displaced bone ends lacerating local vessels
- Nerve injury – the location of the fracture predicts the injured nerve, e.g.
    - Common peroneal nerve is associated with a fibular head fracture and knee dislocations

- The anterior interosseous nerve is most commonly injured in paediatric supracondylar fractures

Early

- Compartment syndrome – this most commonly occurs in men with either tibial or forearm fractures
- Infection – this may occur with open fractures, or incisions through compromised soft tissues as in distal tibial pilon fractures. Often patients need to wait up to 2 weeks after an initial spanning external fixation to allow the soft tissues to recover

Delayed

- Stiffness is common after fractures. It is related both to the trauma of the initial injury itself, and compounded by the surgical treatment. It is a major disability for some fractures and requires aggressive physiotherapy to limit its disabling effect
- Malunion and nonunion may occur due to inadequate reduction, unstable fixation, infection and patient factors such as smoking
- Post-traumatic osteoarthritis may occur in any fracture, particularly where limb alignment or joint congruity are affected
- Chronic regional pain syndrome (CRPS) is also an increasing problem and is recognised in BOAST 7 guidance for fracture clinics. This requires specialist advice from hospital pain services

Further reading

McQueen MM, Christie J, Court-Brown CM. Acute compartment syndrome in tibial diaphyseal fractures. J Bone Joint Surg Br 1996; 78B:95–98.

Related topics of interest

- Topic 14 Compartment syndrome
- Topic 68 Open fractures
- Topic 85 Principles of operative management of fractures

57 Knee – cruciate ligament injuries

Key points
- Early reconstruction of cruciate ligament injuries is critical to reduce the incidence of secondary knee injuries and long term morbidity
- One key to successful surgery is correct anatomical graft placement
- Postoperative physiotherapy is a vital part of the treatment algorithm

Epidemiology

Anterior cruciate ligament (ACL) injuries are one of the most common soft tissue knee injuries. They have an annual incidence of approximately 100,000–200,000 per year in the USA. They are common in many sports especially football, rugby, hockey and basketball – those that involve pivoting and twisting.

Women are 2–6 times more likely to experience this injury compared to men. This is thought to be due to generalised joint laxity, genetic predisposition, hormonal variations, smaller ligaments and higher valgus angle on landing from a jump.

Pathophysiology

The cruciate ligaments are essential to the stability of the knee when pivoting on the leg.

The ACL is comprised of two bundles of fibres (anteromedial and posterolateral bundles) that attach in a fan shape from the medial wall of the lateral femoral condyle and insert into the tibial plateau. The origin of the ACL on the tibial side is in front of the intercondylar eminence where it is in continuation with the anterior horn of the medial meniscus. The ACL functions to resist anterior translation and medial rotation of the tibia in relation to the femur.

The ACL ruptures commonly occur in noncontact injuries while pivoting with axial load. They can occur in isolation or as a combination of ligamentous and meniscal injuries within the knee. The patient will normally develop severe pain and immediate swelling in the knee preventing them from continuing activity. Patients describe the feeling a 'pop' within the knee during the injury.

The posterior cruciate ligament (PCL) originates from the lateral edge of medial femoral condyle and the roof of the intercondylar notch and inserts posteriorly into the nonarticular portion of the tibia. It functions to prevent backwards displacement of the tibia on the femur.

The PCL ruptures can occur from direct force to a flexed knee, often seen in dashboard impact in road traffic collisions. They can also occur from noncontact hyperextension injury of the knee when the leg is planted to the floor.

Clinical features

Patients will present with swollen painful knee secondary to a haemarthrosis. However, in some cases with an isolated complete rupture of the ACL, the knee may be pain free. The anterior draw test can be performed which can give an indication of possible injury. The Lachmann's test (anterior glide of the tibia at 20–30° of flexion) is regarded as the most reliable and sensitive examination for acute ACL ruptures. A pivot shift test may also be performed which indicates instability due to an ACL injury, however, it can be difficult if the patient is not relaxed and is generally more sensitive when performed under anaesthetic. The PCL injuries will demonstrate a posterior sag sign. They may have a positive dial test due to associated posterolateral corner injuries.

The patient may present with an associated meniscal injury (lateral meniscal tear being the most common with up to 50% incidence associated with ACL rupture). This may be elicited with a McMurray's test.

Other associated injuries include medial/lateral collateral ligament injuries and osteochondral defects.

Investigations

Plain anteroposterior and lateral radiographs are commonly performed to help rule out fractures. In a small proportion of ACL injuries there may be a Segond fracture, which is an avulsion fracture of the lateral tibia condyle by the iliotibial tract or joint capsule (**Figure 57.1**). This is pathognomonic for an ACL tear. Radiographs may also show avulsion fractures from the tibial spine (from ACL injury) or the posterior surface of the tibia (with PCL injury).

MRI remains the imaging of choice for ligamentous injuries (**Figure 57.2**). They also provide further information regarding other ligamentous, meniscal and bony injuries that may effect the management of the injury knee.

Classification

The ACL injuries are graded according to stability of the knee (**Table 57.1**).

The PCL injuries are graded according to the position of the tibia against the femur during a posterior draw test.

Treatment

Treatment for acute ACL injuries is dependent on the patient's lifestyle needs. The stability of the knee is fundamental to a sports playing/active patient and would warrant reconstruction. In addition, reconstruction is critical to prevent secondary injuries and long-term morbidity associated with degenerative arthrosis. However, an elderly person or those with light demand lifestyles can be managed nonoperatively.

Nonoperative treatment includes physiotherapy and lifestyle modifications. Physiotherapy can help support the knee by increasing muscle strength and surrounding soft tissue support. Bracing may also help to improve stability of the knee during rehabilitation and for other daily activities.

Operative management is indicated for children, young patients, and those with active lifestyles. Concurrent meniscal tears or associated collateral ligament injuries are indications for surgical intervention.

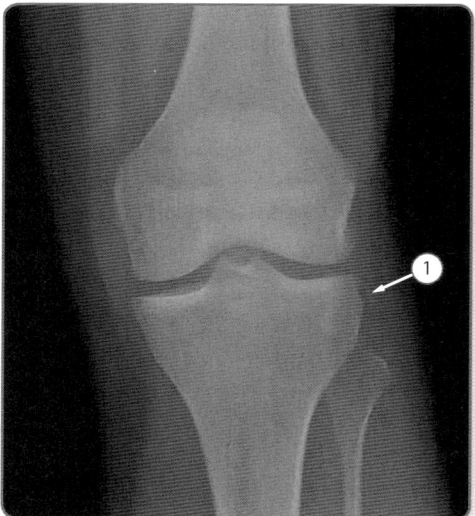

Figure 57.1 Anteroposterior X-ray of the knee, showing a Segond fracture ①.

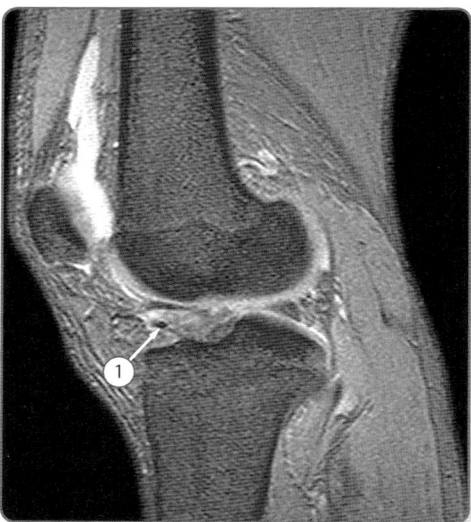

Figure 57.2 Sagittal MRI showing a tear through the anterior cruciate ligament ①, which has been avulsed from its origin at the anterior medial tibia, with loss of the normal 'bundle' morphology.

Table 57.1 The ACL classification according to severity and subsequent stability of the knee

Grade	Features
1	The ligament is stretched but still capable of providing stability to the knee joint
2	The ligament is partially torn and may give a sensation of instability during activities. They may present with a painful knee with an effusion
3	The fibres of the ligament are completely torn into two parts. Clinically, the knee may be less swollen or painful compared to a grade 2 injury. The ligament provides no stability to the knee and there it gives away and feels unstable while performing pivoting activities

Reconstruction aims to restore normal knee kinematics whilst stabilising the knee and preventing arthrosis. Multiple graft options include: (1) quadruple hamstring autograft, (2) bone–tendon–bone (BTB), (3) quadriceps tendon grafts or (4) allograft. BTB autografts are taken from the patella tendon with a bone bridge on either side allow for bone to bone healing and faster incorporation of the graft. This facilitates quicker rehabilitation and return to sport. BTB is associated with anterior knee pain and there is a risk of patella tendon rupture postoperatively. Hamstring grafts are associated with graft site pain and muscle weakness. The incision is smaller, however, there is a weaker fixation to the bone compared to BTB.

Single-bundle reconstruction is the most commonly performed procedure. However, other techniques are used that attempt to mimic the natural ACL with a double-bundle technique. Graft placement is fundamental to the success of the reconstruction. The femoral attachment should be placed posterior near the original attachment on the lateral femoral condyle, and more horizontal to achieve rotational stability by hyperflexing the knee at the time of tunnel placement. Tibial tunnels are placed through the remnant footprint of the old ACL. Grafts can be secured by either cortical suspensory fixation devices, interference screws (either biocomposite or metallic) or staples.

Management of partial tears of the ACL depend on the functional stability of the knee. Stable knees can be treated nonoperatively, with guided rehabilitation. Unstable knees require reconstruction with or without preservation of the partially torn ACL.

Postoperative rehabilitation is focused on physiotherapist guided early weight-bearing with closed-chain activities over a 6–9-month period.

In children, nonoperative management of ACL injuries leads to chronic instability and is associated with meniscal tears and chondral damage. It is possible to perform reconstruction, however, consideration must be taken of the physes, which may still be active. 'All inside' techniques guided by fluoroscopy can be used to prevent untoward damage to the growing physes.

Grade I and Grade II PCL injuries can be managed nonoperatively. The PCL reconstruction is indicated for unstable/Grade III or multiligament injuries. Bony avulsions are amenable to primary fixation. Use of auto and allografts have been used for both single- and double-bundle techniques.

Complications

Complications of nonoperative management of ACL ruptures include on-going instability of the knee. This can lead to secondary injuries, such as complex meniscal tears and long-term degenerative arthrosis. Surgical complications are usually secondary to tunnel placement. Malposition of the tunnels can lead to instability, limited flexion, impingement and ultimately graft re-rupture. Graft site morbidity can be seen with BTB autograft causing anterior knee pain, as well as a risk of patella tendon rupture and patella fracture. Hamstring autografts are associated with knee flexor weakness and there is a risk of damage to the infrapatellar branch of the saphenous nerve.

Further reading

American Academy of Orthopaedic Surgeons (AAOS). Management of anterior cruciate ligament injuries. Evidence based clinical practice guideline. Rosemont, IL: AAOS; 2014.

LaBella CR, Hennrikus W, Hewett TE. Anterior cruciate ligament injuries: diagnosis, treatment and prevention. Pediatrics 2014; 133:e1437–1450.

Unwin A. What's new in anterior cruciate ligament surgery? Orthop Trauma 2010, 24:100–106.

Related topics of interest

- *Topic 59* Knee – meniscal injuries
- *Topic 61* Knee dislocations – multiligament injuries
- *Topic 79* Paediatric tibial fractures

58 Knee – extensor mechanism injury

Key points
- Patella ligament ruptures are more common under 40 years of age, and quadriceps tendon ruptures typically occur over 40 years
- Acute repair of injury is ideal prior to contracture formation and to restore function
- Guided recovery with protection techniques is required to support fixation

Epidemiology

Extensor tendon ruptures of the knee are relatively uncommon injuries. Quadriceps tendon ruptures have an incidence of 1.3% and patella ligament ruptures 0.6%. There is a bimodal distribution according to age and location of the injury. Athletes and young patients (under age of 40 years) more commonly suffer patella ligament ruptures during sporting activities such as high jump, weight lifting and basketball. Patients over the age of 40 years (average age 65 years) commonly present with quadriceps tendon ruptures.

Men are eight times more likely to have an injury compared to females, with the nondominant limb being affected twice as often as the dominant limb. Risk factors for rupture of the extensor mechanism include diabetes, gout, chronic renal failure, endocrine disorders, repetitive microtrauma, fluroquinolone use and systemic steroid use.

Pathophysiology

Disruption of the knees extensor mechanism occurs during a sudden resisted knee extension or passive flexion of the knee with the quadriceps contracted. It may occur at multiple levels: (1) the quadriceps tendon, (2) the insertion of the quadriceps tendon to the proximal pole of the patella, (3) the retinaculum extension, (4) the distal pole of the patella, (5) patella ligament, or (6) its attachment to the tibial tubercle. Fractures of the patella can also be included in extensor mechanism injuries and are covered in Topic 60.

Quadriceps tendon ruptures commonly occur approximately 1–2 cm proximal to the upper patella pole in keeping with the avascular area of the tendon. The tendon is also commonly injured its insertion to the patella and the tear begins centrally then moves to the periphery.

Patella ligament ruptures that occur in younger patients are thought to be the end-stage event of chronic repetitive shearing forces leading to tendinopathy or 'jumper's knee'. In addition, there is some evidence that steroid injections are linked to a higher risk of patella ligament rupture.

Clinical features

The clinical features of extensor mechanism injuries are dependent on the location of the injury. Patients with complete tears at any point of the extensor mechanism will not be able to actively extend their knee (or straight leg raise), this is therefore a crucial part in their examination. A high index of suspicion is crucial during examination to avoid missed diagnosis, which has been reported in 10–50% of cases.

Quadriceps ruptures cause a tearing pain with the knee giving away. This commonly occurs while the patient is trying to regain balance during a fall. They present with a triad of acute pain, inability to actively extend the knee and a palpable suprapatellar gap. This gap can be made more pronounced with flexion of the knee. Partial tears can be difficult to diagnose, clinically as they may be able to straight leg raise and may not have many of the other features associated with a complete tear. An extensor lag may be present if the retinaculum remains intact despite the quadriceps tendon being ruptured.

Patella ligament ruptures present with sudden pain on forced extension of the knee. They present with bruising, swelling, tenderness and a proximally migrated patella (**Figure 58.1**). An infrapatellar gap can sometimes be felt.

Investigations

Plain film radiographs are helpful in ruling out tibial tubercle and patella avulsion fractures. Plain radiographs may also show a haemarthrosis in partial tears and possible soft tissue disruption of the extensor mechanism in keeping with an extensor mechanism injury.

The height of the patella will be affected depending on the location of the injury. The Insall–Salvati method can be used to determine the position of the patella (**Figure 58.2**).

Ultrasonography is commonly used as a quick method to confirm the diagnosis of an extensor mechanism rupture. However, this investigation is user dependent and clinical examination is often sufficient to confirm the diagnosis.

MRI can provide diagnostic imaging and is the most sensitive imaging modality. They can provide more information about the extent of injury, such as whether an injury is an intrasubstance, partial or complete tear (**Figure 58.3**). They also can provide further information regarding any other intra-articular injuries or fractures that are not visible on initial radiographs. This can help guide the surgical strategy, especially when other injuries are suspected.

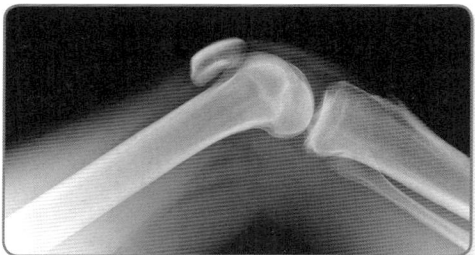

Figure 58.1 Lateral radiograph of a knee showing a high-riding patella (patella alta) in a patient with patella tendon rupture.

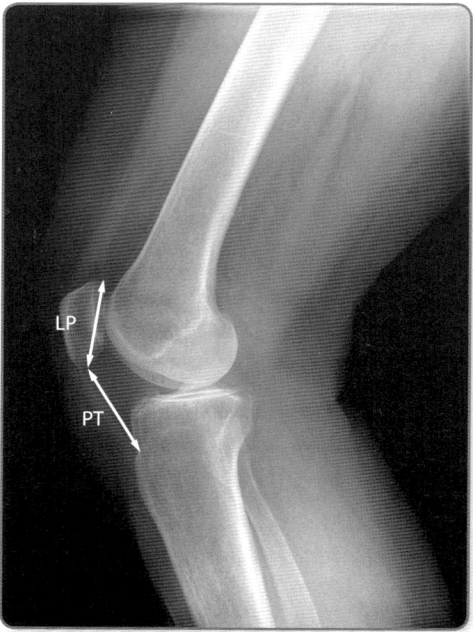

Figure 58.2 Insall–Salvati ratio predicts that the ratio between the patella tendon (PT) and length of patella (LP) are in a ratio of 1:1. Injuries to proximal and including the quadriceps attachment to the patella will lead to a lower patella position (patella infera) with a LP:PT ratio of >1. Injuries distal to the inferior pole of the patella may lead to a high-riding patella (patella alta) with a LP:PT ratio of <1.

Classification

Extensor mechanism injuries can be classified into partial and complete tears. Partial tears allow some function of the extensor apparatus and may be able to be managed nonoperatively. Complete tears prevent the function of the extensor apparatus and require surgical fixation.

Treatment

Complete patella ligament and quadriceps tendon ruptures should be treated promptly with surgical repair. This is to prevent contractures of the extensor mechanism, which can make a tension free surgical repair difficult.

Quadriceps tendon rupture repairs depend on location of the injury. Rarely, a

Knee – extensor mechanism injury

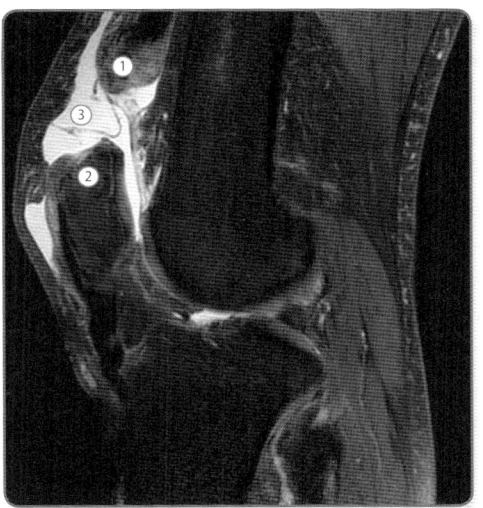

Figure 58.3 Lateral MRI of quadriceps rupture. (1) Quadriceps tendon, (2) patella, (3) suprapatella gap of the quadriceps rupture. Large haemarthrosis can also be seen which can mask the quadriceps rupture gap.

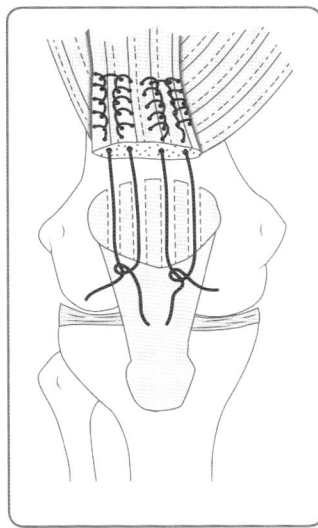

Figure 58.4 Typical fixation of a quadriceps rupture using interlocking sutures and transeosseus fixation via four holes. A three-hole technique can also be used passing the two central strands through the middle hole.

mid-substance tendon tear is repairable end-to-end. A locking stitch (e.g. Krakow) can be thread through both ends of the tendon and secured together. The associated retinaculum tears must also be identified and repaired.

More commonly, an osteotendinous quadriceps rupture can be fixed directly to the patella. Transosseous repair through transpatellar drill holes can provide a secure fixation. The use of a strong suture such as No. 5 Ethibond with locking sutures over the quadriceps tendon is a commonly used technique. Other techniques include the use of suspensory devices (e.g. Endobutton) and suture anchors. The superior pole of the patella is decorticated to encourage tendon to bone healing.

The patella ligament commonly ruptures at its proximal osteotendinous margin. Fixation involves a locking stitch through the tendon fixed to the patella with either suture anchors or via a transosseous method (**Figure 58.4**). All techniques require the fixation to be protected for the first 6 weeks from the strong pull of the quadriceps muscle. This can be achieved with a cylinder cast (which can cause stiffness), a temporary box wire around the proximal pole of the patella and through the tibial tubercle, to fix the patella ligament length, or a hinged knee brace preventing full flexion of the knee. Tibial tubercle fractures are commonly amenable to fixation with lag screws through the fragment. All repairs should be tested intraoperatively to 90° of flexion to test stability of the construct.

Postoperatively, the patients are protected with a brace, which allows limited flexion of the knee and passive extension only. This can be increased over 6 weeks. Nonweight bearing flexion exercises of the knee as tolerated allows for movement to help prevent adhesions and contractures. Active extension can be initiated from 6 weeks onwards with on-going use of the brace for up to 12 weeks whilst weight-bearing.

Partial tendon ruptures and incomplete tibial tubercle fractures can be treated nonoperatively with cylinder cast or brace in extension for 6 weeks. Keeping a low threshold for failure of management helps ensure full recovery is made.

Complications

Postoperative complications include loss of muscle strength and on-going functional impairment. Postoperative stiffness can occur with immobilisation required to protect the repair. Return to sport is dependent of patient factors and fixation. Re-rupture and failure of fixation can occur during recovery or with secondary trauma. Complications are more common in late presenting injuries as well as chronic injuries.

Further reading

Matava MJ. Patella tendon ruptures. J Am Acad Orthop Surg 1996; 4:287–296.

Ramseier LE, Werner CM, Heinzelmann M. Quadriceps and patella tendon rupture. Injury 2006; 37:516–519.

Rasul AT, Fischer DA. Primary repair of quadriceps tendon rupture. Results of treatment. Clin Orthop Relat Res 1993; 289:205–207.

Related topics of interest

- *Topic 60* Knee – patella fractures

59 Knee – meniscal injuries

Key points
- The blood supply of different parts (zones) of the meniscus dictates healing potential
- Examination and MRI form the mainstay of diagnosis and investigation, with arthroscopy reserved for treatment
- Damage or excessive resection of meniscus leads to increased joint contact forces, wear and resultant arthritis

Epidemiology

Meniscal tears are the most common knee injury with an incidence of 60–70 per 100,000 per year. A meniscal tear tends to be more frequent in full contact sports such as rugby or pivoting sports such as football. Tears are more common in men than women, with a quoted ratio of 2.5:1 to 4:1, with men between the ages of 31–40 years old more frequently injuring their meniscus. Women are more likely to tear their meniscus between the ages of 11 and 20 years. A longitudinal tear of the posterior horn of the medial meniscus is the most common isolated meniscal injury tear, with acute ACL injury being more commonly associated with injuries to the lateral meniscus. A chronic ACL injury is usually associated with a medial meniscal tear, alluding to the meniscus' role as a secondary rotational stabiliser of the knee.

Anatomy

The medial and lateral menisci of the knee are semi-lunar wedges of fibrocartilage, located between the femoral condyles and tibial plateau. The medial meniscus is C-shaped and attached along its entire periphery to the joint capsule by the coronary ligament rendering it relatively immobile. The lateral meniscus is O-shaped, with an interruption in its attachment of the joint capsule forming the popliteal hiatus, through which the popliteus tendon passes to its femoral attachment. Contraction by the popliteus during knee flexion pulls the lateral meniscus posteriorly, avoiding entrapment within the joint space. As a result the lateral meniscus is relatively more mobile than the medial.

Both menisci are attached to the tibia at their anterior and posterior horns by entheses, and are attached to each other anteriorly by the transverse ligament. The lateral meniscus alone is attached either anteriorly or posteriorly to the lateral aspect of the medial femoral condyle by ligaments of Humphrey or Wrisberg respectively. The menisci serve to increase tibiofemoral contact area and therefore decrease joint pressures, distributing load evenly across the joint surface. In full extension the menisci transmit 50% of force across the knee, whereas in deep flexion this increases to 90%. They also contribute to anteroposterior joint stability and act as dampeners, shielding articular cartilage from excessive load, as well as distributing synovial fluid, which aids joint lubrication. The menisci along with the cruciate ligaments contribute to proprioception as evidenced by type I and type II nerve fibres within the anterior and posterior horns.

Menisci are composed of an interlocking network of collagen fibres, mostly collagen type I (70%), as well as II, III, V and VI within a matrix of elastin, proteoglycans and glycoproteins. This network of collagen fibres is orientated differently depending on the layer within the meniscus. The superficial surface layer consists of a mesh of fibres primarily orientated radially. The sub surface layer consists of irregularly orientated fibres (i.e. a mix of radial and circumferential) and the middle or deep layer consists of parallel circumferential fibres. This structure allows the menisci to direct compressive loads outwards radially rather than onto the joint surface, minimising contact stresses. Proteoglycans play an important role, with an ability to trap 50 times their weight in water accounting for many of the physical properties of menisci.

Central meniscal blood supply is via the superior and inferior branches of the medial and lateral geniculate arteries via the perimeniscal capillary plexus, with the middle geniculate supplying the horns of the menisci. The peripheral 20–30% of the meniscus in the so called 'red-red zone' within which blood supply is rich and sufficient for healing to take place. The middle third, or 'red-white zone', has a poor vascular supply and limited healing potential and the inner third, or 'white-white zone', is completely avascular, with no healing capacity and relies on synovial fluid for its nutrients. With age, meniscal blood supply and water content decrease, resulting in decreased elasticity and greater susceptibility to deforming forces therefore injury.

Pathophysiology

Injury to the meniscus typically occurs due to rotational forces across a flexed knee joint. Lateral meniscal tears can occur when a valgus force is applied to a flexed knee with a planted foot. Conversely, a medial meniscal tear can result when a varus force is applied to a flexed knee and planted foot.

Clinical assessment

The common symptoms of a meniscal injury are pain, clicking, giving way and especially in the acute presentation – swelling. In cases of large meniscal tears such as bucket handle tears, locking, or a mechanical block to extension may occur due to incarcerated meniscal flaps within the intercondylar notch. Signs associated with meniscal tears include joint line tenderness localised to the medial or lateral side, joint effusion and a positive McMurray's test and/or the Apley grind test.

Investigations

Radiographs can be obtained to rule out other conditions such as fractures or concomitant osteoarthritis. In the UK, it is common to arrange an MRI to confirm the diagnosis, although it may be clear from the history and examination. Recent clinical data shows that MRI and clinical testing are comparable in sensitivity and specificity when looking for a meniscal tear. MRI has an accuracy of diagnosing meniscal tears approaching 95%.

Classification

A meniscal tear can be classified by its anatomic location and associated blood supply, e.g. whether it is located in the 'red-red,' 'red-white,' or 'white-white' zones, or by the tear pattern. A summary of tear patterns is presented in **Figure 59.1**. Ultimately, the purpose of classification is to determine reparability.

Treatment

Nonoperative treatment consists of physiotherapy, supports, rest, analgesia and nonsteroidal anti-inflammatories. Generally, nonoperative treatment is reserved for small stable peripheral tears with no other injury, e.g. ACL rupture. Operative treatment is offered to symptomatic patients who have failed to respond to conservative treatment, or those with a locked knee secondary to displaced meniscal flaps. Operative treatment consists of arthroscopic meniscectomy, menical repair, or meniscal transplants. Arthroscopic meniscectomy is a surgical

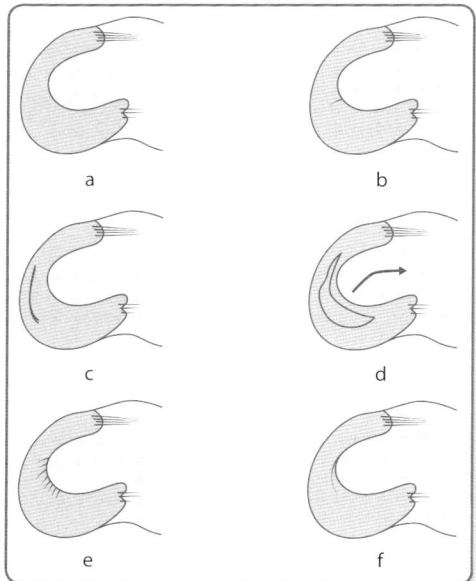

Figure 59.1 Types of meniscal tear. (a) normal, (b) radial, (c) longitudinal, (d) bucket handle tear, (e) degenerate, (f) flap or beak tear.

procedure that partially or completely removes the damaged meniscus. It is not recommended for a degenerative meniscus tear, unless there is locking or catching of the knee.

Complications

Meniscal tears disrupt the physiologically smooth surface of contact with the articular surface generating increased wear in the relevant joint compartment and irreversible damage to the cartilage. This leads to an increased rate of wear within the joint and development of osteoarthritis. Three years postmeniscectomy, 20% of patients will have symptomatic arthritis and 70% will have radiographic changes. Almost all patients will experience arthrosis within 20 years.

Further reading

Baratz ME, Fu FH, Mengato R. Meniscal tears: the effect of meniscectomy and of repair on intraarticular contact areas and stress in the human knee. A preliminary report. Am J Sports Med 1986; 14:270–275.

Salata MJ, Gibbs AE, Sekiya JK. A systematic review of clinical outcomes in patients undergoing meniscectomy. Am J Sports Med 2010; 38:1907–1916.

Smith NA, Costa ML, Spalding T. Meniscal allograft transplantation: Rationale for treatment. Bone Joint J 2015; 97B:590–594.

Related topics of interest

- *Topic 48* Imaging – description and interpretation
- *Topic 57* Knee – cruciate ligament injuries
- *Topic 61* Knee dislocations – multiligament injuries

60 Knee – patella fractures

Key points
- The patella plays an important role in knee extension
- The patellofemoral articulation is subject to the heaviest loads of any joint
- Patella fractures may result from direct or indirect trauma and the associated soft tissue injury can therefore be variable
- The aims of treatment are to achieve anatomical reduction and stable fixation of the joint surface, and to restore the normal extensor mechanism of the knee

Epidemiology

Fractures of the patella account for 1% of all fractures and include a spectrum of fracture patterns. They are mostly seen in those aged 20–50 years and affect men more than women in a 2:1 ratio.

Pathophysiology

The patella is the largest sesamoid bone and has the thickest articular cartilage in the body at 5 mm. It lies within the extensor mechanism of the knee joint. By holding the extensor mechanism away from the centre of rotation of the knee, thereby lengthening its lever arm, it functions to increase the efficiency of the quadriceps during extension. The quadriceps tendon inserts proximally and the patella ligament attaches to the distal pole. The medial and lateral retinaculae – expansions from the quadriceps tendon – are attached to either side of the patella, from where they insert into the proximal tibia.

The patella fractures when subjected to either a direct or indirect force.

Direct trauma to the patella, e.g. a blow against a car dashboard, can result in incomplete, stellate or multifragmentary fractures. In the presence of a wound, this may constitute an open fracture. Displacement of the fragments may be minimal if the retinaculae remain intact.

Indirect trauma to the patella is the more common mechanism of fracture and these fractures are usually closed. Forcible contraction of the quadriceps with the knee in a flexed position typically results in a transverse fracture, when the strength of the bone is exceeded by the strength of the muscular contraction. There may be significant displacement of the fragments as the medial and lateral retinaculae tear, also resulting in loss of active knee extension.

Clinical assessment

The knee is typically swollen painful, and bruised. The patient may be unable to walk. Clinical examination reveals tenderness over the patella and a gap may be felt. The integrity of the retinaculae can be evaluated by asking the patient to actively raise the extended leg. A careful assessment of the soft tissue envelope must be made including prompt identification of any open injury. Neurovascular examination of the leg and foot is mandatory. The remainder of the limb must be examined for any additional injuries.

Investigations

Plain anteroposterior (AP) and lateral radiographs should be obtained. The fracture is usually best demonstrated on the lateral view. On the AP view, a bipartite patella (affecting 8% of the population) can be mistaken for a fracture – comparison views of the contralateral knee may be helpful as this condition is frequently bilateral (50%). A skyline view may reveal osteochondral or vertical fractures.

Classification

Patella fractures can be described as open or closed, and displaced or undisplaced. The pattern of fracture may be transverse, vertical, polar or stellate. Different fracture patterns are shown in **Figure 60.1**.

The AO Foundation's system classifies patella fractures according to the degree of articular involvement, i.e. extra-articular, partial articular and complete articular, and within each category; they can be further

Knee – patella fractures

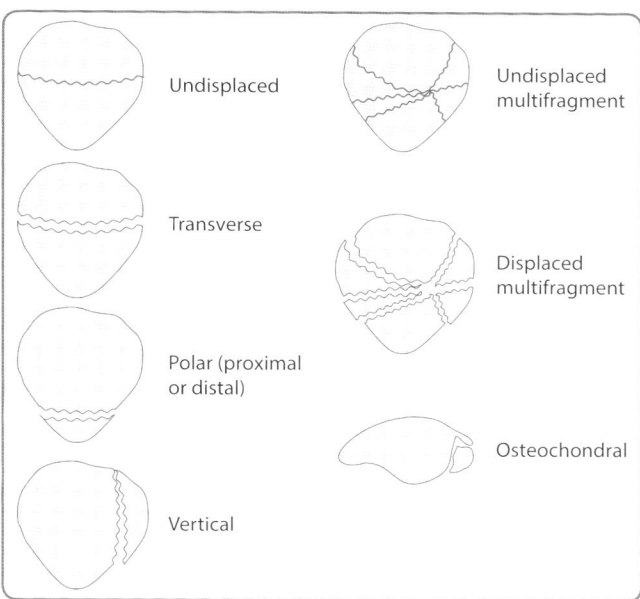

Figure 60.1 Patellar fracture patterns.

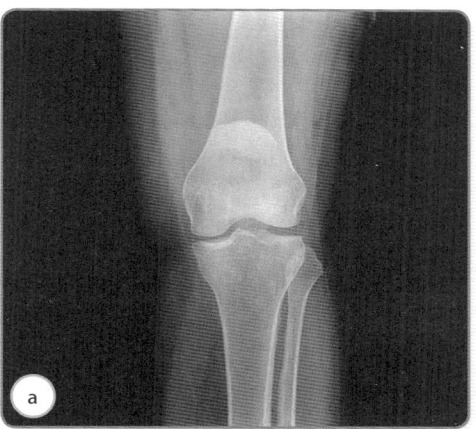
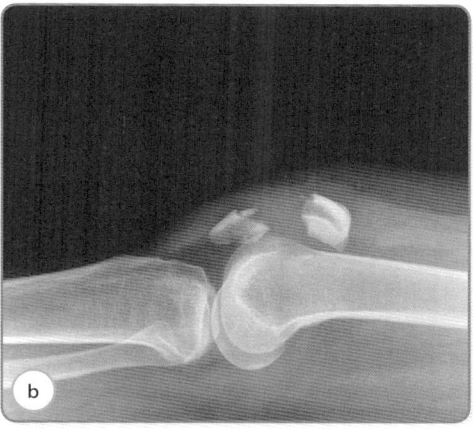

Figure 60.2 (a) AP and (b) horizontal beam lateral radiographs showing an AO/OTA 34-C fracture of the patella.

classified according to the complexity of the fracture pattern. **Figure 60.2** shows an AO/OTA (Orthopaedic Trauma Association) 34-C fracture.

Treatment

Nonoperative

Undisplaced fractures or those displaced <3 mm with <2 mm articular incongruity and an intact extensor mechanism can be treated in an extension brace or cylinder cast for 4–6 weeks, with weight-bearing and quadriceps exercises encouraged from an early stage. Active knee flexion in a hinged knee brace can commence once there is radiographic evidence of healing.

Operative

Open reduction and internal fixation is indicated where active extension is lost,

>2 mm articular incongruity, >3 mm displacement or open fracture. The aim of surgery is to anatomically restore the articular surface of the joint and achieve stable fixation such that early range of movement and rehabilitation can be permitted.

Technique

The patient is positioned supine on the radiolucent table with a sandbag underneath the ipsilateral buttock and a thigh tourniquet applied. A midline longitudinal incision is made over the patella, down through the subcutaneous fat and superficial fascia. The fracture and the extensor mechanism is then examined, including assessment of the retinaculae for any associated tears. The haematoma is cleared from the joint and fracture site, and the articular surface can then be viewed directly. Anatomical reduction with the aid of pointed bone holding forceps can then be achieved. Standard tension band wiring (**Figure 60.3**) or cerclage wiring techniques are then be applied to achieve stable fixation. Lag screws are an alternative method of fixation and transosseous sutures may also be of help, particularly to secure smaller fragments. An on-table assessment of stability of fixation should be made – the knee should be able to bend to 90° without loss of fracture reduction. The medial and lateral retinacular tears must then be repaired prior to layered closure of the wound.

Partial patellectomy has limited indications but may involve excision of unreconstructable polar fragments where there is a larger salvageable fragment.

Total patellectomy is rarely indicated and is reserved for severely comminuted unreconstructable articular fractures. Repair of the retinacular structures is necessary to preserve some extensor function. Notably, the maximum torque of the quadriceps is reduced by around 40% following patellectomy.

Rehabilitation

Gradual increases in flexion may be necessary with the assistance of a hinged knee brace. Generally full weight-bearing in extension is allowed immediately postoperatively.

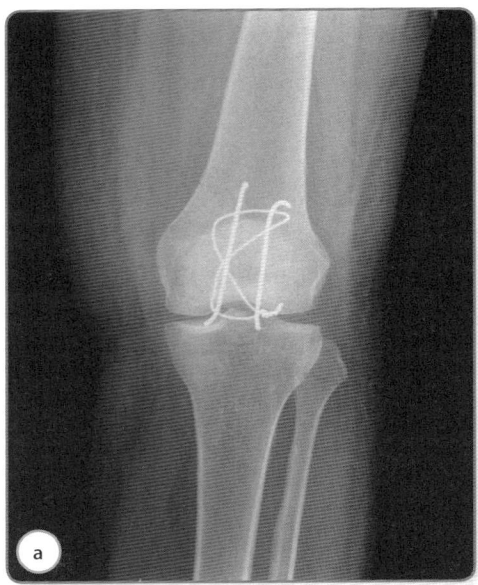

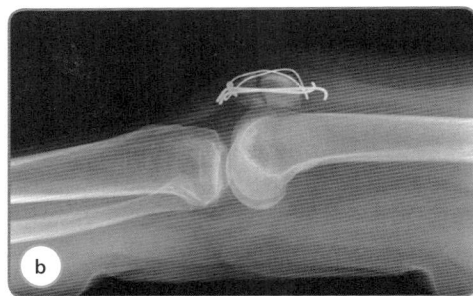

Figure 60.3 (a) AP and (b) lateral radiographs demonstrating standard tension band wiring fixation of a transverse patella fracture (AO/OTA 34-C).

Complications

Early

Although uncommon, infection may follow an open fracture. This requires debridement and antibiotic treatment until resolved. Failure of fixation may occur, particularly in osteoporotic bone, and revision fixation or patellectomy can be salvage options.

Late

Knee range of motion may be reduced, typically following immobilisation or formation of scar tissue. Metalwork may cause irritation to subcutaneous tissues and removal may be required, but this should be left in for at least 9 months where possible to reduce the risk of fixation failure. There is also a small risk of refracture and nonunion (<5%), and a significant (>50%) rate of post-traumatic patellofemoral osteoarthritis.

Further reading

Rüedi T, AO Education AO Foundation. Chapter 6,7. In: AO Principles of Fracture Management, Vol2. Stuttgart: Thieme, 2007.

Wendt PP, Johnson RP. A study of quadriceps excursion, torque, and the effect of patellectomy on cadaver knees. J Bone Joint Surg Am 1985; 67:726–732.

Related chapters of interest

- *Topic 58* Knee – extensor mechanism injury

61 Knee dislocations – multiligament injuries

Key points

- Knee dislocation is a rare but limb-threatening emergency condition
- It typically results from high-energy trauma, but can result from sporting injuries or low energy mechanisms in morbidly obese individuals
- There is a high-rate of associated arterial injury, with all cases requiring immediate vascular assessment

Epidemiology

Knee dislocations represent <0.2% of orthopaedic injuries. Most cases occur in young men.

Pathophysiology

Significant trauma is required to disrupt the soft tissue structures about the knee sufficiently to cause dislocation – generally at least 3 out of 4 of the major ligamentous structures (ACL, PCL, MCL, LCL) of the knee are injured.

Most cases occur during high-energy road traffic accidents, but around one-third are sporting injuries. In a morbidly obese patient, knee dislocation can occur with a low energy mechanism.

Anterior tibiofemoral dislocation, which is most common, occurs with hyperextension of the knee (with or without a varus or valgus force). Posterior tibiofemoral dislocation usually occurs from axial loading on a flexed knee, such as when the proximal tibia strikes a car dashboard during a motor vehicle accident.

Associated fractures of the tibial spines, tibial plateau, proximal fibula, femur and acetabulum may co-exist and must be identified.

Clinical assessment

In an unreduced dislocation there is an obvious, gross deformity of the knee associated with severe swelling, bruising and pain. However, in some cases the dislocation may have spontaneously reduced before medical attention is sought and the findings are less dramatic: rupture of the joint capsule can cause the haemarthrosis to leak into the surrounding soft tissues, and this bruising may be the only sign. Other features may include an effusion, abrasions or pain in the context of a significant mechanism of injury.

The 'dimple' sign, whereby the medial femoral condyle has buttonholed through the medial capsule, suggests posterolateral dislocation and an attempt at closed reduction is contraindicated as this can lead to skin necrosis.

Careful vascular examination is mandatory. The popliteal artery is injured in around 20% of cases. After reduction of the dislocation, the vascular status of the limb – including the dorsalis pedis and posterior tibial pulses as well as capillary refill time – should be examined and the findings clearly documented. An immediate vascular opinion should be sought if there are concerns. Where the limb remains ischaemic after reduction, immediate surgical exploration is indicated. The literature does not support routine angiography in all cases of knee dislocation; however, weak pulses, prolonged capillary refill time or an ankle brachial pressure index measurement of less than 0.9 are indications for vascular imaging.

Neurological examination is also mandatory. The incidence of associated common peroneal nerve injury is around 33% and this is most commonly seen with anterior, posterolateral and medial dislocations; a significant proportion of those will have a complete disruption of the nerve which may require grafting or later tibialis posterior tendon transfer to help restore ankle dorsiflexion.

There is an association with compartment syndrome and a high index of suspicion for this must be maintained when taking care of these patients.

Investigations

Because of the potentially limb-threatening consequences of knee dislocation, reduction is advised prior to imaging. Post reduction plain anteroposterior and lateral radiographs should be taken in the first instance, to assess the reduction and look for any associated fractures.

As above, routine use of angiography for all cases is not supported by the literature; however, if there are any concerns about the vascularity of the limb digital subtraction angiography (DSA) or CT angiography can be undertaken.

MRI is indicated to identify the injured structures and plan suitable reconstructive surgery accordingly.

Classification

The dislocation can be described according to the position of the tibia relative to the femur (i.e. anterior, posterior, lateral, medial, rotational – usually posterolateral) – but in cases where there was spontaneous reduction this can be difficult to determine.

The anatomical classification described by Schenck is more useful as it helps the surgeon to consider which ligamentous structures are injured and require repair (**Table 61.1**).

Treatment
Initial management

The initial management is to reduce the dislocation with axial traction and temporarily splint the knee at 20–30° of flexion. The neurovascular status must then be reassessed and vascular opinion sought if there are concerns about arterial injury.

For grossly unstable knees, those requiring open reduction, or where there is a vascular injury requiring repair, application of a temporary spanning external fixator will provide more reliable and convenient stability.

Nonoperative

The knee can be immobilised in extension in either a long leg cast or external fixator, but whilst prolonged immobilisation leads to marked stiffness, too short a duration of immobilisation can leave residual symptomatic instability. A 6-week period of immobilisation was previously a common treatment for knee dislocation; however, the literature now favours early ligament reconstruction, with this leading to reduced stiffness and instability and consequently improved functional knee scores. There are a few patients who will be unfit for major reconstructive surgery, and in these cases immobilisation may be the only realistic treatment option.

Operative

Multiligament reconstruction requires high surgical skill, and access to resources such as allograft tendons. The timing must be carefully considered, according to whether revascularisation is indicated, the condition of the soft tissues including the presence of an open injury, the severity/extent of the ligament injuries and whether there is an associated periarticular fracture.

Acutely, where revascularisation procedures are carried out, repair of the medial or lateral capsular injury should take place at the same time as this can provide increased stability to protect the vascular graft. External fixation and fasciotomies should also be performed.

Otherwise, timing of ligament reconstruction may be early or delayed. Early (within 3 weeks) surgery has been shown to improve range of motion and have a reduced risk of arthrofibrosis.

Reconstruction of the PCL is key to restoring normal tibiofemoral alignment and this should be done first, because

Table 61.1 The Schenck classification

Classification	Injured structures
KD-I	Either ACL or PCL, in the context of multiligament injury
KD-II	ACL and PCL with collaterals intact
KD-IIIM	ACL, PCL and MCL
KD-IIIL	ACL, PCL and LCL/PLC
KD-IV	ACL, PCL, MCL, LCL, PLC
KD-V	Periarticular fracture-dislocation

ACL, anterior cruciate ligament; LCL, lateral collateral ligament; MCL, medial collateral ligament; PCL, posterior cruciate ligament; PLC, posterolateral corner.

ACL and collateral reconstruction rely on normal tibiofemoral relationship. Ligament reconstruction can be achieved by open or arthroscopic methods, using autografts or allografts (Achilles tendon, patella tendon, hamstring, synthetic grafts). Early reconstruction of the posterolateral corner is recommended as delayed reconstruction can be extremely difficult.

Intensive postoperative rehabilitation is key in reducing the severity of joint stiffness, but this must be judiciously supervised in a hinged knee brace to reduce the risk of graft (including vascular graft) failure.

Complications
Immediate
Arterial injury occurs in a significant proportion of patients and is limb-threatening. Without appropriate, prompt treatment this can lead to amputation.

Nerve injury, particularly of the common peroneal nerve is also reasonably prevalent and may require later grafting or tendon transfer to restore dorsiflexion. Where the nerve is not completely disrupted, recovery is possible but can take many months.

Early/late
Function does not usually return to pre-injury levels after knee dislocation even following surgical reconstruction and intensive rehabilitation.

Stiffness and limited range of motion is the most common complication and results from scar tissue formation and arthrofibrosis. Early surgery to reconstruct damaged ligaments followed by intensive rehabilitation may reduce this compared to delayed surgery or nonoperative treatment, but once established the stiffness can be very difficult to treat.

Ligamentous laxity may occur but is not usually sufficient to cause recurrent dislocation. Meticulous surgical reconstruction and appropriate rehabilitation including quadriceps strengthening exercises help to reduce the impact of this.

Complications of surgery can include graft failure, infection and stiffness.

Post-traumatic osteoarthritis is present in up to 50% of patients.

Further reading

Fanelli GC. The multiple ligament injured knee. Berlin: Springer, 2013.

Robertson A, Nutton RW, Keating JF. Dislocation of the knee. J Bone Joint Surg Br 2006; 88B:706–711.

Related chapters of interest

- *Topic 57* Knee – cruciate ligament injuries
- *Topic 58* Knee – extensor mechanism injury
- *Topic 59* Knee – meniscal injuries
- *Topic 60* Knee – patella fractures

62 Major trauma – Advanced Trauma and Life Support principles

Key points
- Major trauma is associated with a trimodal distribution of death
- A systematic approach to clinical examination and intervention is required
- Assessments should be repeated to ensure appropriate response to any intervention performed
- Classification systems correlate severity of injury with outcome

Epidemiology

The World Health Organization reported in 2010 that more than 9 people died every minute globally from violence or injury. The main causes of death were road traffic accidents, suicides and homicides. The introduction of major trauma centres in the USA has reduced mortality rates in severely injured patients by up to 25%.

Major trauma is the leading cause of mortality in people aged <45 years old in the UK. Major trauma centres were introduced to the United Kingdom in 2012. They are the focal point of trauma networks and offer consultant-led multi-specialty hospital care with the aim of reducing mortality rates.

Pathophysiology

There is a trimodal death distribution associated with major trauma. The first is associated with the severity of the trauma itself, e.g. it is unsurvivable. The second peak is known as the golden hour and occurs within minutes to hours after the trauma. Patients in this category will die, usually from haemorrhagic shock, unless they receive urgent clinical intervention and resuscitation. The third peak occurs days to weeks after trauma and most commonly is due to multi-organ dysfunction or sepsis. The chances of a positive outcome at this stage relate to the quality of care received at the preceding stages.

The purpose of major trauma centres is to positively impact on the outcomes of patients in peaks 2 and 3. Mortality rates will only reduce in peak one if public health and prevention methods are introduced such as air bags and lower speed limits.

Clinical assessment

Clinical assessment takes a systematic approach [A(cc)-B-C-D-E], identifying and addressing the most serious life-threatening conditions first.

First and most important is securing the patient's airway (A). Coupled with this is cervical spine control (C) and control of exanguinating haemorrhage. Both unstable cervical spine injuries and uncontrolled massive haemorrhage can cause death rapidly.

The airway can be assessed by simply asking the conscious patient to state their name, or by opening the jaws and looking inside the oral cavity if the patient is obtunded. Suction catheters can be used to aid removal of blood, mucus and vomit which prevents the patient from aspirating. The cervical spine should be managed with a hard collar to maintain anatomical alignment and prevent neurological injury. Control of major haemorrhage can be achieved either through direct external pressure to the area, or through the application of a trauma tourniquet to control arterial bleeding. The time at which this is applied should be written on the tourniquet so everyone is aware of the ischaemia time.

Hypoxia is the next biggest threat to life; therefore, high flow oxygen should be administered via a nonrebreathe reservoir mask. An assessment of the respiratory system (B) should then be undertaken and consists of tracheal position, respiratory rate, oxygen saturation, chest expansion, percussion of the anterior thorax and auscultation for added or reduced breath sounds.

The circulatory system (C) should then be assessed. Monitoring should be applied in the form of ECG leads, blood pressure cuff and pulse oximeter to support the clinical assessment. Peripheral and central refill, patient warmth, rate, volume and strength of the radial pulse, and auscultation of heart sounds should be performed. Patients suspected of sustaining a pelvic injury should have a pelvic binder fitted. In the trauma setting patients are most likely to be hypotensive and tachycardic secondary to haemorrhagic shock, they should receive blood transfusions rather than successive boluses of crystalloid or colloid solutions, which dilute the blood volume further and have no oxygen-carrying capacity. The grade of haemorrhagic shock can be determined using **Table 62.1**.

The neurological system (D) should be assessed and is most easily performed using the Glasgow Coma Scale (**Table 62.2**). A full neurological assessment should be undertaken as part of the secondary survey. For patients with spinal injuries the American Spinal Injury Association (ASIA) impairment scale should be completed and the severity of the spinal injury graded.

Lastly the patient should be completely exposed (E) to look for any occult injuries. They should then be recovered and warming devices applied to prevent hypothermia.

This clinical examination should be revisited regularly to ensure that the patient is responding appropriately to any intervention.

Investigations

Intravenous access should be gained in the first instance. This should be achieved with wide bore cannulas allow for blood samples to be sent for full blood count, urea and electrolytes, group and save, clotting screen,

Table 62.1 Grading of haemorrhagic shock

	Grade 1 shock	Grade 2 shock	Grade 3 shock	Grade 4 shock
Blood loss (% total volume)	<15	15–30	30–40	>40
Blood loss (mL)	<750	750–1500	1500–2000	>2000
Heart rate (bpm)	<100	100–120	120–140	>140
Blood pressure	Unchanged	Unchanged	Decreased +	Decreased ++
Pulse pressure	Unchanged or increased	Decreased +	Decreased ++	Decreased +++
Respiratory rate (bpm)	Unchanged	20–30	30–35	>35
Urine output (mL/h)	>30	20–30	5–15	<5
Mental status	Normal	Anxious	Confused	Obtunded

Table 62.2 Glasgow Coma Scale: the three scores are totalled (maximum 15)

Eyes (maximum score: 4)	Voice (maximum score: 5)	Motor (maximum score: 6)
Open spontaneously (4) Open to voice (3) Open to pain (2) Do not open (1)	Normal speech (5) Confused speech (4) Inappropriate speech (3) Incomprehensible sounds (2) No sounds made (1)	Normal movements and follows commands (6) Localises to pain (5) Withdraws to pain (4) Abnormal flexion to pain – decorticate posturing (3) Abnormal extension to pain – decerebrate posturing (2) No movements (1)

and venous blood gas (VBG). The VBG offers basic biochemistry and haematology results, as well as lactate. Serial lactates evidence a patient's response to fluid resuscitation and an important physiological marker in deeming if patients are fit for theatre. Female patients should also have a beta-human chorionic gonadotropin (β-HCG) test.

Generally urgent plain radiographs of the neck, chest and pelvis should be avoided in favour of a CT scan. The CT scan should include the entire body from head to lesser trochanters of the femur. If there are no contraindications, contrast for vascular assessment should be included in the CT. Ideally a senior radiologist should report the CT scan within an hour.

Chest X-rays may be requested after intervention such as a chest tube for pneumothorax, although clinical response is the best indicator of a successful treatment. Plain pelvic radiographs can be undertaken after the CT scan if there is any suspicion of ligamentous injury. This should be done with the pelvic binder taken off as part of the secondary survey.

Classifications

The injury severity score (ISS) is an anatomical grading system that provides an overall score for patients with multiple injuries. It correlates with morbidity, mortality and severity of injury. Six anatomical regions: (head and neck, face, chest, abdomen, limbs, external) are assigned an abbreviated injury score (AIS). The AIS is graded between 1–6, with 6 marking an unsurvivable injury. The three highest scores are squared and added together to give an ISS between 0 and 75. Any anatomical region scoring an AIS of 6 automatically scores an ISS of 75.

The mangled extremity severity score (MESS) was designed to assist in the care of patients with limb-threatening injuries, although it's ability to predict amputation is still contested. Four criteria are scored: skeletal/soft tissue injury; limb ischaemia; shock and age. If the limb is ischaemic for >6 hours, the overall score is doubled.

Treatment

The primary aim of treatment is to resuscitate the patient rapidly and prevent the lethal triad of hypothermia, acidosis and coagulopathy. Interventions are administered in parallel with the clinical assessment. Thus, a definitive airway should be acquired, oxygenation and ventilation assured, and cardiac output maintained. This may necessitate intubation of the airway, performance of a cricothyroidotomy, decompression of a tension pneumothorax and subsequent chest drain insertion. The trauma surgeon should be competent to perform these interventions if required.

A 'code red' alert may be put out either before the arrival or at any stage thereafter for patients who are in haemorrhagic shock and require a massive transfusion. This ensures patients receive red blood cells, fresh frozen plasma and platelets, usually in a 1:1:1 or 2:1:1 ratio. A thromboelastogram can be obtained to determine the adequacy of resuscitation. A systematic clinical assessment should be undertaken concurrently to identify and treat the cause of shock.

Complications

Complications can arise in any of the peaks of trauma previously described. The trauma itself can result in either loss of life or limb, or permanent disability, e.g. secondary to spinal or neurological injury. Complications can also arise secondary to the trauma, e.g. pneumonia secondary to dyspnea and pain on inspiration and coughing. Inadequate care can also negatively impact upon the patient, e.g. failing to secure and stabilise an unstable cervical injury.

Major trauma centres aim to reduce these complications through consultant-led care and having all necessary multi-disciplinary professionals on site to offer the rehabilitation required.

Further reading

World Health Organization (WHO). Injuries and violence: the facts. Geneva: WHO; 2010.

Related topics of interest

- *Topic 17* Damage control orthopaedics and trauma physiology
- *Topic 37* Guidelines in trauma
- *Topic 38* Gunshot injuries
- *Topic 45* Head injury
- *Topic 86* Resuscitation and massive transfusion

63 Major trauma networks

Key points

- The organisation of trauma services into a countrywide network with centralisation of specialist care is associated with a reduction in death and disability
- A major trauma network requires a multidisciplinary approach along the entire care pathway
- Systematic data collection is of major importance in order to audit, standardise and improve the quality of care (QoC) in major trauma patients

Definition

Trauma is the leading cause of death among children and young adults of 44 years and under. In addition, trauma leaves many thousands of people severely disabled for life.

The term 'major trauma' is used to define a patient who has suffered significant trauma and presents with multiple injuries to the same or different body regions or systems. The injury severity score grades the clinical significance of the injuries, and although it has some recognised limitations, it is regarded as the 'gold standard' for trauma severity grading. An injury severity score greater than 15 qualifies as major trauma.

A major trauma centre (MTC) is a hospital capable of providing total care for every aspect of injury, from resuscitation through to rehabilitation. MTC trauma services represent the organisational infrastructure that assures holistic care for the individual patient. In the UK, MTCs are supported by a network of trauma units (TUs) and local emergency care centres, rehabilitation units and ambulance services.

History

Reports in 1988 from the Royal College of Surgeons of England and in 1989 from the British Orthopaedic Association (BOA) identified and raised awareness of deficiencies regarding the management of seriously injured patients in the UK. Many hospital units receiving seriously injured patients were too small and often the initial resuscitation was performed by inexperienced staff. Lack of intensive care facilities, deficiencies in equipment and in general the lack of resources was concerning. There was no explanation in regards to variations of mortality in different hospitals, significant delays in patient transfers when needed, and too few consultants with a special interest in trauma. The data collection was performed in a local manner, with no regional or national communication or analysis of this data. Three pre-existing large centres were used as models in 1988 for the future network: the Royal London Hospital in London, the John Radcliffe Hospital in Oxford and North Staffordshire Hospital in Stoke.

A later report in 1997 by the BOA concluded that patients in the UK were not receiving the QoC available in many developed countries, including Germany, Switzerland and the USA. In the BOA's view, the QoC would only be achieved by:

- Taking patients to hospitals most suited to the nature of their injuries, rather than to the nearest hospital
- Centralising expertise in the management of severe injuries
- A multi-disciplinary team approach with the integration of hospitals into a system of care, and direct involvement of senior clinicians

The need of a national strategy for care of the severely injured was reported in 2000, but it was only in 2010 when the planning and designing of a national integrated system began. The final implementation took place in 2011 with the establishment of a national major trauma network. There are currently 27 MTCs in the UK.

Rationale

The aim of implementing a major trauma network is to improve the QoC for severely injured patients. This includes not only decreasing mortality, but also to improving the quality of life in the survivors with rehabilitation pathways to give the patients the best chance of recovery following surgery.

A trauma system combines the cooperation of prehospital, hospital, and rehabilitation facilities within a defined geographic area integrated with a regional health system. When designing a trauma network, a multidisciplinary approach and integration along the entire trauma care pathway is a priority, and the standard of care must be coordinated nationally. Countries like the USA, Australia, Denmark and Canada have established trauma networks and report benefits both on mortality and morbidity.

The ideal trauma system includes:
- Prevention of trauma
- Pre-hospital care
- In-hospital care
- Rehabilitation facilities
- Internal and external quality control
- Education and research programs

The UK trauma network

The fundamental components of the regional trauma system were initially based on the US model, although this model could not be fully extrapolated to the UK due to the presence of many densely populated areas, shorter transportation distances and the already existing infrastructure of district general hospitals.

The system started in London and then went live for the whole of England in April 2012, when the National Health Service in England introduced the trauma network system, centralising the care in each region. 22 MTCs were initially designated across England. This subsequently expanded to 27.

In England, patients who are seriously injured are treated in integrated trauma networks comprising ambulances services, TUs and MTCs. These services are bound by protocols governing arrangements for triage, transfer, and treatment, backed by governance and benchmarking processes, to ensure that the right patient gets to the right hospital at the right time.

Data collection

Collecting information on care is essential for monitoring and improving services. In the UK, the Trauma Audit and Research Network (TARN) is responsible for collection, analysis and publication of data from the network, including audit and analysis. These data are used to evaluate the QoC as well as providing a source for hypothesis-generation for research in trauma. Compliance with data collection plays an important role too, the performance of the hospitals that do not submit data to TARN cannot be measured.

Outcomes

The 16,000 life-threatening major traumas are the biggest cause of death in children and adults under the age of 40 years annually in the UK. In all, some 37,000 are seriously injured in England each year. Trauma Networks have improved outcomes for trauma patients across the country.

Fewer patients require secondary transfer from other hospitals following the launch of the trauma network. Previously these patients

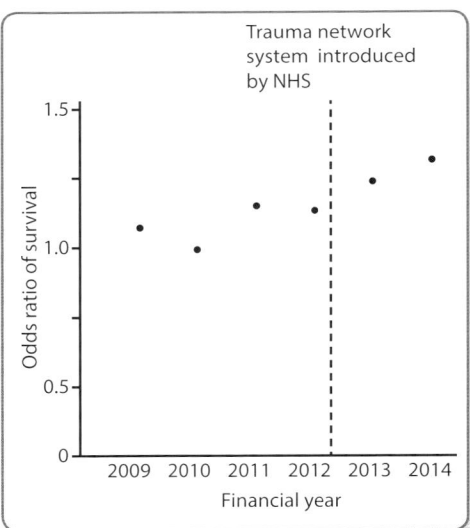

Figure 63.1 Survival rates after major trauma in England. $n = 62, 290, p = 0.014$.

often waited 7–10 days in a local hospital before being transferred to a specialist surgical unit for treatment of complex injuries to their spine, pelvis or limbs. Over 90% of patients are transferred within 2 days, treated and then go home promptly or move to a hospital close to their home to complete their recovery.

Although the UK network has only been functioning for over 2 years, preliminary data show that the proportion of patients coded as having a good recovery at discharge has increased significantly.

Results from the TARN national audit reported by NHS England show that 1 in 5 patients who would have died before the networks are now surviving severe injuries. Patients in England have a 30% improved chance of surviving severe injuries after the introduction of regional trauma networks across England in April 2012 (**Figure 63.1**).

Further reading

Darzi A. High Quality Care for All, NHS Next Stage Review – Final Report. London: Department of Health, 2008:1–92.

Metcalfe D, Bouamra O, Parsons NR, et al. Effect of regional trauma centralization on volume, injury severity and outcomes of injured patients admitted to trauma centres. Br J Surg 2014; 101:959–964.

NHS England. NHS saves lives of hundreds more trauma victims just two years after changes to care. NHS news. London: NHS England, 2014.

Related topics of interest

- *Topic 62* Major trauma – Advanced Trauma and Life Support principles
- *Topic 65* Multiple casualties
- *Topic 86* Resuscitation and massive transfusion

64 Malunion and deformity correction

Key points

- Knowledge of the normal mechanical/anatomical axes of the limb is essential for understanding malunion and deformity assessment
- Altered distribution of weight-bearing stresses leads to abnormal force concentration across joints
- The principles of deformity correction are to restore length, alignment and rotation, whilst maintaining normal joint orientation

Malunion

Following fracture healing, the morphology of the involved bone is sometimes altered to a degree in which efficient function of the limb is impaired. Alterations of length, angulation, rotation and translation are generally well tolerated by patients but sometimes these changes need correcting. The most significant problems are functional impairment, cosmesis and long-term effects of malalignment on joint integrity due to altered distribution of load across the joint.

A thorough understanding of the biomechanics and its alterations as well as a preoperative plan are imperative in the treatment of malunions. Both patient and surgeon must fully understand and consider the risks and benefits of this treatment, its complexity and the complications that may arise as a result of it.

Deformity assessment

The mechanical axis of a bone is defined by the line that connects the center points of the proximal and distal joints. The anatomical axis is the diaphyseal line (**Figure 64.1**).

In the lower limb, the mechanical axis passes from the femoral head to the center of the ankle in the frontal plane. This axis crosses the knee 10 mm medial to its frontal plane centre. In the sagittal plane, the mechanical axis from the center of the femoral head to the

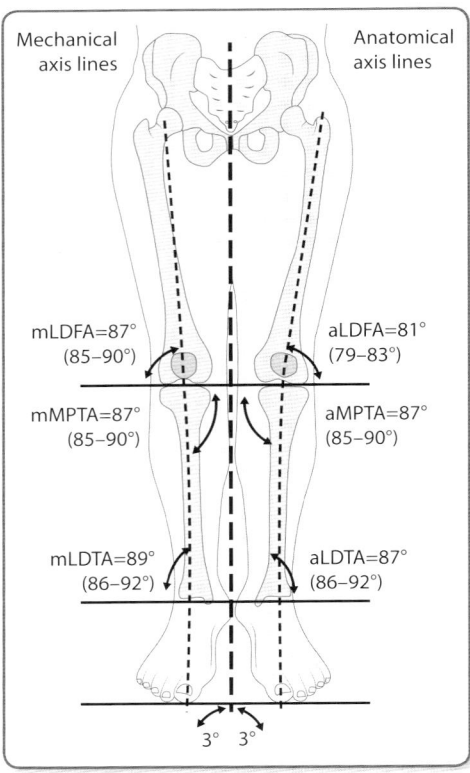

Figure 64.1 Mechanical and anatomical axes. The lower limbs are in the 'at attention' standing position. Note that the alignment of the lower limbs to the ground changes when the feet are together ('at attention' position) and when the feet are separated at a distance equal to the width of the pelvis ('at ease' position). mLDFA, mechanical lateral distal femoral angle; mMPTA, mechanical medial proximal tibial angle; mLDTA, mechanical lateral distal tibial angle; aLDFA, anatomical lateral distal femoral angle; aMPTA, anatomical medial proximal tibial angle; aLDTA, anatomical lateral distal tibial angle.

centre of the ankle lies anterior to the center of rotation of the knee joint, allowing passive locking of the knee in full extension.

Deformity assessment of the lower limb:
- Leg length discrepancy (LLD) – this can be estimated using calibrated blocks to

level the anterior superior iliac spines on palpation. The contribution of the tibia to the discrepancy can be estimated clinically by positioning the patient prone with 90º of knee flexion. The difference in height can usually be attributed to the tibia, with the reminder accounted for by the femur. Radiographically, the assessment is more precise, with leg-length radiographs or with computer tomography
- Limb rotation – it can be estimated by comparing maximal internal and external rotation of the lower limbs
- Angular deformity – once proximal and distal anatomical axes are defined, the point of intersection of both axes is defined as centre of rotation of angulation (CORA). The CORA will be found in the apex of the deformity in cases of pure angulation, but moved away from the site of maximal angular deformity when the angulation is combined with a rotational deformity. The plane of maximal angular deformity can be assessed quantitatively: by rotating the limb into a plane in which no angular deformity is seen on fluoroscopy, orthogonal to this plane is the plane of maximal angular deformity
- Effect of the deformity on the joint mechanics
- Symptoms – careful evaluation of ligamentous stability, local muscle strength, range of motion, degenerative changes of the involved joints and gait analysis

Surgical indications

Conservative treatment is the first line when addressing malunion. The use of shoe orthoses, lifts, load transferring braces and analgesics should be tried before considering surgical treatment.

When the malunion requires surgical management, an osteotomy must be designed following the principles of deformity correction: restore normal alignment, length, rotation and horizontal joint line orientation. Some complications associated with an abnormal alignment of the limb such as muscle weakness, joint fibrosis and articular degenerative changes are not generally improved with corrective surgery and must be considered during decision making.

Indications for surgery:
- LLD >2 cm
- Varus malalignment of the knee or ankle >10º
- Valgus malalignment of the knee or ankle >15º
- >20 mm medial shift in the mechanical axis
- Ligamentous instability on the convex side of the deformity
- Inability to place foot in plantigrade position
- Unicondylar arthritis of the knee

Osteotomy

Location

Location and type and method of osteotomy are the steps that follow the decision of proceeding with surgical treatment.

Ideally, the angular correction is centred coincident with the CORA. If it is moved from the CORA, a residual translation deformity remains. This must be anticipated and corrected.

Biologic factors such as bone quality and soft-tissue compromised areas have to be considered and may modify the initial planned location of the osteotomy.

The plane of the deformity must be defined, depending on the deformity this being angular in the frontal or sagittal plane, rotational, oblique, translational, or frequently a combination of these. The need of lengthening or shortening must also be taken into account.

Type

The different osteotomy types include opening wedge, closing wedge, oblique, dome and distraction osteogenesis. Each type has its own characteristics, advantages, disadvantages and complications. Opening wedge osteotomies restore length and can be performed percutaneously but can potentially provoke triangular defects. Closing wedge osteotomies achieve bone contact and can be applied directly to the CORA; however, they need greater surgical exposure and can potentially lengthen tendons and ligaments that cross the osteotomy.

Fixation methods

Intramedullary devices can be used if the medullary canal remains. Modern intramedullary nail designs allow the surgeon not only to stabilise the osteotomy but also to lengthen or shorten the bone.

Plate fixation was the gold standard of osteotomy stabilisation before the modern external fixators appeared. This method requires open exposure and is especially advantageous when stabilising short metaphyseal segments.

External fixators play an important role in deformity correction, especially where limb elongation and rotational correction is required. The use of this hardware is on the rise again, as it was before World War II and again in the seventies and early eighties. A wide variety of fixators with articulations and pin-grippers are available nowadays. The constructs have evolved, and based on the Ilizarov circular fixators new modern and more advantageous designs are in the market. Designs like the Taylor Spatial Frame or the TL-Hex use struts to connect Ilizarov type rings, which can be independently lengthened or shortened, and the relationship between rings can be altered. Mathematically the path that the displaced bone fragment must travel is defined, and the correction is performed precisely and in a controlled fashion.

Advantages of circular external fixators:
- Minimally invasive
- Can promote bony tissue generation
- Often require only minimal soft tissue dissection
- Versatile
- Can be used in the face of acute or chronic infection
- Allow for stabilisation of small intra-articular or periarticular bone fragments
- Allow for simultaneous bony healing and deformity correction
- Allow for immediate weight-bearing
- Allow for early joint mobilisation

Fixator-associated problems:
- Pressure necrosis of the skin and undue or excessive pain
- Pin site infection
- Pin or wire breakage
- Disruption of patient's lifestyle, psychosocial problems
- Multiple follow-ups, prolonged period of treatment

Further reading

Paley D. Principles of deformity correction. Heidelberg, Berlin: Springer-Verlag, 2002.

Related topics of interest

- Topic 67 Nonunion of fractures
- Topic 85 Principles of operative management of fractures
- Topic 91 Soft tissue coverage in trauma

65 Multiple casualties

Key points
- Mass causality incidents have the potential to overwhelm standard resources
- A coordinated, multi-agency response and preparedness is essential in achieving the best outcome
- Rapid triage is casualties critical

Background

A multiple casualty or mass casualty incident (MCI) is a single event or simultaneous events in which the standard resources of the responding emergency services provider are overwhelmed by the number of casualties. Services have to be significantly augmented to provide a sustainable response.

Conventional incidents are those that do not involve chemical, biological, radiological or nuclear (CBRN) aspects. Such events include building collapse, terrorism events, and mass transit accidents. Complex incidents are defined as mass numbers of casualties over a large geographic scale with potential CBRN elements. Recent examples from around the world include the Boxing Day tsunami in the Indian Ocean in 2004, the attack on the World Trade Center in New York in 2001, the Boston marathon bombings in 2013, the multiple bombing attacks on the Madrid transport system in 2004, and the 7th July bombings in London in 2005. All these examples required an unprecedented level of preparedness.

Historically, civilian medical personnel have little experience in treating patients in such extreme circumstances. The increased threat from terrorism and chemical, biological and nuclear attacks have forced most western cities (and hospitals) to enhance their frameworks for responding to MCIs. Furthermore, the diverse causes of MCIs require adequate flexibility within organisational planning. This chapter uses the UK's NHS arrangements to illustrate the principles of planning and coordinating responses to MCIs. Other countries have similar systems and processes in place.

Governance

In the UK, the Civil Contingencies Act (CCA) 2004 outlines the responsibilities of those involved in preparations for MCI. Planning is multi-layered and ranges from individual hospital major incident planning to national frameworks.

NHS England helps to establish the precise organisational management and training involved in preparing for MCI. The Emergency Preparedness Division of the UK Department of Health published the 'NHS Emergency Planning Guidance' in 2005 and the 'MCIs– a framework for planning' in 2007 to provide specific guidance for the health service in preparing for MCIs beyond the capacity of local major incident plans. Testing of these protocols at a local and national level is essential in ensuring preparedness.

Definitions

An emergency is defined by the CCA in 2004 as 'an event or a situation which threatens serious damage to human welfare in a place in the UK, the environment of a place in the UK, all war or terrorism which threatens serious damage to the security of the UK'. The term 'emergency' is used interchangeably with 'incident'.

The term 'major incident' is the pluralistic term used in the UK National Health System (NHS). It is defined by the NHS Emergency Planning Guidance document as 'any occurrence which presents serious threat to the health of the community, disruption to the service or causes (or is likely to cause) such numbers or types of casualties as to require special arrangements to be implemented by hospitals, ambulance trusts or primary care organisations'. There are three scales of major incidents in the NHS (**Table 65.1**).

A MCI is defined as 'A disastrous event or other circumstances where the normal major incident response of NHS organisations must be augmented by extraordinary measures

Table 65.1 NHS categories for major incidents

Category	Description
1	Rapid triage of casualties is critical to management
2	Incidents requiring collaboration of neighbouring NHS trusts and ambulance services. Potentially hundreds of casualties, major facility evacuation and service disruption lasting many days, e.g. building collapse, fire and contamination
3	Incident causing severe disruption of healthcare services exceeding capability of collective effort of neighbouring NHS trusts

in order to cope'. MCIs are distinguished from typical major incidents by their scale, duration and also by the additional challenges of potential loss of infrastructure or services.

Types of mass casualty incident

- 'Big bang' incidents – a sudden incident such as a building collapse, explosion, mass transit accidents or a series of smaller incidents
- 'Rising tide' incidents – an evolving incident such as an outbreak of infectious disease, power shortage, crisis of capacity or a major event elsewhere requiring preparatory action
- CBRN incidents – these pose a different set of challenges. A specialised team is required and rapid control of the site with mass decontamination facilities is essential

Multi-disciplinary team

The best outcome for causalities is achieved with careful planning, cooperation and coordination of the emergency services, transport and government agencies. Essential personnel and agencies include:
- Emergency medical technicians and paramedics – to triage and treat at the scene
- Land and air ambulances – to evacuate casualties from scene
- Police officers: to secure the scene
- Fire fighters – to extricate casualties and for fire suppression and prevention
- Transportation agencies – to augment services and offer assistance as required
- Primary and tertiary medical personnel – to receive, triage and treat causalities
- Specialised teams to neutralise biological, radiological or chemical hazards
- Charitable and nongovernment organisations – to provide manpower and shelter
- Media – to inform and advise the public

At the scene

Declaring a mass casualty incident

In Big Bang incidents, the first responder to a scene is usually the ambulance services. The initial assessment is feedback and a system is triggered leading to a declaration of a MCI. In the UK, e.g. the London Ambulance Service would attend an incident in London, NHS London is notified of a potential MCI and the Mass Casualties Framework would be activated.

Specific responsibilities of the ambulance services include:
- Alerting the most appropriate receiving hospital
- Notification of the police and fire services of the extent and circumstance of the incident
- Communicating with the wider community

In rising tide incidents, the ambulance services may not be directly involved initially. Government organisations such as the Strategic Health Authority in the UK and National Incident Management System in the USA, take responsibility for the implementation of command and control mechanisms along with the appropriate deployment of resources.

Triage

During an established MCI, patient care is the priority based on requirement. The first responders to the scene are essential in triaging the casualties. Triage should be rapid and consist of assessment for life-threatening conditions.

An easy and widely utilised triage system in MCI is the Simple Triage and Rapid Treatment (START) system. The three parameters of respiration, perfusion and mental status (RPM) are assessed using this system and a colour-coded triage level is given (**Figure 65.1**). The highest priority of triage (immediate treatment/red tag) is assigned to casualties with salvageable major life-threatening injuries. The second highest level of triage (delayed treatment/yellow tag) is assigned to casualties with nonlife-threatening injuries and stable cardiovascular/respiratory function. Reassessment of such casualties is required as they can often decompensate. The second lowest level in triage priority (walking wounded/green tag) is assigned to individuals with minor injuries and the ability to vacate the scene to a place of safety/medical assistance without assistance. The lowest level of triage (deceased or nonsalvageable/black tag) is assigned to casualties who are deceased at the scene and those requiring artificial ventilation or cardiopulmonary

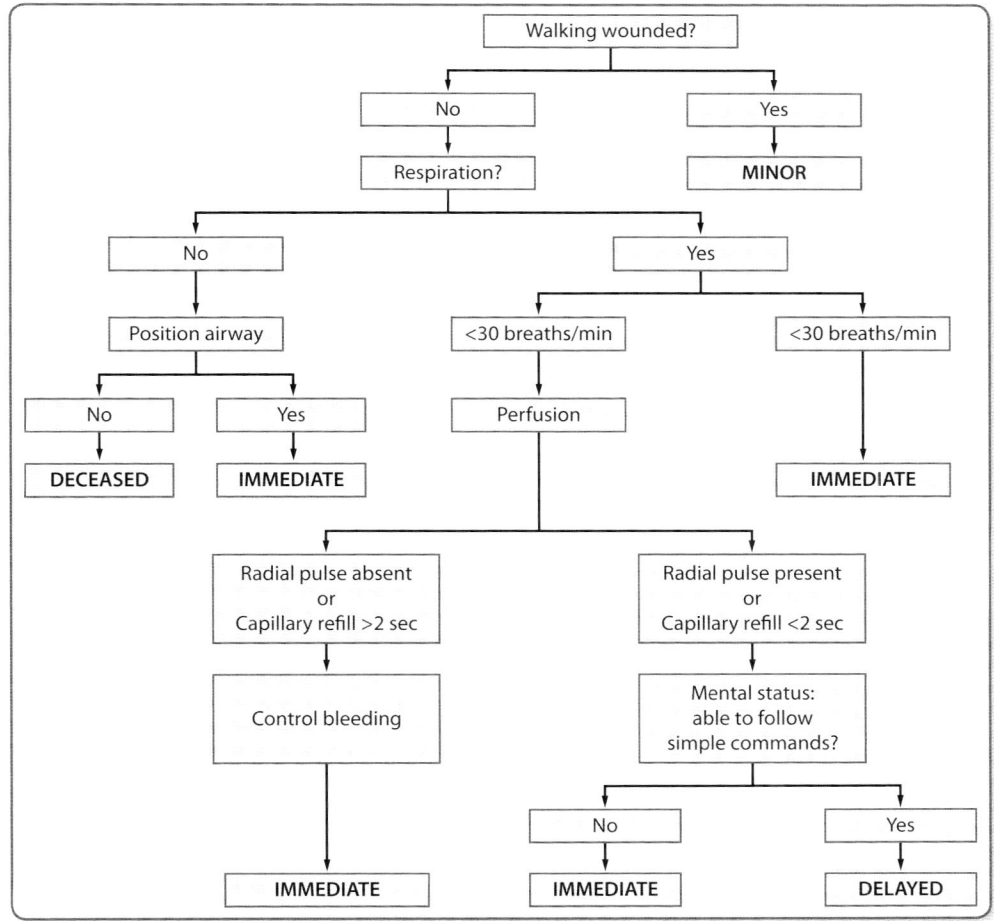

Figure 65.1 The Simple Triage and Rapid Treatment (START) system.

resuscitation. The London Ambulance Service has an additional priority level to differentiate nonsalvageable casualties from the deceased (**Table 65.2**).

In the context of a CBRN incident a clear zone which ranges from the most contaminated to the clean areas must be established. The hot zone is the contaminated site of the incident, the warm zone is where decontamination occurs and the clean zone/cold zone(s) are uncontaminated areas usually uphill and upwind of the hot zone.

As soon as more responders arrive, casualties are treated and transported according to their triage level with the highest priority patients taking precedence. Care delivered at the scene of a MCI is usually not definitive. Temporary treatment centres are usually erected and permanent nonhospital buildings can be converted to treatment centres to cope with the demands of a MCI.

Hospital planning and preparedness

Expanding the workforce and increasing capacity pose great challenges to responding appropriately in an MCI. Major cities across the world have implemented frameworks to prepare and respond to MCIs. In the UK, the NHS Emergency Planning Guidance of 2005 makes the Chief Executive Officer of each NHS organisation responsible for guaranteeing that their organisation has a Major Incident Plan in place. The underpinning principles are:
- Co-operation with partners
- Risk assessment
- Emergency planning
- Communicating with the public
- Information sharing

As part of their preparedness, acute NHS hospitals are mandated to identify additional suitable facilities for critically ill casualties. Further measures to increase capacity include cessation of all elective activity, rapid discharge of appropriate patients, and identification of nonpatient care areas within the hospital, which are suitable for conversion. Incident planning should also include workforce contingency planning for the recruitment of additional clinical and nonclinical staff throughout a potential MCI. Every member of staff should be aware of the hospital reporting policies along with their roles and responsibilities during such incidents.

Aftercare
Mass fatality

In some MCIs, temporary facilities to handle the deceased at the scene must be considered to ensure dignity and prevent disease outbreak. The police usually manage such facilities at the scene. Hospitals should also have policies in place in conjunction with the local authorities and police to cope with additional fatalities, especially in incidents involving CBRN.

Recovery

A significant MCI could affect regional services, healthcare provision and infrastructure for a prolonged period. A multi-agency group is required in the recovery from such an event. Senior representatives

Table 65.2 Combination of London Ambulance Service and START casualty triage

Category	Priority	Order of treatment	Description	START tag
Immediate	Priority 1	1	Unstable casualties needing immediate life-saving intervention	Red
Urgent	Priority 2	2	Stable casualties needing early treatment	Yellow
Delayed	Priority 3	3	Stable casualties for which treatment can be delayed	Green
Expectant	Priority 4	4	Severely injured and unlikely to survive	Black
Dead	Priority 5		No further medial intervention required	Black

from the relevant response agencies and government officials will contribute to the recovery group and the initial focus will be the response to the incident. The Healthcare services usually have a protracted recovery due to augmentation of services. Further long-term challenges include re-development of damaged infrastructure and helping survivors to regain normality.

Further reading

Born CT, Briggs SM, Ciraulo DL, et al. Disasters and mass casualties: I. General principles of response and management. J Am Acad Orthop Surg 2007; 15:388–396.

Mass Casualty Incidents: A framework for planning. London: UK Department of Health, Emergency Preparedness Division, 2007.

The NHS Emergency Planning Guidance. London: UK Department of Health, Emergency Preparedness Division, 2005.

Related topics of interest

- *Topic 17* Damage control orthopaedics and trauma physiology
- *Topic 62* Major trauma – Advanced Trauma and Life Support principles
- *Topic 99* Trauma scoring systems

66 Nailbed injuries

Key points
- Nailbed injuries are common and the spectrum of injuries covers a wide range
- Appreciation of the anatomy is essential for management and outcome prediction
- Early anatomical repair of the nailbed reduces the likelihood of deformity

Epidemiology

The nailbed is frequently injured because the fingertip is the point of contact between the body and the surrounding world in most activities of daily living. The fingernail (plate) protects the nailbed. The fingernail is important in modern human function: it is used to scratch, it contributes to tactile sensation and it protests the fingertip; its loss can be aesthetically displeasing.

Nailbed injuries occur in all age groups. Injuries to the nailbed most often involve the fingertip instead of the nailbed in isolation. These injuries are the most common hand related trauma presentation to accident and emergency departments. Hand trauma accounts for 10% of trauma presentations. It is most common in children, the younger male population (<30) and in occupations involving manual labour. The exact prevalence is unknown as a significant proportion of nailbed injuries do not seek medical attention. The middle finger (longest finger) nailbed is most likely to be injured followed by the ring, index, little finger and thumb.

Anatomy

The nailbed lies between the nail plate and distal phalanx. Understanding the anatomy of the nailbed and surrounding tissue is essential in treating subsequent injuries (**Figure 66.1**). The key anatomical components of the fingertip are:
- Nail plate – hard multi-layered sheets of keratinised squamous cells
- Paronychium – lateral nail folds
- Hyponychium – junction between the skin if the fingertip and nailbed. It is a physical and immunological barrier. The nail plate becomes nonadherent beyond this point
- Nail fold – the skin overlying the proximal nail plate
- Eponychium (cuticle) – the distal part of the nail fold which attaches to the nail plate
- Lunula – the semi-circular pale part the nail plate just distal to the eponychium
- Nailbed – soft tissue under the nail plate bound to periosteum of distal phalanx. It is composed of a germinal (proximal to lunula) and sterile (distal to lunula) matrix
- Perionychium – the nail plate, nailbed and nail folds

The nailbed is highly vascularised and supplied by anastomoses of two terminal branches of the volar digital arteries. Radial and ulnar digital nerves innervate the nailbed and fingertip. Nail formation occurs predominantly at the germinal matrix. The proximal nail fold produces cells that give the nail its gloss, paronychia provides lateral

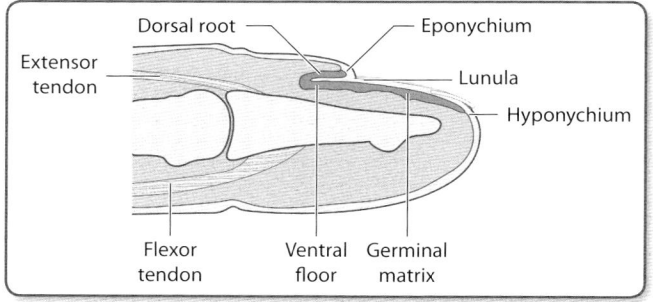

Figure 66.1 Anatomy of the nailbed and fingertip.

restraints and the sterile matrix adheres the nail plate to the nailbed. Fingernails grow distally within the confinement of the nail folds at approximately 0.1 mm/day and complete nail growth takes 3–6 months. Growth can be arrested for up to 1 month after injury.

Pathophysiology

Nailbed injuries can be caused by blunt or sharp trauma to the nail plate. Injuries can range from simple subungal haematoma, to lacerations and avulsion injuries. Nailbed injuries are most often caused by crush injuries. A direct blow with a hammer and catching the fingertip in a closing door the most common causes of crush injuries. In such injuries the nailbed is pinched between the hard nail plate and the distal phalanx. Simple or stellate (complex) lacerations may occur depending of the magnitude of force. Up to 50% of crush injuries causing nailbed laceration have an associated fracture of the distal phalanx. Sharp objects such and knives, saws and drills can also cause injury to the nailbed. High-energy avulsion injuries of the nail plate result in partial or complete loss of the nailbed.

Clinical features

Clinical assessment should include a detailed history including the mechanism of injury, the time of injury, initial management, hand dominance (in finger injuries), tetanus status, occupation and past medical history.

After excluding other injuries, specific assessment and documentation is required for presence subungal (under nail plate) haematoma, deformity, presence of contaminants, active bleeding, surrounding tissue injury, neurological status of the fingertip distal to the injury and distal tendon function (specifically extensor tendon). In practice a digital block is required for complete assessment.

Investigations

Plain film anteroposterior, oblique and lateral radiographs of the injured digit should be obtained to determine associated phalangeal fracture or foreign body (**Figure 66.2**). Further imaging is rarely required.

Diagnosis

The presence of subungal haematoma indicates damage to the nailbed. A haematoma occupying >50% of the visible nail plate is suggestive of a nailbed laceration. The nail plate should be removed is such a scenario to facilitate assessment and repair of the nailbed. Associated nail plate fracture, surroundings tissue damage, fracture and tendon injury should be noted as it may alter management.

Treatment

The aim of treatment is to relieve pain, restore function and reduce nail deformity. Treatment is determined by the size of the underlying haematoma with an intact nail plate. Sharp trauma causing laceration to the nail plate or avulsion injuries usually requires surgical intervention (**Table 66.1**).

Nonoperative

Pressure of the haematoma on the nailbed can cause severe throbbing pain. Small painless haematoma resulting from a crush injury underlying <50% of the nail plate usually requires no treatment. Painful haematomas can be drained to relieve pain. After appropriately cleaning the injured digit, trephination of the nail plate is classically performed using a sterile needle. Handheld disposable cautery devices are available in most emergency departments and are a safer way to achieve the same end. Immediate relieve is achieved from escape of the pressurised haematoma and patients can be discharged with analgesia and light dressings (**Figure 66.3**).

Operative

Nailbed laceration

Haematoma occupying 50% or more of the nail plate or associated distal phalanx fracture usually indicates a significant nailbed laceration and requires removal of the nail. Preoperative antibiotics and tetanus boosters

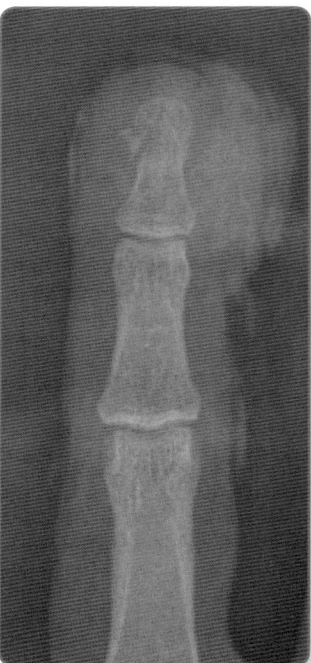
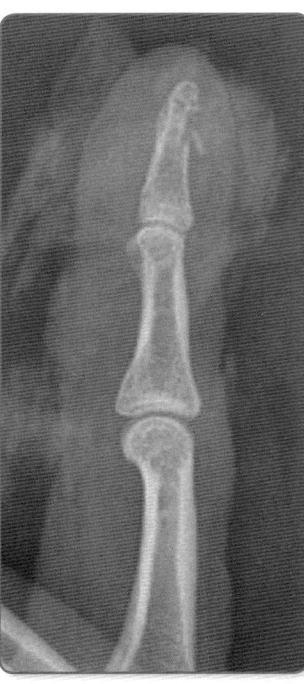

Figure 66.2 Fracture distal phalanx.

Table 66.1 Management of nailbed injuries

Injury	Management
Painful subungal haematoma (<50%)	Drainage of haematoma
>50% haematoma Nail bed laceration Haematoma + fracture	Removal of nail plate, washout and repair of nailbed
Avulsion injury/loss of nailbed	Split thickness skin graft or free graft of nailbed from other digits. Consider referral

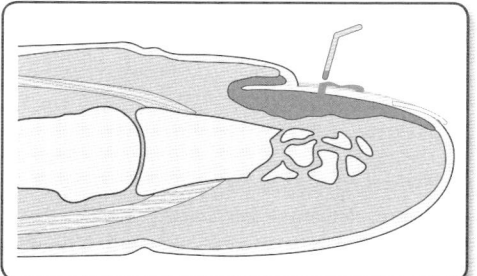

Figure 66.3 Drainage of a subungal haematoma.

are given when appropriate. Principles of treatment include evacuation of haematoma, minimal debridement, preservation of soft tissue, tension free approximation of the lacerated nailbed and splintage.

- In adults and cooperative children repair can be performed under a digital block. 1% lignocaine combined with bupivacaine hydrochloride provides up to 8 hours of anaesthesia
- The limb is prepared with povidine-iodine, sterile draping and a digital tourniquet is applied
- Fine curved scissors are slid under the nail plate and gently opened to separate the nail from the nailbed. The nail fold and paronychium is undermined to allow detachment of the nail
- The nail is inspected, the dorsal surface of the nail plate is cleaned and any attached nailbed to the volar surface of the nail is preserved especially in avulsion injuries
- The nailbed is irrigated and the nailbed is inspected. Careful handling is required to prevent further damage

Nailbed injuries

- In associated fracture, crushed or infolded nailbed should be elevated to prevent entrapment within the fracture
- Using magnifying loupes, lacerations should be repaired as anatomically as possible without tension. Inversion or eversion can lead to permanent deformity. Absorbable suture material – 6/0 gauge (or smaller) is ideal. Tissue adhesive can also be successfully used
- Associated soft injuries such as pulp laceration often require debridement and repair before addressing the nailbed
- Severely displaced distal phalanx fractures can be fixed with a K-wire
- The nail plate with a hole for drainage should be placed back under the nail fold. It secured in position with nonabsorbable monofilament suture (5/0 gauge). The nail plate acts as a biological dressing protecting the nailbed repair and providing a template for growth. It also stabilises fractures and prevents scarring between the eponychium and nailbed
- With loss of the nail, adequate splints can be made from plastic syringes or aluminium suture packaging. The digit is dresses with nonadherent dressings

Nailbed avulsion

Severe fingernail avulsion injuries with significant loss of the nailbed cannot be anatomically repaired. Nailbed grafts can be obtained from uninjured parts of involved digits or from the great toe. Most of these severe injuries require specialist input from a dedicated hand or plastic surgery unit.

Table 66.2 Post-traumatic nail deformities

Deformity	Pathology
Split nail	Minor scarring within the germinal matrix
Hook nail	Inadequate bony support of the matrix
Nonadherent nail	Scarring in the sterile matrix
Absent nail	Severe scarring in the germinal matrix
Linear ridging	Associated bone or soft tissue injury
Pincer nail	Damage to paronychium
Dull streaks/lack of gloss	Scarring to dorsal roof of nail fold

Complications

- Infection is uncommon in nailbed injuries.
- Early anatomical reconstruction yields excellent cosmetic results. Severe crush injuries with associated fractures and avulsion injuries with significant nailbed loss have the worst outcome
- The damaged part of the perionychium and subsequent scarring corresponds to deformity observed (**Table 66.2**). Referral to a hand surgeon should be considered a year after injury if outcome is not satisfactory. Delayed reconstruction or revision surgery is invariably less effective than appropriate initial intervention

Further reading

Krull E, Zook EG, Baran R, et al. Nail surgery: A Text and Atlas. Philadelphia, PA: Lippincott Williams & Wilkins; 2001.

Strauss EJ, Weil WM, Jordan C, Paksima N. A prospective, randomised, controlled trial of 2-octylcyanoacrylate versus suture repair of nail bed injuries. J Hand Surg Am 2008; 33:250–253.

Zook EG, Guy RJ, Russell RC, et al. A study of nail bed injuries: causes, treatment and prognosis. J Hand Surg Am 1984; 9:247–252.

Related topics of interest

- *Topic 41* Hand and wrist – metacarpal fractures
- *Topic 42* Hand and wrist – phalangeal fractures

67 Nonunion of fractures

Key points
- Nonunion represents the failure of a fracture to unite within the timeframe expected for that fracture in that patient
- The aetiology of nonunion is multifactorial
- Identifying and managing the cause(s) of nonunion are key to successful management

Epidemiology

Delayed fracture healing has been shown to occur in 5–10% of all fractures based on multiple small scale, retrospective series. Nonunion is the failure of a bone to heal where the cellular processes which create bone healing have ceased and is estimated to have a prevalence of 2.5%. There is no strict timeframe to define a nonunion, as it varies on the bone, the part of the bone and the host (patient) status. The risk of nonunion increases in high energy injuries; open fractures of the tibia demonstrate nonunion rates of up to 20–48% dependent on the extent of soft tissue stripping. Recent epidemiological studies estimate the incidence of nonunion requiring inpatient care to be closer to 20/100,000 population and each episode is projected to cost between £7000 and £79,000 per patient.

Pathophysiology

Host factors

Any systemic condition which affects the microcirculation and which adversely impacts on immunocompetence can affect fracture healing. Diabetes mellitus is the most commonly encountered and has also been associated with increased soft tissue complications and increased infection rates after surgery. Vascular disease is also implicated in the cause of nonunion. Any catabolic state including malignancy, malnutrition and vitamin deficiencies (especially B6) may add to the risk of nonunion. Many drugs are associated with nonunion. Corticosteroids show reversible inhibition of union in spinal fusion by lowering insulin-like growth factor-1 (IGF1) and transforming growth factor β (TGF-β) levels and nonsteroidal anti-inflammatory drugs (NSAIDs) have been shown to reduce angiogenesis and thus bone healing in vitro. The effect of smoking, specifically the effect of nicotine, adversely influences outcomes after osteotomy and fracture healing (30% of smokers demonstrated delayed or nonunion), through impaired collagen and ALP synthesis. High dose radiation therapy decreases the cellularity of bone, delaying union.

Fracture factors

Certain bones and certain locations within bones are often more prone to nonunion. Often this is due to poor local blood flow, which commonly arises from soft tissue attachments. Examples include the proximal pole of the scaphoid, talar neck, metaphyseal-diaphyseal junction of the 5th metatarsal base, and the tibial subcutaneous border.

The mechanism of injury also plays a part. Open high-energy injuries are associated with soft tissue and periosteal stripping which delays union. Closed high-energy injuries may hide disruption to the endosteal and periosteal blood supply that leaves the fracture fragments at risk of nonunion despite no apparent damage to the soft tissue envelope. Bone loss at the fracture site, or soft tissue interposition reduces bone-bone contact and also implies a significant open injury, both of which are associated with nonunion.

Fixation factors

Fractures require an appropriate strain environment in which to heal, i.e. the choice of fixation construct must match the surgeon's planned mode of fracture healing. Fractures which require primary bone healing need to be stabilised to provide gap free compression with rigid internal fixation to encourage cutting cones to cross the fracture site and allow Haversian remodeling to begin. By contrast, fractures in the diaphysis of long bones need more micromotion (0–2% strain environment) to induce union as the bone unites through callus formation. Excessive motion leads to osteoprogenitor cells entering the fibroblast lineage (fibrous nonunion) and if left without intervention, an eventual pseudarthrosis. Iatrogenic stripping of the periosteum at the time of surgery can further damage the blood supply, as can disruption by the direct contact between the plate and bone. Modern approaches include the use of low-profile plates such as the limited contact dynamic compression plate (LC-DCP) and minimally invasive percutaneous osteosynthesis (MIPO) techniques to enhance fracture healing by minimising soft tissue disruption.

Infection

Any delay in bony healing may be due to infection. Although bone can heal in an infected environment, the consequences of osteomyelitis not only make nonunion more likely, but complicate operative management. Devitalised remnants of bone separate and form sequestra surrounded by a sclerotic margin that reduces antibiotic delivery. The most common infective organisms are *Staphylococcus* species, including methicillin-resistant *Staphylococcus aureus*, and coagulase-negative staphylococci. Less commonly found are *Coliforms* and *Pseudomonas* species.

Clinical assessment

Nonunion causes pain, sometimes with detectable movement at the fracture site, months after the initial fracture or surgery with no evidence of bony union on imaging. It is crucial to learn as much information as possible about the initial injury from the history, including the mechanism, associated soft tissue injuries (especially if soft tissue cover was required) and whether secondary debridement was necessary for infection. In common with all orthopaedic injuries, it is important to ascertain the occupation and functional status of the patient and to explore their expectations for the future before embarking on a potentially complex management plan.

Many patients who present with established nonunions have had several attempts at operative intervention, either to improve the mechanical environment (e.g. dynamisation or implant exchange) or to supplement the biological environment (e.g. bone grafting or infection management). Understanding why these procedures have failed helps in formulating a new surgical plan.

Investigations

On plain radiographs, fracture union is most typically defined by the appearance of bridging callus on three cortices on orthogonal views. Radiographs may also demonstrate hardware failure around a nonunion site such as broken screws or bent/broken implants. Multiplanar CT provides useful information in quantifying the percentage of bridging callus as compared to the total diameter of bone. Bone scans are relatively nonspecific as there is sometimes intense tracer uptake both at nonunion and healing fracture sites. MRI is used in the management of established, infected nonunions in monitoring chronic osteomyelitis and aiding in surgical planning. Blood tests are useful to identify raised inflammatory markers indicating potential infection, and vitamin D/calcium levels should also be checked.

Classification

Aseptic nonunions were initially classified by Judet et al. (1958) and subsequently by Weber and Cech (1976) into hypertrophic/hypervascular and atrophic/avascular dependent on their radiological and histological appearance. The hypertrophic/hypervascular groups were subdivided into:
- 'Elephant's foot' highly hypertrophic, abundant callus – good blood supply but inadequate fracture immobilisation leading to failed enchondral ossification (**Figures 67.1** and **67.2**)
- 'Horse's hoof' moderate hypertrophy formation, poor callus formation – due to inadequate fracture fixation
- Oligotrophic nonunion, inadequate reduction at the fracture site leading to

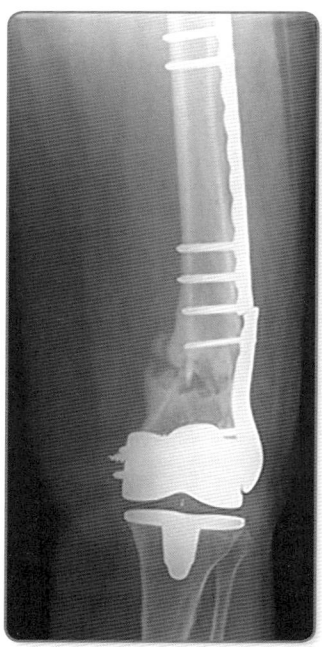

Figure 67.1 Hypertrophic nonunion in a distal femoral fracture. The plate has suffered a fatigue failure. Callus formation is present and the classical 'elephants foot' shape to the nonunion can be seen.

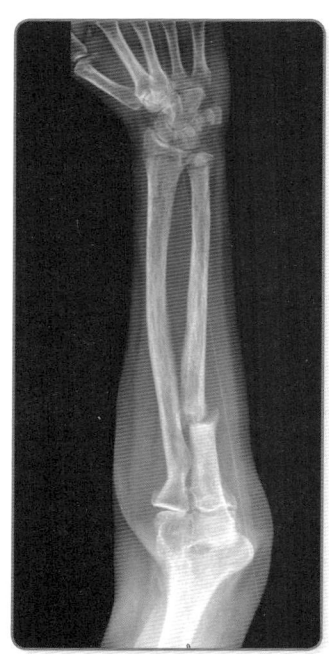

Figure 67.2 Hypertrophic nonunion of the ulna.

distraction with no callus formation and no hypertrophy

Atrophic/avascular nonunions are classified as:
- Torsion/wedge
- Comminuted with interposed necrotic bone
- Defect nonunions with bone loss through an open fracture
- Atrophic nonunions have avascular nonviable bone ends with a porotic, fragile appearance (**Figure 67.3**)

Umiarov's classification of septic nonunions (1986), grades 1–4 is based on an assessment of bone viability, limb shortening, bone loss and soft tissue defect.

Treatment

Nonoperative

Indirect interventions include smoking cessation, correcting endocrine disturbances, stopping harmful medications (such as steroids and NSAIDs) and improving nutritional status. Provided that there is no unacceptable malalignment, weight-bearing provides a safe method to

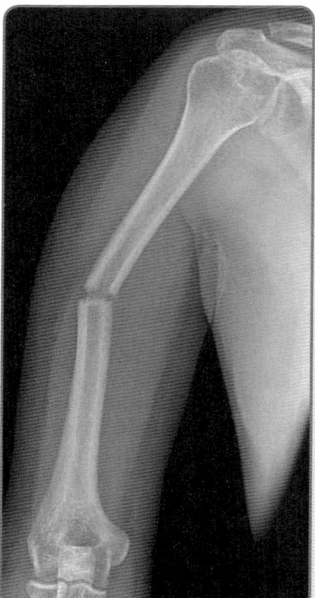

Figure 67.3 Atrophic nonunion of the humerus – there is no callus formation seen on the radiographs.

stimulate osteoblast activity. Other external interventions such as ultrasound and piezoelectric stimulation may play a role in reducing healing times, although prospective double blind randomised controlled trial data is lacking to support this theory currently.

Operative

Surgery aims to restore mechanical alignment and optimise the biological and mechanical environment in order to produce fracture healing.

- *Hypertrophic nonunions*: These fractures have the biological capability to heal, but have not previously had the mechanical stability needed to produce mature healed bone. These fractures may not require debridement of the nonunion site or bone grafting. Treatment is focused on improving the strain environment by more rigid fixation such as plate fixation or increasing the internal diameter of an intramedullary nail
- *Atrophic nonunions*: These fractures lack the blood supply and biological environment to heal and so require debridement back to bleeding bone ends and possible bone grafting. Autogenous bone graft supplies osteogenic and osteoconductive material and provides an osteoinductive scaffold for new bone growth. Autogenous bone graft can be harvested from the femoral canal using the RIA (Reamer-Irrigator-Aspirator, Synthes) or alternatively from iliac crest
- *Oligotrophic nonunions*: These require a combined approach, improving both the strain environment and blood supply and may also require significant debridement and grafting along with implant exchange
- *Segmental loss*: Techniques such as primary shortening followed by lengthening or alternatively bone transport are commonly described. Recently, the Masquelet technique has gained favour, whereby the segmental loss is filled with PMMA cement which over 4–6 weeks is enveloped in an osteogenic membrane of bone morphogenetic protein 2 (BMP-2) rich synovium like material. The cement is subsequently removed and replaced with cancellous bone graft
- *Infection*: Serial debridement and removal of hardware with subsequent external fixation fixed outside the zone of infection is usually required. Samples taken in theatre guide eradication intravenous antibiotic therapy which last at least 6 weeks via peripheral long lines. For diaphyseal long bone nonunions, antibiotic eluting nails have been show to aid fracture healing
- The use of BMPs (rhBMP2, rhBMP7) remain under investigation as adjuncts to bone healing

Complications

- Malunion can result from inadequate reduction or failure to correct a deformity prior to treatment of the nonunion
- Infection may persist, even in healed fractures leaving ongoing sinuses or intermittent flare of redness and pain
- Chronic (especially neurogenic) pain may persist and necessitate amputation of the limb. This requires a considered multidisciplinary approach involving psychological support and liaison with post amputation rehabilitation services

Further reading

Perren SM. Evolution of the internal fixation of long bone fractures. J Bone Joint Surg Br 2002; 84B:1093–1110.

Redento Mora. Nonunion of the Long Bones. Milan: Springer-Verlag Italia; 2006.

Related topics of interest

- *Topic 68* Open fractures
- *Topic 85* Principles of operative management of fractures

68 Open fractures

Key points

- Open fractures occur when there is a break in the skin associated with a fracture that allows communication between the bone and the external environment
- They are significant, potentially limb threatening injuries
- Timely expert care, including initial management in the emergency department, improves outcome and in the UK is guided by the BOAST 4 recommendations
- The most severe fractures should be managed in centers with combined orthoplastic capacity

Epidemiology

Open long bone fractures are estimated to occur with a frequency of approximately 11.5/100,000 persons per year with a bimodal distribution between young, mostly male adults involved in road traffic accidents and the elderly sustaining low energy injuries. The tibia is the most common site for open long bone fractures. Historically reported rates of complications of open fractures included nonunion (50%), deep infection (30–60%), compartment syndrome (0–20%), indicating just how severe these injuries are. For the most severe grade of open tibial fracture (Gustilo-Anderson IIIc), the reported rate of amputation reaches 64–86%. More modern series demonstrate improved outcomes but these injuries still command respect in all aspects of their management.

Classification systems

In a retrospective study of the management of 673 long bone fractures between 1955 and 1968, Gustilo and Anderson identified that intravenous antibiotics reduced infections in extensive open injuries however primary fracture fixation and primary wound closure of high-energy segmental fractures were associated with high infection rates. In response, they designed a protocol for treatment that focused on early debridement, copious irrigation and antibiotic therapy for 3 days following surgery with primary closure reserved only for small open wounds. Their subsequent prospective ($n = 352$) study separated the most severe (type III) open fractures into three subgroups. This grading is dictated by the intraoperative findings and can only be confirmed in theatre (**Table 68.1**).

BOAST 4

In 2009, the British Orthopaedic Association (BOA) and the British Association of Plastic, Reconstuctive and Aesthetic Surgeons (BAPRAS) issued joint guidance as regards the management of open tibial fractures. These were derived from evidence base and expert opinion and contain fifteen 'standards for practice'. This guidance emphasised the importance of 'timely, specialist surgery rather than emergency surgery by less experienced teams' and has driven the move from open fractures being managed as surgical emergencies within 6 hours of injury, to planned trauma lists with senior orthopaedic and plastic surgery input.

These guidelines are summarised below:

1. Intravenous antibiotics should be administered within 3 hours of injury (co-amoxiclav or cefuroxime) and are continued until wound coverage. Clindamycin is used in those with penicillin allergy.
2. The vascular and neurological status of the limb is assessed systematically and repeated after reduction of fractures or the application of splints.
3. Vascular impairment requires immediate surgery, ideally within 3–4 hours, with a maximum acceptable delay of 6 hours warm ischaemia.
4. Compartment syndrome requires immediate surgery, with four compartment decompression via two incisions.
5. Urgent surgery is needed in some multiply injured patients with open fractures or

if the wound is heavily contaminated by marine, agricultural or sewage matter.
6. A combined plan for the management of both the soft tissues and bone should be formulated by both plastic and orthopaedic surgical teams and clearly documented.
7. In the emergency department, the wound is handled only to remove gross contamination and to allow photography, then covered in saline soaked gauze and an impermeable film to prevent desiccation.
8. The limb, including the knee and ankle, is splinted.
9. Centres that cannot provide combined plastic and orthopaedic surgical care for severe open tibial fractures should have protocols in place for the early transfer of the patient to an appropriate specialist centre.
10. Primary surgical treatment (wound excision and fracture stabilisation) of severe open tibial fractures only takes place in a nonspecialist centre if the patient cannot be transferred safely.
11. The debridement should be performed by senior plastic and orthopaedic surgeons working together on scheduled trauma operating lists within normal working hours and within 24 hours of the injury. Coamoxiclav and Gentamicin are administered at debridement and continued for 72 hours or definitive wound closure, whichever is sooner.
12. If definitive skeletal and soft tissue reconstruction is not to be undertaken in a single stage, then vacuum foam dressing or an antibiotic bead pouch is applied until definitive surgery.
13. Definitive skeletal stabilisation and wound cover should be achieved within 72 hours and should not exceed 7 days.
14. Vacuum foam dressings are not used for definitive wound management in open fractures.
15. The wound in open tibial fractures in children should be treated in the same way as adults.

Further considerations

- The debridement of an open fracture of the lower limb should include wound extension along fasciotomy lines, to avoid damaging the vascular perforators that may be required for later definitive soft tissue coverage procedures (**Figure 68.1**)
- Both ends of the bone should be delivered and cleaned thoroughly. Pulsed lavage is not recommended
- The debridement of an open fracture should be systematic, from superficial to deep or vice versa and include an assessment of all related structures. Nonviable bone fragments – those that fail the 'tug' test and have no soft tissue attachment, should be removed
- An assessment of the fractured pelvis should include a vaginal and rectal examination to elicit blood or bone fragments in the vagina or rectum. An open pelvic fracture may require a temporary colostomy to divert faeces away from the fracture site and avoid catastrophic contamination

Table 68.1 The Gustilo–Anderson grading system

Grade	Description
I	<1 cm, no sign of crush or contusion
II	>1 cm, no extensive soft tissue damage
III	All high-energy injuries Extensive soft tissue damage to skin, muscle and neurovascular structures, with periosteal stripping. Significant contamination, high risk from farmyard debris
IIIa	Sufficient soft tissue cover to permit tension free wound closure
IIIb	Periosteal stripping, soft tissue loss requiring plastic surgical techniques to achieve coverage (**Figure 68.2**)
IIIc	Any open fracture with vascular damage requiring repair

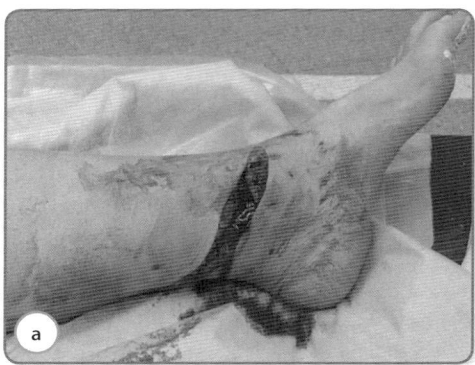 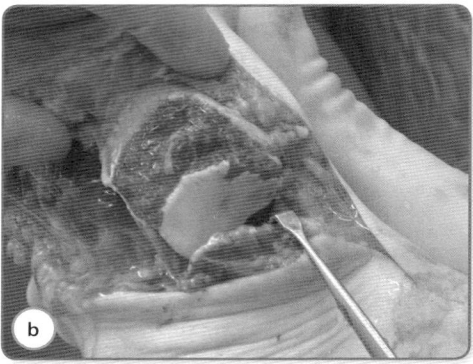

Figure 68.1 (a) Gustilo 3A distal tibial ankle fracture. Note the importance of delivery of the bone end, allowing for full debridement and cleaning. (b) The articular cartilage in this case can also be assessed.

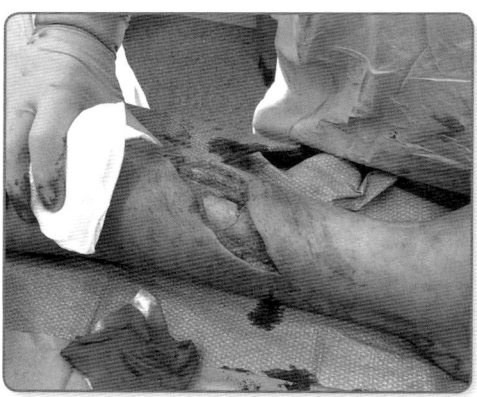

Figure 68.2 Tibial fracture, after debridement and intramedullary nailing, now requiring free tissue transfer to cover.

Further reading

British Orthopaedic Association (BOA) and the British Association of Plastic, Reconstuctive and Aesthetic Surgeons (BAPRAS) Standards for Trauma-BOAST 4 Summary 2009. London: BOA, BAPRAS, 2009.

Chang Y, Kennedy SA, Bhandari M, et al. Effects of antibiotic prophylaxis in patients with open fracture of the extremities. A systematic review of randomized controlled trials. J Bone Joint Surg Rev 2015:6.

Gustilo RB, Anderson JT. Prevention of infection in the treatment of one thousand and twenty-five open fractures of long bones: retrospective and prospective analyses. J Bone Joint Surg Am 1976; 58:453–458.

Related topics of interest

- *Topic 14* Compartment syndrome
- *Topic 67* Nonunion of fractures

69 Osteoporosis

Key points

- Osteoporosis is defined as a reduction in bone mass
- Prevention of future fractures and modifications of fracture risk is essential
- Atypical fractures may result from treatment of osteoporosis

Epidemiology

Osteoporosis affects an estimated 300 million people worldwide and around 3 million in the UK. All fragility fractures in the elderly, excepting pathological fractures, can be regarded as osteoporotic fractures. As an example, 300,000 fragility fractures are recorded in the UK annually with hip fractures accounting for 1.8 million bed days. It places a significant burden on the wider health economy; for example, hip fractures cost the UK's National Health Service (NHS) approximately £1.9 billion and this does not include the additional social care costs required by many individuals following a fragility fracture.

Up to 30% of postmenopausal women have osteoporosis with around 40% of women and 15–30% of men sustaining at least one fragility fracture in their lifetime. A fragility fracture is a major risk for having new fractures – the lifetime risk is increased by 86%.

Hip and vertebral fractures are associated with an increase in mortality and morbidity. For hip fractures, the 1 month mortality is between 5–10% and up to 38% at 1 year. Only around 54% of hip fracture patients are independently mobile at 1 year and around 20% will require nursing home placement having previously lived at home; for men this figure may be as high as 50%.

Pathophysiology

Osteoporosis is a disease characterised by low bone mass and associated micro-architectural changes that result in a high-risk of fracture. After the age of 30 years bone density gradually declines due to an increased imbalance between the rate of resorption and formation. Trabecular bone is the more metabolically active type of bone with 25% being reabsorbed and replaced annually compared to 3% of cortical. Following the menopause, oestrogen deficiency causes, predominantly, the loss of trabecular bone leading to an increased incidence of distal radius and vertebral fractures in the 6th and 7th decade.

Risk factors and secondary causes of osteoporosis

There are a number of clinical risk factors associated with osteoporosis. Some act independently of bone mineral density to increase fracture risk including:
- Age
- Female sex
- Alcohol >3 units/day
- Smoking
- BMI <19
- Early menopause
- Current glucocorticoid treatment (any dose for >3 months)

Table 69.1 Causes of secondary osteoporosis

Causes	Examples
Endocrine disease	Type 1 diabetes, hyperthyroidism, hyperparathyroidism, hypogonadism, Cushing's syndrome
Rheumatologic disease	Rheumatoid arthritis
Respiratory disease	COPD
GI disease	Chronic liver disease, Malabsorption syndromes (e.g. Coeliac disease)
Renal disease	Chronic kidney disease
Organ transplantation	Solid organs
Haematological disease	Multiple myeloma, thalassaemia
Medication	Steroids, barbiturates, lithium

- Previous fragility fracture
- History of parental hip fracture and
- History of falls.

There are also a number of conditions that cause secondary osteoporosis (Table 69.1).

Diagnosis

Osteoporosis is diagnosed when the bone mineral density is 2.5 standard deviations below the young female adult mean (T-score ≤ –2.5; Table 69.2). Dual-energy X-ray absorptiometry (DEXA) scan is considered the gold standard for diagnosing osteoporosis. It evaluates the amount of radiation that passes through the tested bone. The risk of fracture increases approximately two-fold for each standard deviation decrease in bone mineral density (BMD).

The aims of investigation in osteoporosis are to identify the cause of osteoporosis and any underlying clinical risk factors, exclude other pathology (e.g. osteomalacia, myeloma), assess future fracture risk and guide treatment choice. Therefore, the need for any further investigation will depend on the clinical history and physical examination.

Routine investigations should include:
- Bloods tests – full blood count, urea and electrolytes, liver function tests, bone profile, thyroid function tests, erythrocyte sedimentation rate and C-reactive protein
- Assessment of BMD: DEXA scan

Other investigations, when indicated, may include:
- Myeloma screen
- Vitamin D
- Parathyroid hormone
- Serum prolactin
- Dexamethasone suppression test
- Urinary calcium excretion

Male hormone screen (testosterone, sex hormone binding globulin, follicle-stimulating hormone, luteinising hormone)
- Coeliac screen – tissue transglutaminase antibodies
- Markers of bone turnover

Assessing the risk of future fragility fracture

There is no screening programme for osteoporosis in the UK; however, National Osteoporosis Guideline Group (NOGG) and National Institute for Health and Care Excellence (NICE) guidelines suggest a case finding strategy. This involves the identification of individuals that have had a previous fragility fracture or have one or more clinical risk factor (see p.261). Women with a previous fragility fracture should be considered for pharmacologic treatment without measuring the bone mineral density. However, postmenopausal women and men >50 with significant clinical risk factors should be assessed using a risk assessment tool.

Risk assessment tools recommended by NICE include FRAX and Qfracture. FRAX combines clinical risk factors with or without BMD at the femoral neck to provide a 10-year probability of major osteoporotic fracture (clinical vertebral, hip, wrist or proximal humerus). It is freely available on the internet and is central to the current NOGG guidelines. The results are displayed on a graph with a recommendation of treatment, reassurance or DEXA scan shown.

Treatment

Although osteoporosis is diagnosed following a DEXA scan it is the combination of the T-score and other risk factors that determine whether pharmacologic treatment is necessary. The aim of management is to reduce fracture risk.

Current UK guidelines on the assessment of fracture risk and osteoporosis management include the NICE guidelines (CG146, 2012) and the NOGG who updated their guidance

Table 69.2 World Health Organization diagnostic thresholds for bone mineral density at the spine hip or distal forearm

Diagnosis	Bone mineral density T-score (SD units)
Normal	≥1
Osteopenia	<1 but >2.5
Osteoporosis	≤2.5
Severe osteoporosis	≤2.5 plus one or more fragility fracture

Table 69.3 Effect of major pharmacological interventions on fracture risk when given with calcium and vitamin D in postmenopausal women with osteoporosis

	Vertebral fracture	Nonvertebral fracture	Hip fracture
Alendronate	↓	↓	↓
Denosumab	↓	↓	↓
Strontium ranelate	↓	↓	↓
Raloxifene	↓	No clear evidence	No clear evidence
Teriparatide	↓	↓	No clear evidence

Compston J, Cooper A, Cooper C. UK clinical guideline for the prevention and treatment of osteoporosis. SpringerLink, Archives of Osteoporosis (online), 2017.

in January 2016 (**Table 69.3**).

Nonpharmacologic treatment of osteoporosis should include a falls risk assessment and prevention plan for all patients at risk of fragility fracture and lifestyle modification. Maintenance of mobility, correction of nutritional deficiencies (especially calcium, vitamin D and protein) and treatment of secondary causes is advised.

Pharmacologic treatments include supplements, antiresorptive agents, formation-stimulating agents and strontium ranelate. The major pharmacological interventions are described below.

Calcium and vitamin D

Calcium and vitamin D are used as an adjunct to other pharmacological treatments for osteoporosis because the clinical trials for all other treatments were performed in patients who were calcium and vitamin D or were known to be replete. A recent study suggested calcium supplements are associated with an increased cardiovascular risk; therefore, individuals who have an adequate oral calcium intake should have vitamin D alone.

Bisphosphonates

Bisphosphonates are structural analogues of inorganic pyrophosphate they bind to bone mineral and inhibit resorption. Alendronate (weekly, oral), ibandronate (monthly, oral or intravenous injection), risedronate acid (daily or weekly, oral) and zoledronic acid (annual, intravenous injection) are all used in the treatment of osteoporosis. There are a number of factors that need to be taken into account when choosing which bisphosphonate to use including: gender, the presence of upper gastrointestinal (GI) disease and the underlying cause of osteoporosis.

Oral bisphosphonates are contraindicated in the presence of upper GI disease and all bisphosphonates are contraindicated in the presence of hypocalcaemia and significant renal impairment. To be taken safely orally the patient must be able to take them on an empty stomach, 30 minutes before food or drink and then remain upright for 30 minutes.

The NOGG have published guidance in January 2016 for the monitoring of patients on bisphosphonates.

Denosumab

Denosumab is also an antiresorptive agent. It is a fully human monoclonal antibody that inhibits osteoclasts by targeting the RANK ligand. Unlike bisphosphonates denosumab does not accumulate in the bone. It is given as a 6-monthly subcutaneous injection. It is contraindicated in the presence of hypocalcaemia and calcium must be adequately replaced prior to injection.

Complications of biphosphates and denosumab

Major potential complications of both bisphosphonates and denosumab include atypical fractures and osteonecrosis of the jaw (ONJ).

Atypical fractures

These are femoral fractures that mainly affect the subtrochanteric and diaphyseal region and have been reported following the, usually prolonged, use of bisphosphonates and denosumab. They are often associated with minimal trauma and a prodromal

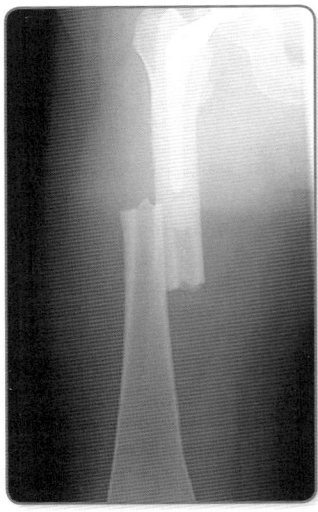

Figure 69.1 A typical bisphosphonate induced fracture. This has occurred in the femoral shaft distal to a hip replacement. There is a characteristic transverse fracture with sharp well defined edges, and a thickened lateral cortex. Fractures typically occur in the subtrochanteric region – in this case, this region was protected by the joint replacement and thus the fracture occurred distal to the tip of the implant.

thigh or groin pain. The pathology is usually bilateral; therefore, the contralateral femur should be assessed in all femoral shaft fractures associated with bisphosphonates or denosumab. Radiographic features include transverse or oblique fracture, cortical thickening, cortical 'beaking' adjacent to the fracture line and a prominent lateral cortical 'spike' (**Figure 69.1**).

Strontium ranelate

The pharmacology of strontium ranelate is not fully understood, however, it has the dual effect of promoting bone formation while inhibiting bone resorption. It is contraindicated in women of a childbearing age and patients with an increased cardiovascular risk. It should be used with caution in those renal impairment and those at increased risk of venous thromboembolism. As a consequence recommendations state it should only be prescribed by a specialist and when there is no other possible treatment option and individuals should be regularly reviewed by their doctor for potential risk.

Raloxifene

Raloxifene is a selective oestrogen receptor modulator that has been shown to significantly decrease the incidence of vertebral fracture in postmenopausal women. Although it is associated with an increase in BMD at the femoral neck is has not been shown to decrease the incidence of nonvertebral fractures. It is contraindicated in women of a childbearing age, patients at increased risk of venous thromboembolism, patients with unexplained uterine bleeding and those with hepatic or significant renal impairment.

Teriparatide

Teriparatide is a recombinant form of parathyroid hormone with anabolic properties that lead to increased bone formation. It is a daily subcutaneous injection and can be given for a maximum of 18 months. It is approved for the treatment of severe osteoporosis in men and postmenopausal women. Contraindications include hypercalcaemia, other metabolic bone disease and severe renal impairment.

Further reading

National Institute of Health and Care Excellence (NICE). Osteoporosis: assessing the risk of fragility fracture (CG146). London: NICE; 2012. Updated 2017.

Compston J, Cooper A, Cooper C. UK clinical guideline for the prevention and treatment of osteoporosis. SpringerLink, Archives of Osteoporosis (online), 2017.

70 Paediatric clavicle fractures

Key points
- Paediatric clavicle fractures are common in infants
- The majority of childhood clavicle fractures can be managed nonoperatively

Epidemiology
The prevalence of paediatric clavicle fractures is approximately 7%. It accounts for up to 90% of obstetric fractures. This injury occurs in normal deliveries (0.5%) as well as breech deliveries (1.6%). Boys have a bimodal distribution whereas girls have a unimodal distribution, with an initial peak in prevalence at the age of 6 years. It is the most common fracture seen in the 0–1-year age group, along with distal humeral fractures.

Pathophysiology
The clavicle is the first bone to ossify and forms by undifferentiated cells aligning in layers; intramembranous ossification. The secondary ossification centres develop by enchondral ossification. The majority of growth (80%) takes place at the medial epiphysis.

The mechanism of injury is most commonly a result of direct trauma, usually to the clavicle or the lateral aspect of the acromion. Indirect trauma involves a fall onto an outstretched hand.

Medial clavicle injuries, such as periosteal sleeve avulsions, are more common than sternoclavicular joint dislocations. These injuries are usually Salter–Harris type I or II fractures. Medial clavicular fractures are rare.

Clinical features
Fractures at birth usually present with an asymmetrical palpable mass overlying the fracture site. There may be tenting of the skin, ecchymosis and crepitus. Neurovascular status should be evaluated and carefully documented as brachial plexus injuries and upper extremity vascular injuries can result. Differential diagnoses can include cleidocranial dysostosis, which results in the absence of part or the whole clavicle and is the result of a defect in intramembranous ossification. Congenital pseudoarthrosis occurs due to the failure of union between the medial and lateral ossification centres.

Investigations
Ultrasound is used for diagnosis in neonates. A single anteroposterior radiograph is sufficient to diagnose clavicle fractures. Other views are performed when the diagnosis is in question. A cephalic tilt view of 35–40° minimises overlapping structures to show the degree of displacement. Radiographs of the chest should be taken if breathing difficulties develop to exclude possible pneumothoraces. Medial injuries can be assessed with serendipity views and/or a CT scan.

Classification
Fractures of the clavicle can be classified descriptively. The location, whether the fracture is open or closed, displacement and angulation are all described individually. The Allman classification describes fractures of the middle third (type I), lateral third, i.e. lateral to the coracoclavicular ligaments (type II) and medial third fractures (type 3). This was further subdivided according to the probability of nonunion by Robinson et al.

Treatment
Nonoperative treatment dictates middle third clavicle fractures. Studies comparing a simple sling with a figure-of-eight splint for middle third clavicle fractures demonstrate similar outcomes in both groups. Hence the complications associated with the figure-of-eight splint, such as compression of the

axillary vessels and brachial plexopathy, can be avoided. Operative indications include severely displaced and irreducible fractures that threaten skin integrity, open fractures, concomitant vascular injury and compromise of the brachial plexus function.

Distal clavicle fractures are considered a childhood equivalent to adult acromioclavicular joint (ACJ) injuries. The clavicle displaces away from the physis and periosteal sleeve, which remains intact and attached to the ACJ and coracoclavicular ligaments. These are described as pseudodislocations of the ACJ. Once again, the majority are managed nonoperatively. Types IV, V and VI distal clavicle fractures (Dameron and Rockwood classification) remains controversial.

The majority of medial clavicular fractures are fractures through the physis. Undisplaced medial physeal fractures can be managed symptomatically. Anterior displaced medial clavicular fractures and sternoclavicular dislocations should be reduced with gentle posterior pressure over the fracture site to encourage reduction. Posteriorly displaced medial fractures or sternoclavicular joint dislocations require assessment of injury to the airway and great vessels. Urgent reduction under general anaesthesia should be performed. Both closed and open methods of reduction need to be prepared for.

Complications

Severe displacement of clavicle fractures can cause neurovascular compromise, however, this is rare as the periosteum is thick and protects the underlying structures. Compression of the great vessels and trachea is also a major complication requiring urgent expedient surgical reduction. Malunion is once again rare as the clavicle has a high remodelling potential. Pulmonary injury such as a pneumothorax can occur with high-energy trauma.

Further reading

Tennent TD, Pearse EO, Eastwood DM. A new technique for stabilizing adolescent posteriorly displaced physeal medial clavicular fractures. J Shoulder Elbow Surg 2012; 21:1734–1739.

Related topics of interest

- Topic 13 Clavicle fractures
- Topic 76 Paediatric humeral fractures
- Topic 77 Paediatric physeal fractures
- Topic 84 Principles of nonoperative management of fractures

71 Paediatric distal tibial and ankle fractures

Key points

- In paediatric distal tibial and ankle fractures, understanding of fracture types and use of appropriate investigations is key to management
- Age, fracture pattern and severity of injury determine management options
- Some injuries and their treatment may affect growth, thus long-term follow may be essential

Epidemiology

Ankle injuries represent approximately 5% of all paediatric fractures and 15% of physeal injuries. The peak incidence of these injuries occurs between the ages of 8 and 15 years. Risk factors predisposing children to ankle fractures include obesity and the participation in sporting activities.

Pathophysiology

Injuries to the ligamentous structures in the paediatric patient are rare, owing to the fact that the ligaments are generally stronger than the bone and its open physes. An understanding of anatomy in the paediatric ankle is key to interpreting certain fracture patterns. Accessory ossification centres may mimic the appearance of a fracture. In adolescents, the distal tibial physis closes over a period of 18 months first centrally, then medially, and finally laterally Closure of the physis is seen at the age of 15 years in girls and 17 years in boys

Strain of either the anterior inferior tibiofibular ligament or the posterior inferior tibiofibular ligament may result in avulsion fractures or Salter–Harris II fractures in younger patients. As the physis closes in young teenagers (medially to anterolaterally), ankle injuries may often lead to transitional fracture patterns such as tillaux and triplane injuries.

Tillaux fractures (Salter–Harris III) occur when the anterior inferior tibiofibular ligament avulses the anterolateral portion of the distal tibia. These fractures are most common children between the ages of 12–14 years.

Triplane fractures (Salter–Harris IV) have components in the sagittal, coronal, and transverse planes. These fractures are considered to be transitional fractures, but may occur in younger children. Triplane fractures usually involve both a posterior metaphyseal fragment and a lateral epiphyseal fragment.

Clinical features

Thorough history taking and examination are required. Nonaccidental injury or a pathological fracture should be considered if there is an inconsistency between the mechanism of injury and the fracture pattern. High-energy injuries such as those sustained in road traffic accidents may lead to physeal crush injuries which are not always evident on initial X-rays.

Other concomitant injuries must be ruled out and the sensory and motor status must be clearly documented before and after any intervention performed. The status of the skin surrounding the injury must be thoroughly assessed and urgent reduction performed when the soft tissue envelope around the fracture is under threat.

Investigations

Three radiographic views of the ankle can be used in the diagnostic process: anteroposterior, lateral and mortise views. Transitional fracture patterns may be missed when only two views are used. Subtle changes such as soft tissue swelling may be the only radiographic abnormalities detected in Salter–Harris I fractures. Stress views and weight-bearing views are not routinely performed, but may be useful in adolescents.

Injuries through anatomical variations (such as accessory ossicles) must be noted and correlated with the findings of the clinical examination.

The use of CT scan is helpful in the diagnosis of complex intra-articular and transitional fracture patterns. It may be essential for accurate preoperative planning and assessment of fracture reduction. The use of MRI is more controversial. It can prove valuable in the detection occult fractures or in the diagnosis of persistent sources of pain following fracture union.

Classification

The two most common classification schemes in paediatric ankle fractures are the Salter–Harris and Dias–Tachdjian systems. The former is easily reproducible and describes a fracture according to its relationship with the physis.

- Type 1 – These represent fractures that occur through the zone of hypertrophy in the physis
- Type 2 – The fracture extends through the physis and exits in the metaphysis. In these fractures, the periosteum may become interposed in the fracture site
- Type 3 – In this instance, the fracture exits through the epiphysis. They may be associated with a step in the articular surface
- Type 4 – These fractures cross the metaphysis, physis and epiphysis, entering the joint
- Type 5 – A compressive force occurs across the physis itself. These fractures are difficult to detect and the diagnosis is often made retrospectively
- Type 6 – A late addition to the classification system which describes open injuries with physeal loss

The Dias–Tachdjian system describes the position of the foot at the time of injury and the direction of the force applied to it. It is useful when planning fracture reduction.

Treatment

Treatment of these fractures depends on the fracture type and the amount of fracture displacement. The objective of treatment is to restore the alignment of the physis and the congruity of the joint.

Type 1 and 2 injuries: Displaced fractures should be reduced and immobilised in order to prevent growth deformity. This should be done under general anaesthetic and the attempted number of reductions kept to a minimum. Open reduction should be attempted if closed reduction is difficult. It is usually necessary when the reduction is impeded by a structure such as the periosteum. Reduction is usually followed by a period of immobilisation of at least 4 weeks in a below-knee cast. Internal fixation is rarely necessary except for large Salter–Harris II fracture fragments.

Type 3 and 4 injuries: These fractures involve the articular surface. An articular step-off may be present. The majority of intra-articular fractures require anatomic reduction and absolute stability. Joint incongruity or growth disturbance may result from inadequate reduction. Nonoperative treatment consists of a nonweight-bearing cast for 4 weeks followed by a weight-bearing cast for 2. It is reserved for patients with nondisplaced fractures. Regular radiographic follow-up is necessary in the first few weeks after injury.

Open reduction and internal fixation is recommended in displaced fractures. Smooth wires and screws may be used in fixation but must always avoid the growth plate where possible. Fixation pins which cross the growth plate must be removed within a few weeks (as soon as the fracture in stable).

Type 5 injuries: These fractures are rare and difficult to diagnose. If they are identified early then they may be treated by guided growth techniques. The overall prognosis is poor and the mainstay of treatment is around correction of any limb length and angular deformities that occur.

Type 6 injuries: These open injuries are extremely serious. Appropriate input from vascular and plastic surgeons must be sought. The acute management involves antibiotic and tetanus prophylaxis in addition to washout and debridement of nonviable tissue. Open reduction and fixation of fractures must be followed by soft tissue reconstruction.

Complications

Growth arrest
This is caused by premature closure of the physis and may cause both angular deformity and leg length discrepancy. The degree of physeal involvement and the age of the child at the time of injury determines the magnitude of the acquired deformity. The treatment involves ranges from guided growth techniques with epiphysiodesis to corrective osteotomies and limb lengthening.

Chondral injury
Injury to the cartilage of the talar dome may be detected with MRI. Open or arthroscopic surgery may be used to treat these injuries with either stabilisation or microfracture. Arthritis is a recognised complication of chondral injury. Its incidence as a late complication is reduced by early anatomical reduction of intra-articular fractures.

Compartment syndrome
Extensor retinaculum syndrome is a rare but serious complication. Patients present with severe pain and swelling. A hypoasethetic first web space, weakness of the extensor hallucis longus/digitorum communis, and pain on passive toe flexion may all be detected. It may be treated with extensor retinaculum release and fracture fixation.

Reflex sympathetic dystrophy
This serious complication is often diagnosed late. Early recognition is essential to improve outcomes. The condition presents with pain out of proportion to the severity of the injury and with signs of autonomic dysfunction. Physiotherapy, effective analgesia, psychological counselling and sympathetic blockade may all play a role in the management of this complex condition.

Further reading

Blackburn EW, Aronsson DD, Rubright JH, Lisle JW. Ankle fractures in children. J Bone Joint Surg Am 2012; 94:1234–1244.

Dias LS, Giegerich CR. Fractures of the distal tibial epiphysis in adolescence. J Bone Joint Surg Am 1983; 65:438–444.

Kay RM, Matthys GA. Pediatric ankle fractures: evaluation and treatment. J Am Acad Orthop Surg 2001; 9:268–278.

Related topics of interest

- *Topic 74* Paediatric fractures – nonaccidental injury
- *Topic 77* Paediatric physeal fractures
- *Topic 79* Paediatric tibial fractures

72 Paediatric femoral fractures

Key points
- The treatment of paediatric femoral fractures remains controversial
- Modalities of treatment vary according to age, fracture pattern and site
- Always consider nonaccidental injury

Epidemiology

Femoral fractures are among the most common fractures of long bones. The incidence of these fractures is equal in both genders in the first year of life, it is found to increase in males, who are 4.7 times more likely to sustain a femoral fracture at by the age of 14 years. There is as yet no evidence to support any particular explanation for this difference.

Injury during the summer months is twice as common and is thought to be related to an increased level of outdoor activity. Nonaccidental injury was occurs in 1.3% of all cases. This figure rises to 8.5% in children aged 1 year or under. The single best predictor of whether or not a paediatric femoral fracture is caused nonaccidentally is the child's ability to walk.

Pathophysiology

Fractures to both the proximal and the distal femur are rare. The former represent <1% of all paediatric fractures. These are usually the result of high-energy injuries. Injuries to the distal femur carry a significant risk of injury to the growth plate.

Fractures of the femoral shaft are most common. The properties of the paediatric femur vary with age. The thick, vessel-rich periosteum in the young child has implications on the amount of remodelling that occur following injury.

The strength of the paediatric femur increases with age. This is due to a change in structure from primarily weak woven bone to stronger lamellar bone. More energy is therefore required to produce a femoral fracture in adolescence.

Clinical features

Thorough history taking and examination are key to an accurate diagnosis. Nonaccidental injury or a pathological fracture should be considered if there is an incongruence between the mechanism of injury and the fracture detected. The fracture must be considered within the context of the patient as a whole. Advanced Trauma Life Support principles must be followed.

Clinical examination may be difficult, particularly in younger children. A thorough examination must focus not only the femur but on the hip and knee.

Both the sensory and motor status must be clearly documented before and after any intervention performed. Careful circumferential examination of the skin surrounding the fracture must be carried out.

Investigations

Plain films form the basis of investigation in these injuries. Anteroposterior and lateral films must be performed both before and after any intervention. More advanced imaging (CT/MRI) may be useful in proximal and distal femoral fractures which involve the hip/knee joints.

Classification

The AO Pediatric Expert Group and the AO Pediatric Classification Group have formulated a comprehensive classification system for the description of paediatric long bone fractures. This is based on the Müller AO classification for adults and considers features which are child-specific.

Fractures of the distal femur are considered using the Salter–Harris classification system and fractures of the proximal femur are traditionally classified using the Delbet's system. The latter relates the fracture position to the physis, the neck and the trochanters. It is used to predict the likelihood of avascular necrosis.

Treatment

Multiple factors influence the management of these fractures: their location within the femur, the age and size of the patient, as well as the fracture configuration.

Proximal and distal femoral fractures

These are increasingly managed with internal fixation. Nonunion and malunion are prevented with the use of modern angular stable implants. Distal femoral fractures may be managed nonoperatively by casting for a minimum of 4 weeks if they are undisplaced. Salter–Harris I fractures, which are thought to be displaced and unstable are reduced in a closed manner and fixed with anterograde crossed Kirschner wiring. A minimum of 4 weeks in a cast is then required. The wires may be removed once this period has elapsed.

Salter–Harris II fractures are usually managed operatively. The size of the fragments involved determines the method of fixation. Wires are used with smaller fragments while screws are preferred when the fragment is larger. Preoperative planning may be assisted by the use of CT. Type 3 and 4 fractures are transphyseal and intra-articular, therefore are almost always managed surgically with open reduction and internal fixation.

Femoral shaft fractures

The neonate and infant

Neonates can be managed with immobilisation in a Pavlik harness for up to 3 weeks. Management options for the fracture in this age group tend to be noninvasive and include either traction or hip spica casting. Skin traction in smaller children (<12 kg) should be in the form of Gallows traction.

Young children and toddlers (18 months to 5 years)

Noninvasive management forms the main basis of treatment. Balanced traction systems (such as Hamilton–Russell traction) are suitable for definitive management. The amount of weight needed is usually one pound of weight and 1 week of traction per year of age. Hip spica casting may also be used in this age group. It does not have to be applied in the acute setting. It may be initiated following an initial period of traction.

Children aged 5–12 years

An increasing period of immobilisation is required for nonoperative management in older children. It is in this age group that management options begin to steer towards surgical as they allow for earlier return of function.

Operative management may take the form of intramedullary fixation, or the use of plates or external fixators.

The use of flexible intramedullary nailing is currently the technique of choice in the management of most femoral diaphyseal fractures in this age group (**Figures 72.1** and **72.2**). They are favoured because they allow an early return to function and create little damage to the soft tissues. Plates still retain a role as young patients heal rapidly and the complication of plate failure is rarely seen. External fixators are primarily reserved for use in the polytrauma setting or for patients with extensive soft tissue damage.

The older child and the adolescent

Intramedullary fixation is primarily used. The key determinant for the choice of treatment is the size of the child. Younger/smaller patients may still be treated with elastic nailing whereas older/larger children require the use of more rigid nails. The risk of avascular necrosis associated with the use of the latter must be considered. Plating may be of use in comminuted fracture patterns.

Complications

Fractures of the proximal femur

Fractures of the proximal femur carry a risk of both avascular necrosis and post-traumatic arthritis. Both the proximity of the fracture and increasing age lead to higher rates of complication. Displacement of the fracture

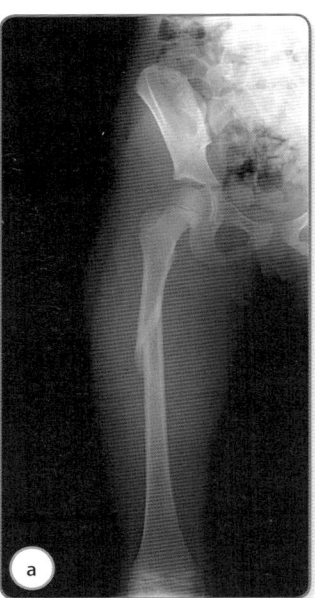

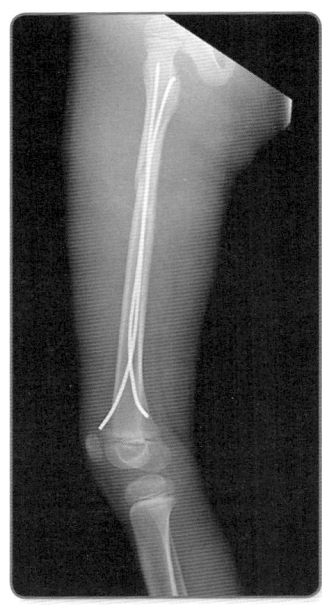

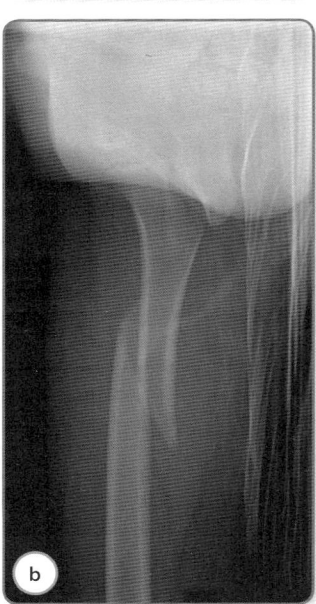

Figure 72.1 (a) Anteroposterior and (b) lateral views of a spiral fracture of the femoral diaphysis in a young child.

Figure 72.2 The spiral fracture (same case as Figure 72.1) has been treated with flexible intramedullary nails.

and delay to reduction also predispose to the risk of developing avascular necrosis. It is thought that open, anatomical reduction and internal fixation reduces this risk.

Fractures of the distal femur

Fractures of the distal femur are associated with a high rate of complications. Growth arrest is a serious problem with these injuries and may be associated with up to 52% of distal femoral fractures. The risk of growth arrest increases with fracture displacement and proxima comminution.

Femoral shaft fractures

Differences femoral length, rotation and angular deformity are all recognised complications of femoral shaft fractures. Care must be taken in their management to correct for these. Prevention of these complications is best achieved at the time of injury and with the acute management. Osteotomies may be used in the chronic setting to correct these deformities.

Further reading

Brousil J, Hunter JB. Femoral fractures in children. Current opinion in pediatrics 2013; 25:52–57.

Harvey AR, Bowyer GW, Clarke NMP. The management of paediatric femoral shaft fractures. Current Orthop 2002; 16:293–299.

Hunter JB. Femoral shaft fractures in children. Injury 2005; 36:86–93.

Related topics of interest

- *Topic 74* Paediatric fractures – nonaccidental injury
- *Topic 77* Paediatric physeal fractures
- *Topic 84* Principles of nonoperative management of fractures

73 Paediatric forearm fractures

Key points

- Paediatric forearm fractures are extremely common
- The forearm has some scope for remodelling but this decreases with age
- Surgical stabilisation may be necessary in certain situations, for example open fractures and unstable fracture patterns

Epidemiology

Paediatric forearm fractures account for 41.1% of all fractures in children. The majority of these are fractures of the distal radius and ulna. The incidence of fractures increases with age, falls from below bed height (<1 m) being the most common cause. Incidence is increasing due to increased sporting activity and increasing body weight.

Fractures of the radius and ulna diaphysis have a bimodal distribution for both males and females with the first peak at 6 years. Fractures of the distal and proximal forearm have linear relationship with a peak at 12 years.

Pathophysiology

Diaphyseal fractures of the forearm usually occur as a result of indirect trauma. The spectrum of injuries ranges from plastic deformation to complete unstable fractures where there is no continuity of either cortex, with periosteal disruption. Plastic deformation results when the load applied exceeds the elastic limit of bone. In this instance, there is no cortical disruption, however there is microscopic failure on the tension side, which does not propagate to the compression side. When there is increased bending force, there is a continuum of plastic deformation to fracture. The tension side fails and results in fracture but this does not propagate to the compression side, resulting in a greenstick fracture.

The most common mechanism of forearm fractures is a fall onto an outstretched hand. The position of the hand and forearm is critical to the resulting deformity. If the hand is in pronation, at the time of impact, the forearm will rapidly supinate, which will result in a dorsally angulated fracture. If the forearm is in supination at the time of impact, there will be rapid pronation of the forearm resulting in a volar angular deformity.

Clinical features

Children usually present with clinical deformity, pain and reduced range of movement. The attending orthopaedic surgeon should carefully note the mechanism of injury, as high-energy injuries should be managed with Advanced Trauma Life Support principles. Analgesia should be prescribed as soon as possible to facilitate a full history, examination and further investigations. Prior to splinting the limb, a full examination, including a circumferential investigation of the surrounding skin to exclude an open fracture is mandatory. Ipsilateral concurrent supracondylar fractures occur in 15% of injuries and should always be suspected. A careful neurological examination and vascular examination should be performed and recorded. Compartment syndrome may occur.

Investigations

Standard anteroposterior (AP) and lateral radiographs of the whole forearm, including wrist and elbow joints, usually allow for an accurate diagnosis. Assessment of the distal radioulnar joint is important to exclude a Galeazzi fracture dislocation, as is inspection of the radiocapitellar joint to exclude a Monteggia fracture. Comparing the cortical widths both sides of the fracture assesses rotational deformity. With normal rotational alignment on the AP radiograph, the bicipital tuberosity and radial styloid should be 180° from each other. The relationship of the coronoid process and ulnar styloid should once again be 180° from each other on the lateral radiograph. The mid-axis line of the radius should intersect the capitellum in all views.

Classification

Paediatric forearm fractures are classified by four main features:
- Anatomical location
- Fracture pattern
- The presence of associated injuries to the joints of the forearm units (Monteggia's and Galeazzi's fractures)
- Displacement

Remodelling

Before discussing treatment options, it is important to understand the remodelling potential in children. The remodelling capacity in children's fractures is dependant on several factors, including the distance from the fracture to the physis, the amount of growth remaining, and plane of remodelling required. Rotation has poor remodelling potential. Seventy-five percent of growth takes place in the distal radial physis. The potential for remodelling of diaphyseal fractures is not as great as in distal radial fractures.

Angulation for acceptable remodelling is understandably different for different age groups and distal and diaphyseal fractures (Table 73.1). As a general rule, 'after eight, the radius should be straight.'

Treatment

The majority of paediatric forearm fractures can be managed with closed reduction and application of a cast. Redisplacement however occurs in up to 32% of fractures. The redisplacement is related to fracture site stability, quality of the reduction and cast application. Application of a well-moulded cast with three-point fixation is critical when managing these injuries; the cast index diameter is measured at the fracture site and is the sagittal width inside the cast, divided by the coronal width in the cast. A cast index of <0.7–0.8 has been shown to prevent loss of reduction.

The incidence of surgical stabilisation of paediatric forearm fractures has increased from 10–30% over the last 10 years. There are various reasons for this, but a lower risk of redisplacement postoperatively is an important factor. Shorter periods in a cast and less intensive periods of follow-up are additional reasons.

Indications for surgical reduction and stabilisation include open fractures, fractures in which the surgeon is unable to achieve satisfactory alignment through closed means and unstable fractures in which adequate alignment cannot be maintained by closed methods.

Kirschner-wire fixation may be required to stabilise distal radial fractures if it is shown to be unstable following reduction, or where nonoperative management has failed. Shaft fractures that are irreducible or unstable, require closed +/– open reduction and intramedullary nailing. Open reduction and internal plate fixation is reserved for older children and fractures of the distal shaft. The principles of management in this age group are anatomical reduction, absolute stability and early mobilisation.

The gold standard surgical tool for paediatric forearm fractures requiring fixation is elastic stable intramedullary nailing (ESIN). The success of these nails is based around the respect of the biology and growing bone. The periosteum is more biologically active in children than in adults and is a rich source of blood supply to cortical bone. Disruption has a deleterious effect on healing. The ESIN is more biologically friendly than plate fixation.

The intramedullary nails are inserted to achieve three-point fixation and to achieve this, the nails are prebent (pretensioned). The bend should be three times the diameter of the long bone at its isthmus. The curvature of the nail is achieved by bending them beyond

Table 73.1 Acceptable angulations for shaft and distal forearm fractures		
Age (years)	Shaft fractures	Distal radius/ulna
<10	15°	30° (dorsal)
>10	10°	15° (dorsal)

their elastic limit. In their new position of stability, they resist the tendency to straighten thus creating tension within the construct. Each nail used must have a diameter that is 40% of the intramedullary canal at the level of the isthmus. Once in the canal the nails resist angular, compressive and rotational forces. The elasticity of the construct allows for ideal micromotion for rapid fracture healing.

Complications

Immediate complications include nerve injury. Neurological function should be documented before and after any intervention. The majority are a neurapraxia but the incidence is said to be as high as 8.5% in surgically stabilised fractures. Early complications include compartment syndrome, the risk of which increases with multiple attempts at closed reduction and prolonged operating time. Loss of reduction has been reported in the literature to be as high as 33% for distal fractures and 27% for diaphyseal fractures. Infection is a rare complication.

Late complications included malunion, which if significant can lead to reduced pronation and supination. Refracture carries a risk of 7% irrespective of the fracture being managed with operative or nonoperative means. Avoiding repeated attempts at manipulation, and manipulation after 7 days can reduce incidence of growth arrest. Synostosis is rare.

Further reading

Colaris JW, Allema JH, Biter LU, et al. Re-displacement of stable distal both-bone forearm fractures in children: a randomised controlled multicentre trial. Injury 2013; 44:498–503.

Kosuge D, Barry M. Changing trends in the management of children's fractures. Bone Joint J 2015; 97B:442–448.

Patel A, Li L, Anand A. Systematic review: functional outcomes and complications of intramedullary nailing versus plate fixation for both-bone diaphyseal forearm fractures in children. Injury 2014; 45:1135–1143.

Related topics of Interest

- *Topic 9* Bone structure and physiology
- *Topic 52* Implants – nails
- *Topic 74* Paediatric fractures – nonaccidental injury
- *Topic 77* Paediatric physeal fractures

74 Paediatric fractures – nonaccidental injury

Key points

- Knowledge and understanding of risk factors and certain injury patterns are essential in assessing any child with suspected nonaccidental injury
- Skin lesions, followed by fractures are the most common manifestation of nonaccidental injury
- Treatment includes a multidisciplinary approach with all specialties including paediatricians, radiologists and orthopaedic surgeons, with referral to the relevant safeguarding lead and social services

Epidemiology

Nonaccidental injury (NAI) was first described by Caffey in 1946. There is a wide variation in the reported incidence of NAI in the literature. Values ranging from 0.47 per 100,000 to 2000 per 100,000 have been quoted. Although some studies declare there is more than a 50% decrease in fractures resulting from NAI over the last two decades, other sources have shown there is an overall increase in the number of children being referred to social services. There also has been an increase in the number of children becoming the subject of a child protection plan.

Pathophysiology

The clinical history of a suspected NAI includes a vague unwitnessed mechanism of injury inconsistent with the clinical findings and developmental age. When the history given by the caregiver does not match the suspected mode of injury, this should alert the attending physician to possible NAI. One should be diligent for seeking out changes in the history between carers or on repeated telling. If no plausible history for the injury can be given, NAI should be suspected. Any physician dealing with NAI should be aware of normal motor and social developmental milestones as inconsistencies can be sought

Table 74.1 Developmental milestones

Age	Motor skills	Social skills
3 months	Lifts head up when prone	Smiles when spoken to
6 months	Sits with support Head steady when sitting	Laughs and smiles spontaneously
9 months	Sits without support	Waves 'bye-bye' Vocalises 'ma-ma' 'da-da'
1 year	Walks with one hand support	Starts cooperating with dressing
2 years	Runs forward	Use three word sentences Matches colours Ask for food
3 years	Jumps in place	Dresses self Puts own shows on Dry throughout night Interactive play with other children Learn to help
5 years	Hops	Names four colours Counts ten objects correctly
6 years	Skips	Does small buttons on shirt Ties bows on shows

out, e.g. a 2-month-old child will not be able to physically roll off a bedside (**Table 74.1**). Delays in seeking medical attention may occur alongside aggressive parental responses. Timing of the injury given in the history may differ from the timing derived from the radiographs. A social history and previous attendances to the emergency department should be obtained.

Risk factors are a lower socioeconomic class, preterm baby, twins and unplanned birth. Children with special needs are also at increased risk. Many studies have shown that the younger the child, the greater the likelihood of abuse.

Clinical features

Bruising is the most common manifestation of NAI. Isolated or multiple posterior rib fractures are the most specific type of injury for NAI. Other associated fractures with a high specificity include scapular, lateral clavicle, digital (in nonmobile children), vertebral and complex skull fractures. As previously mentioned, fractures at inappropriate ages are also highly specific, for example lower limb fracture in a non-ambulatory child. Frequently encountered fractures include mid-clavicular fractures, simple linear skull fractures and single long-bone fractures, but these have a low specificity.

Systemic findings of failure to thrive, seizures, apnoea or difficulty breathing should be excluded. Bruising is very common in the ambulatory child, however bruises away from bony prominences and clusters of bruising is not characteristic of accidental injury. When a child is assessed for NAI, underlying metabolic bone disease of prematurity and osteogenesis imperfecta should be excluded as these conditions can cause recurrent low-energy fractures.

Investigations

Any child who is seen with suspected NAI should be admitted for further assessment. The lead paediatric safeguarding consultant should be notified and the named safeguarding nurse should be made aware of the child's admission. Diagnostic imaging including anteroposterior and lateral radiographs of the injured limb should be obtained. Assessment of the joints above and below should be completed.

A bone profile and metabolic markers including calcium, phosphate, alkaline phosphate, copper, caeruloplasmin, vitamin D, parathyroid hormone and magnesium need to be completed to exclude metabolic bone disease.

A skeletal survey is the standard imaging of choice for any child suspected of NAI. The Royal College of Radiologists, the Royal College of Paediatrics and Child Health and the American College of Radiology have produced a joint document with an agreed policy for suspected NAI. Full skeletal surveys should be done in all children under the age of 2 years where the history is not reliable. A dedicated paediatric musculoskeletal radiologist should report the images. The skeletal survey comprises high-quality radiographs of the entire skeleton, which includes separate views of all four limbs, the chest, spine, skull, abdomen, pelvis, hands and feet. A single total body radiograph must not be performed. A senior radiographer and radiologist should supervise the radiographs in case additional coned views are required.

Skeletal injury associated with nonaccidental injury

Rib fractures

Rib fractures are very uncommon, even following high-energy major trauma. They are rarely seen even after cardiopulmonary resuscitation (CPR); when they do occur during CPR they tend to be multiple and anterior. Thus rib fractures, particularly those that present without a clear history, have a 100% positive predictive value for NAI when all other causes have been excluded. These fractures tend to be bilateral and may become flail segments. The mechanism of action is an anteroposterior compression of the chest.

Metaphyseal fractures

Metaphyseal fractures are relatively rare in infants and are highly specific for NAI. These fractures are transmetaphyseal disruption through the weak zone of provisional calcification of the physis. Centrally, the fracture abuts the chondro-osseous junction and peripherally it turns away from the physis and undercuts a larger peripheral fracture fragment. Therefore, the peripheral fracture is thicker than central fractures, which includes the subperiosteal bone. Position and projection influence the appearance of the fracture line on the radiographs resulting in the characteristic metaphyseal fractures. The crescent-shaped fragment may be named a 'bucket handle' fracture if radiographs are angled cranially or caudally. If viewed at right angles, the peripheral thicker fragment is viewed as a triangular shaped fragment and named a 'corner' fracture.

Long bone fractures

Femoral fractures are more commonly seen in NAI than either tibial or fibular fractures, with the mid-shaft being the most prevalent site. The younger the child the more likely it is the fracture was caused by NAI. Spiral pattern fractures are the most common abuse-related femoral fracture in children under the age of 15 months. However, there is no association between specific fracture patterns and NAI. Spiral fractures generally require rotational force, whereas a transverse fracture is usually a result of indirect bending force or direct blow to the bone. Femoral fractures below the age of 12 months and tibial fractures below the age of 18 months, regardless of type, are highly suggestive of NAI.

Skull fractures

In both abused and nonabused children, skull fracture is most common under the age of three. It is frequently reported following nonabusive trauma. There is a strong association between skull fractures and intracranial pathology including intracranial haemorrhage. For children subjected to nonaccidental injury, those with skull fractures have the highest mortality rate.

Treatment

A multi-disciplinary team approach is utilised for the management of NAI. There should be a local policy and guideline in the local institution. This will provide a wealth of information on whom to contact. The paediatricians will be intrinsically involved in the care, as will the radiologists. The named consultant and nurse for child safeguarding should be notified as should social services. Documentation and communication is of paramount importance in managing NAI. It is important to make an assessment of any other child living within the premises of the child whom NAI is suspected. If this is the case, social services should remove this child to a place of safety as they are also at risk. The re-injury rate of a battered child has been quoted up to 50% and the risk of death is between 6 and 10%.

Each fracture should be treated on their own merits. The child's age and weight are important factors to consider when treating paediatric femoral shaft fractures.

Further reading

Alshryda S, Jones S, Banaszkiewicz PA. Postgraduate Paediatric Orthopaedics: The Candidate's Guide to the FRCS (Tr and Orth) Examination. Cambridge: Cambridge University Press, 2014:249–252.

Jayakumar P, Barry M, Ramachandran M. Orthopaedic aspects of paediatric non-accidental injury. J Bone Joint Surg Br 2010; 92:189–195.

Kosuge D, Barry M. Changing trends in the management of children's fractures. Bone Joint J 2015; 97B:442–448.

Related topics of interest

- Topic 70 Paediatric clavicle fractures
- Topic 72 Paediatric femoral fractures
- Topic 75 Paediatric humeral condylar fractures
- Topic 77 Paediatric physeal fractures

75 Paediatric humeral condylar fractures

Key points

- Displaced condylar fractures are articular fractures and must be treated with anatomic reduction and rigid internal fixation
- Complication rates can be as high as 20%
- Management of these fractures is complex and controversial

Epidemiology

Lateral humeral condyle fractures are the second most common type of elbow fractures, representing 10–20% of all paediatric elbow injuries. Diagnosis and assessment of epiphyseal extension and displacement may be difficult because the capitellum is largely cartilaginous in young children and not always visualised on plain radiographs. They commonly occur in the 5- to 10-year age group.

Medial condylar fractures comprise up to 10% of elbow injuries in children. Diagnosis can be difficult because the trochlea ossifies much later than the capitellum and is not completely ossified till the age of 9 years. Most reported fractures occur between the ages of 9 and 14 years, with the peak incidence occurring at 11–12 years of age. Boys constitute the majority with a male to female ratio of 4:1. 50% of such injuries are associated with elbow dislocations of which a proportion go unrecognised due to spontaneous relocation. In 15%, the fragment may become entrapped in the joint.

Pathophysiology

Both medial and lateral condylar fractures are Salter–Harris type IV injuries. Physeal injury is a potential outcome. There are pull-off and push-off theories describing the mechanism of injury for both fracture variants.

The most common mechanism of injury of lateral condylar fractures is a violent varus force with the elbow in extension. The condyle is avulsed by the lateral ligament and the extensor muscles (pull-off). Fall onto an outstretched hand can also cause impaction of the radial head into the lateral condyle causing fracture (push-off).

Medial condylar fractures are thought to be caused by a valgus force on an extended elbow with the force transmitted via the olecranon or coronoid process into the medial condyle (push-off). Alternatively, this fracture occurs as an avulsion of the condyle by the action of the forearm flexors (pull-off). With large enough energy forces, the medial condylar fracture can extend through the lateral wall of the trochlea and disrupt the soft tissues causing a fracture dislocation (**Figure 75.1**).

Clinical features

Due to the challenges of radiographic evaluation, a thorough physical examination is paramount. Children will not usually move the elbow if a fracture is present. On examination, swelling is a telling feature. Vascular and neurological assessment is essential as neurovascular injuries can occur before and after reduction.

Compartment syndromes are rare but can occur.

Investigations

Anteroposterior (AP) and lateral radiographs are the most important initial views. Often the views obtained are not ideal because it may be difficult to position the injured extremity. CT scan should be considered if a diagnosis is not possible from the radiographs. Arthrogram, prior to internal fixation is well described but mandates and anaesthetic.

Classification

Roly Jakob performed an anatomical study and a clinical review of lateral humeral condyle fractures in 1975 in an attempt to

Paediatric humeral condylar fractures

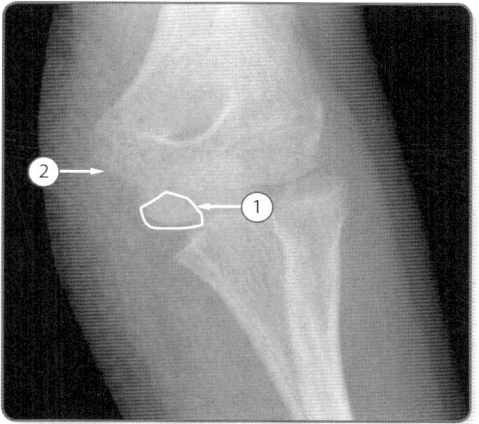
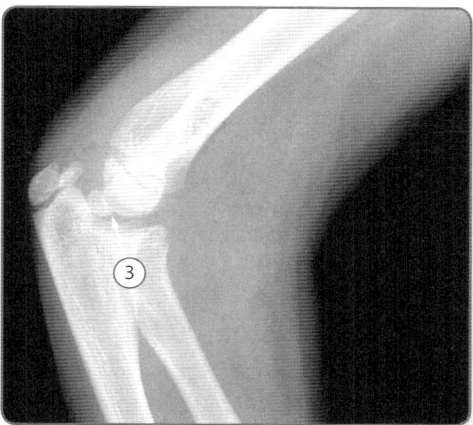

Figure 75.1 (a) Anteroposterior elbow radiograph showing a medial condylar fracture. The medial epicondyle ① has fractured and displaced from its anatomical position ②. The fragment now sits in the elbow joint. (b) Lateral radiograph of medial epicondylar fracture the epicondyle ③ now sits in the elbow joint.

describe the mechanism of injury and propose a method of classification. He concluded that the level of displacement was correlated to the integrity of the preosseous cartilage of the humeral epiphysis. In undisplaced fractures, the cartilage is intact acting as a hinge but allowing the fracture to open like a book but preventing gross displacement and rotation of the condyle. As soon as the hinge was divided, the fracture became unstable and the condyle could then be displaced and rotated without difficulty (**Figure 75.2**).

Medial condylar fractures are quantified by the amount of displacement (**Figure 75.3**). Bensahel et al. proposed a classification system based on this and the amount of rotation present (**Table 75.1**). It is important to remember that medial condylar fractures are associated with 50% of elbow dislocations; most of which spontaneously relocate and can often go unrecognised.

Treatment

Controversy and debate still exists about the definitive management of these fractures.

Displaced lateral condyle fractures

Surgery is accepted as the treatment of choice for lateral condyle fractures displaced >2 mm.

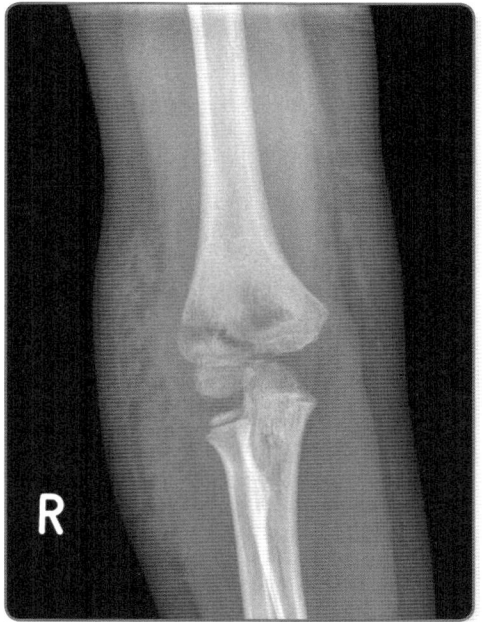

Figure 75.2 A Jakob type 2 lateral condyle fracture.

The aims of surgery are anatomical reduction of the articular surface and stable internal fixation (**Figure 75.4**). The reduction should be performed open via a direct lateral approach. The amount of displacement often determines

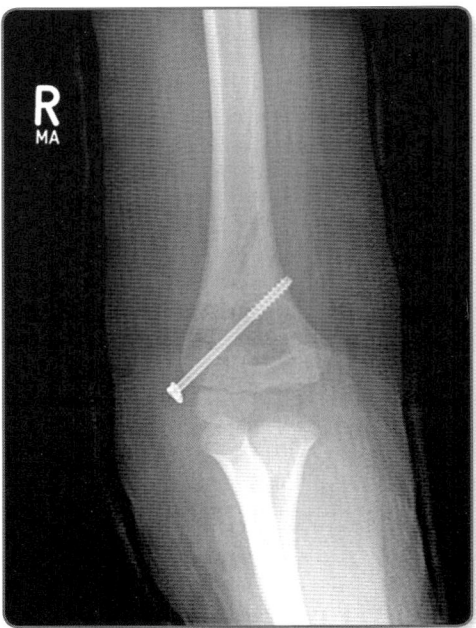

Figure 75.3 Fixation of a Jakob type 2 lateral condyle fracture.

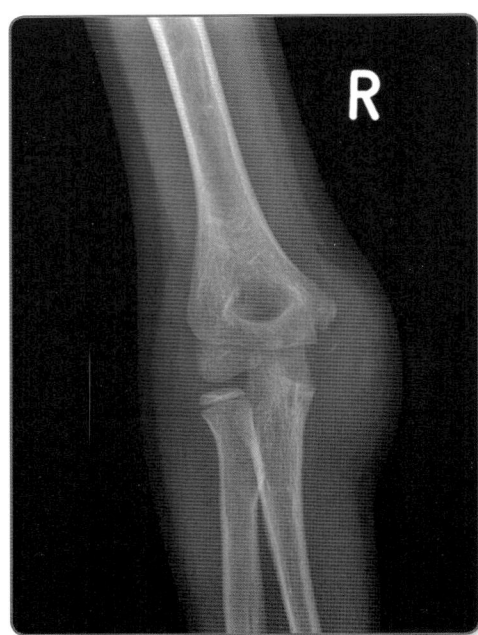

Figure 75.4 A displaced medial condyle fracture with significant soft tissue swelling raising suspicion of an associated elbow dislocation.

Table 75.1 Bensahel classification of medial condyle fractures

Classification	Description
Type 1	Minimally displaced
Type 2	Displaced but minimally rotated
Type 3	Significantly displaced and rotated

the ability to reduce the fracture closed and it is very hard to gauge accurate reduction. Methods of stabilisation are determined by surgeon preference and the literature reports the use of 2 or 3 Kirschner (K) wires or screws. Surgical stabilisation is followed up with immobilisation in an above elbow cast for up to 6 weeks and subsequent implant removal.

Undisplaced lateral condyle fractures

For nondisplaced and minimally displaced (<2 mm displacement) fractures, both nonoperative treatment with plaster immobilisation and surgical stabilisation have both been proposed. Launay et al. compared outcomes of both these treatment modalities.

Of the 17 treated nonoperatively, 5 displaced at the fracture site of which 4 required operative stabilisation. The rate of displacement is significant occurring within the first 2 weeks in nonoperatively managed injuries. This is related to whether the cartilaginous bridge is intact or not. Patient compliance to follow-up for weekly serial radiographs especially within the first 2 weeks is of utmost importance. Total immobilisation in an above elbow cast is required for 6 weeks. There is a significant risk of nonunion and malunion in patients managed purely nonoperatively.

All 13 patients with undisplaced lateral condyle fractures managed operatively achieved union although 2 patients malunited due to loss of reduction related to surgical technique.

An accepted treatment algorithm for these injuries is to offer nonoperative management to compliant patients with undisplaced fractures followed up with serial radiographs to assess for displacement and nonunion. If features consistent with displacement and nonunion arise, operative intervention should be considered.

Undisplaced medial condyle fractures

It is described that medial epicondyle fractures with <5 mm of displacement can be treated nonoperatively with plaster cast immobilisation in an above elbow plaster cast with the elbow at 90° for 2–3 weeks followed by early mobilisation.

Displaced medial condyle fractures

There is controversy surrounding the management of fractures with >5 mm of displacement. Numerous investigators report that these fractures should be treated by open reduction and internal fixation but other authors have reported that nonsurgical treatment yields results that are similar to or better than those of surgical treatment. Relative indications for surgical intervention include suspicion of ulnar nerve entrapment and elbow instability in young athletes.

The aim of surgical management is anatomical reduction of the articular surface and stable internal fixation. Open reduction is achieved using an anteromedial approach and internal fixation using 2 or 3 K-wires for small fragments or cannulated screws for larger fragments.

Complications

Immediate
- Nerve injury – ulnar nerve injury can occur during medial condyle fixation

Early
- Wound infection after operative management

Late
- Elbow deformity and instability due to nonunion, malunion or growth arrest resulting in restriction of strength and range of motion
- Chronic pain and post-traumatic osteoarthritis

Further reading

Jakob R, Fowles JV, Rang M, Kassab MT. Observations concerning fractures of the lateral humeral condyle in children. J Bone Joint Surg Br 1975; 57:4:430–436.

Kamath AF, Baldwin K, Horneff J, Hosalkar HS. Operative versus non-operative management of paediatric medial epicondyle fractures: a systematic review. J Child Orthop 2009; 3:345–357.

Launay F, Leet AI, Jacopin S, et al. Lateral humeral condyle fractures in children: a comparison of two approaches to treatment. J Pediatr Orthop 2004; 24:385–391.

Related topics of interest

- *Topic 70* Paediatric clavicle fractures
- *Topic 77* Paediatric physeal fractures
- *Topic 78* Paediatric supracondylar humeral fractures

76 Paediatric humeral fractures

Key points
- In children, proximal humeral fractures commonly involve the physis
- Nonaccidental injuries must always be considered
- Acceptable degrees of deformity decrease with age

Epidemiology
Paediatric humeral fractures (metaphyseal and diaphyseal) account for <3% of all paediatric fractures. These follow a unimodal distribution. There is a gradual increase in incidence up to the age of 12–14 years in both sexes, with a later decrease in incidence, particularly in girls.

Pathophysiology
Humeral fractures are a common birth-related injury. Larger size and breech presentations have been associated with increased incidence in humeral fractures. Trauma can be direct or indirect and are often metaphyseal, physeal or both. A humeral diaphyseal fracture under the age of 3 years should alert the attending orthopaedic surgeon of nonaccidental injury. Older children sustain transverse fractures as a result of a direct blow. Pathological fractures through simple bone cysts are common.

Clinical features
Humeral fractures, both metaphyseal and diaphyseal can present with a pseudoparalysis. Movement of the shoulder girdle exacerbates pain. The upper limb is held in internal rotation due to the pull of pectoralis major on the distal fragment. The rotator cuff produces abduction and external rotation of the proximal fragment. Associated injuries should be excluded. High-energy injuries of the proximal humerus may be associated with a concomitant dislocation of the glenohumeral joint. Neurological injury to the brachial plexus can occur.

Investigations
The proximal humeral epiphysis is not visible on plain X-rays until 6 months of age, in which case ultrasound can be used. The vanishing epiphyseal sign indicates posterior displaced physeal fractures. Two X-rays perpendicular to each other are usually diagnostic. A true anteroposterior view of the shoulder and an axillary lateral view should be performed. The axillary lateral is often difficult to obtain due to the acute fracture hence a scapula-Y view is performed. CT scan may be useful in diagnosing posterior dislocations and complex fractures.

Classification
Fractures of the proximal humerus can involve the metaphysis and physis. Fractures involving the physis are classified according to the Salter–Harris classification. Neer–Horowitz classified proximal humeral fractures according to the degree of displacement with respect to the shaft diameter.

Humeral diaphyseal fractures are classified according to the location (proximal, middle, distal, diaphyseal metaphyseal junction), the pattern (spiral, transverse, oblique) and the direction of displacement. Segmental fractures or associated glenohumeral dislocations should be noted. Ipsilateral forearm fractures result in a floating elbow.

Treatment
The proximal humerus has great potential for healing and remodelling. Obstetric fractures infrequently require fixation. Children <11 years have excellent outcomes despite the degree of displacement. Children >11 years who have grossly displaced angulated fractures may require closed or open

reduction and stabilisation as the remodelling potential decreases with increasing age. The majority of proximal humeral fractures will be managed in a shoulder immobiliser or keeping the limb splinted against the chest. Several methods of reduction are available, such as direct manual manipulation. Despite all these manoeuvres, some fractures cannot be reduced. Anatomical structures preventing reduction include the periosteum, shoulder joint capsule and biceps tendon. Should this occur, a limited deltopectoral approach is utilised.

Indications for surgical fixation are open fractures, neurovascular compromise, the polytrauma patient and significant displacement in older adolescents. Fixation options include plating, screw fixation and intramedullary fixation. Percutaneous Kirschner wire and external fixation may be alternatives.

The humerus is not a weight-bearing bone and does not require precise anatomical alignment. With marked mobility of the shoulder axial and rotational deformities can be well tolerated. Guidelines have been published for acceptable alignment and are based on the patient's age (**Table 76.1**).

Table 76.1 Acceptable angulation and displacement for paediatric humeral fractures

Age (years)	Acceptable angulation and displacement	
	Angulation	Displacement
<5	70°	Any
5–12	40–50°	50% of width of shaft
>12	20°	<30% of width of shaft

Complications

Proximal humeral varus, a rare complication, causes a decrease in neck shaft angle to 90^0 with shortening and loss of glenohumeral abduction. Osteotomy may be required to correct this. Growth arrest may occur if the physis is crushed or significantly displaced. Axillary nerve injury can occur in fracture dislocations. Osteonecrosis may occur with disruption of the anterior circumflex artery. Early complications of humeral fractures include radial nerve palsy. Compartment syndrome and vascular injuries both require immediate surgical intervention. Late complications include malunion.

Further reading

Caviglia H, Garrido CP, Palazzi FF, Meana NV. Peadiatric fractures of the humerus. Clin Orthop Relat Res 2005:49–56.

Kraus T, Hoermann S, Ploder G, et al. Elastic stable intramedullary nailing versus Kirschner wire pinning: outcome of severely displaced proximal humeral fractures in juvenile patients. J Shoulder Elbow Surg 2014; 23:1462–1467.

Related topics of interest

- *Topic 13* Clavicle fractures
- *Topic 70* Paediatric clavicle fractures
- *Topic 77* Paediatric physeal fractures
- *Topic 84* Principles of nonoperative management of fractures

77 Paediatric physeal fractures

Key points
- Physeal injuries account for 15–30% of musculoskeletal trauma in children
- The Salter–Harris classification describes fracture pattern and guides management and prognosis
- The outcome is determined by any interruption of vascular supply to the physis

Epidemiology

Physeal injuries account for 15–30% of all musculoskeletal injuries in children. Approximately, 80% of physeal injuries occur between the ages of 10 and 16 years. Physeal injuries are more frequent in boys than in girls due to an increased overall incidence of musculoskeletal injuries. The incidence peaks at age 12–14 years in boys and age 11–12 years in girls. The age difference is due to the physes closing at an older age in boys than girls.

The most common causes of physeal fractures are acute trauma and chronic overuse. Accidents during sport are the most common cause of trauma.

Pathophysiology

The term 'physis' comes from the Latin term for growth, thus it is also known as the growth plate. The physis is made of cartilage and is the anatomical region responsible for the longitudinal and circumferential growth of bone. Long bones have primary growth centres in the diaphyseal region and one or more secondary ossification centres in the epiphysis.

The physis is connected to the epiphysis and metaphysis by the zone of Ranvier and perichondral ring of LaCroix. It is primarily responsible for longitudinal growth whilst the zone of Ranvier contributes to circumferential growth. Osteoblasts, chondroblasts and fibroblasts make up the zone of Ranvier. The perichondral ring of LaCroix is fibrous in nature and is continuous with the fibrous region of the zone of Ranvier and with the periosteum.

The microscopic anatomy of the physis consists of columns of chondrocytes in various stages of maturity and bony transformation. There are five zones within an extracellular matrix. These are illustrated in **Figure 77.1**. The first three zones are sensitive to trauma and injury here can have serious

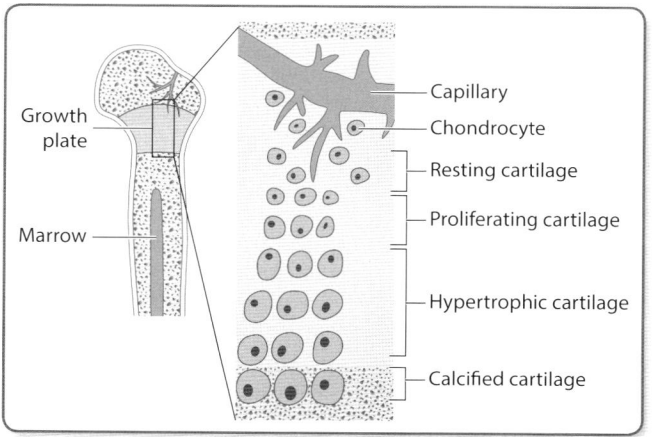

Figure 77.1 Anatomy of the growth plate and its different layers.

consequences to future growth. Listed in order from the epiphysis to the metaphysis, they are:
1. **Resting zone:** cells are irregular in shape and are responsible for storing nutrients
2. **Zone of differentiation:** cells divide, differentiate and orientate into columns. Cells produce matrix
3. **Zone of proliferation:** chondrocytes rapidly increase in number. The first three layers are relatively strong and resistant to shear forces
4. **Zone of hypertrophy:** this is an avascular region where cells are responsible for elongation of bone. Cells enlarge by cytoplasmic and nuclear swelling. They follow a cycle of programmed cell death. There is a lack of matrix making this zone susceptible to shear forces
5. **Zone of provisional calcification:** mineralisation of the matrix occurs here. This provides increased resistance to shear. This zone overlaps the metaphysis and is invaded by osteoblasts to eventually become replaced by bone

The nutrient blood supply to the first three layers of the physis comes from the epiphyseal arteries. Vessels do not cross from the metaphyseal side into the epiphysis. They form loops that end in the hypertrophic zone. The zone of Ranvier is supplied by the periosteal artery.

Normal growth and maturation at the physis is dependent on this intact vascular pathway.

Clinical assessment

Children generally have increased ligamentous strength versus adults resulting in mechanical forces stressing the integrity of the physis. Thus, a mechanism of injury that would cause a sprain in adults can cause physeal injuries in children.

A thorough history and examination are vital to establish a proper diagnosis. With all paediatric trauma it is important to exclude nonaccidental injury.

Investigations

Plain film radiography is usually sufficient to guide management in combination with a good history and examination. These can be challenging to interpret due to the radiolucent nature of the physes thus orthogonal views are pertinent.

CT and MRI can be used as adjuncts in complex intra-articular fracture patterns. A common example for which CT can guide management is the triplane ankle fracture.

Classification

The Salter–Harris classification system (**Figure 77.2**) is most commonly used to describe physeal injuries. This was first described in 1963 by Robert Salter and Robert Harris from Toronto, Canada. It is based on the involvement of the physis, epiphysis and joint (**Table 77.1**). The system is prognostic – the higher the Salter–Harris classification of the fracture, the greater the likelihood of interruption of the vascular supply to the physis, and thus the greater likelihood of physeal arrest and joint incongruity.

Treatment

The Salter–Harris classification offers a guide to management and prognosis. Salter–Harris I and II are extra-articular fractures with the epiphyseal blood supply intact. Type I fractures and undisplaced type II fractures can be managed with splintage. Displaced type II fractures can be managed

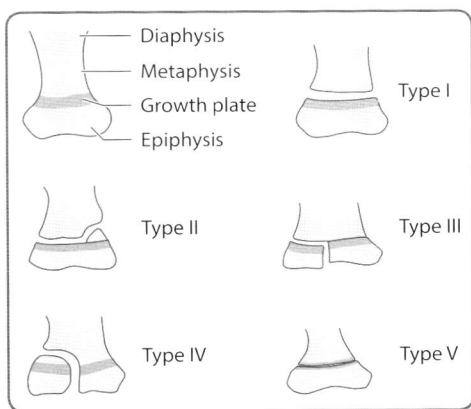

Figure 77.2 The Salter–Harris classification of growth plate injuries.

Table 77.1 The Salter–Harris classification of physeal fractures

Salter–Harris type	Incidence	Fracture pattern and pathology	Mnemonic
I	6%	Separation of the epiphysis from the metaphysis through the hypertrophic zone of the physis. The growing cells remain on the epiphysis and the nutrient blood supply is intact	S – Separation
II	75%	The fracture line runs through the hypertrophic zone of the physis and then out through a segment of metaphyseal bone. The growing cells remain on the physis and their nutrient blood supply is intact	A – Above the physis and away from the joint
III	10%	An intra-articular fracture of the epiphysis with extension through the hypertrophic cell layer of the physis. The greater the displacement increases the risk of disruption of blood supply	L – Lower (below the physis and away from the joint)
IV	10%	The fracture line originates at the articular surface, crosses the epiphysis, extends through the physis and exits through the metaphysis. Displacement governs the likelihood of blood supply disruption	TE – Through Everything (the epiphysis, physis and metaphysis)
V	1%	Caused by axial compression crushing the physis and injuring the resting and proliferative zones. The blood supply is disrupted	R – Rammed (crushing of the physis)

with closed reduction and splintage. The prognosis for both these types of injuries is excellent.

Type III and IV fractures are intra-articular fractures and should be managed as such with anatomical reduction and stable internal fixation to maintain blood supply and joint congruity. These injuries, even with a good reduction carry a significant risk of growth disturbance.

Type V injuries carry the worst prognosis and commonly affect the lower extremities. The diagnosis is often made in retrospect once a bone growth abnormality is identified. Fortunately, these fractures are rare. These are usually managed by casting and keeping the patient nonweight-bearing.

Complications

Most physeal injuries heal without complications. A thorough understanding of growth plate anatomy and function can optimise patient outcomes. The major complication that can occur is growth arrest. This can have devastating effects on function, comfort, cosmetic appearance and quality of life. Children should be followed up for long enough to ensure growth disturbance has not occurred.

Further reading

Dodwell ER, Kelley SP. Physeal fractures: basic science, assessment and acute management. Orthop Trauma 2011; 25:377–391.

Perron A, Miller M, Brady M. Orthopedic pitfalls in the emergency department: Pediatric growth plate injuries. Am J Emerg Med 2002; 20:50–54.

Salter RB, Harris WR. Injuries involving the epiphyseal plate. J Bone Joint Surg Am 1963; 45:587–622.

Related topics of interest

- Topic 71 Paediatric distal tibial and ankle fractures
- Topic 74 Paediatric fractures – nonaccidental injury
- Topic 75 Paediatric humeral condylar fractures

78 Paediatric supracondylar humeral fractures

Key points

- Paediatric supracondylar fractures are a relatively common injury comprising a large proportion of paediatric fractures
- Neurovascular injury is associated with the more severe variants and must be identified, documented and managed in a timely fashion
- Restoration of alignment, rotation and reduction of angular deformity influences functional outcome

Epidemiology

Paediatric supracondylar fractures account for up to 65% of all paediatric fractures and tend to occur in children between the ages of 5 and 7 years, with an equal incidence between boys and girls.

Pathophysiology

Characteristically, the child falls on to an extended arm, frequently on a trampoline or similar. The resultant injury usually arises from a mechanism of extension with axial loading. At around 6–7 years of age, increased laxity of the ligaments about the elbow is common. Nerves at risk of damage include the anterior interosseous branch of the median nerve, the posterior interosseous branch of the radial nerve and the ulnar nerve, in decreasing order of frequency. Ulnar nerve injury is usually associated with rarer, flexion-type injuries. In most cases any neuropraxia will recover without intervention. Vascular injury is rare with an incidence in the order of 1%.

Clinical assessment

A thorough history should be taken which includes the circumstances and timing of injury and any subjective neurological disturbances. Examine for associated injuries such as an ipsilateral distal radius fracture. It is vital to assess and document neurological status. In a child typically this involves checking the 'OK' sign for anterior interosseous nerve function, crossing index and middle fingers for the ulnar nerve function and 'thumbs up' for posterior interosseous nerve. The radial pulse and capillary refill time of the fingers should then be checked. A cold, pale, pulseless hand is a surgical emergency and prompt reduction and stabilisation are mandatory. If perfusion is not restored, exploration in conjunction with vascular or plastic surgeons is required. A warm, pink pulseless hand may be due to vasospasm but should be discussed urgently with vascular or plastic surgeons.

Investigations

Orthogonal radiographs of the elbow required to classify the fracture and plan its management. In subtle injuries, a fat pad sign may be seen on the lateral radiographs, suggestive of an acute fracture around the elbow. The anterior humeral line should intersect the middle third of the capitellum, so if it crosses, it more anteriorly some posterior angulation of the fragment is present. Baumann's humeral-capitellar angle, measured between the line perpendicular to the long axis of the humeral shaft and the physis of the lateral condyle on the anteroposterior (AP) radiograph, should be between 15–20° (**Figure 78.1**). A deviation of 5° or less from that of the uninjured side is acceptable.

Classification

Classification is most commonly by Gartland's system as modified by Wilkins:
- 1 – undisplaced fracture
- 2a – displaced fracture, posterior cortex intact, no rotational deformity
- 2b – displaced fracture, posterior cortex intact with rotational deformity or fragment translation

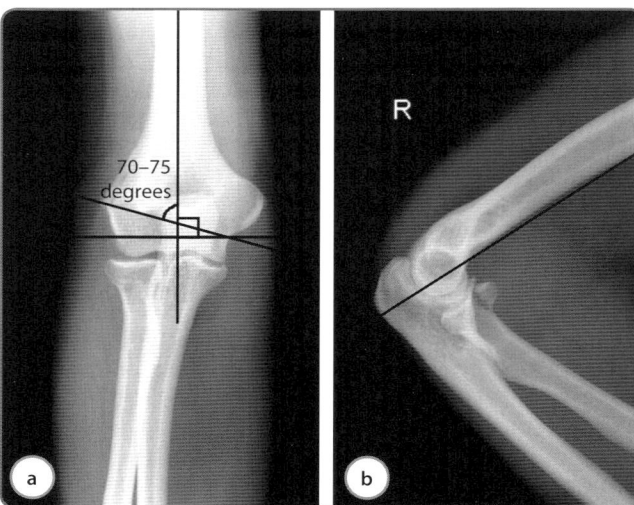

Figure 78.1 AP and lateral radiographs showing (a) Baumann's angle and (b) anterior humeral line.

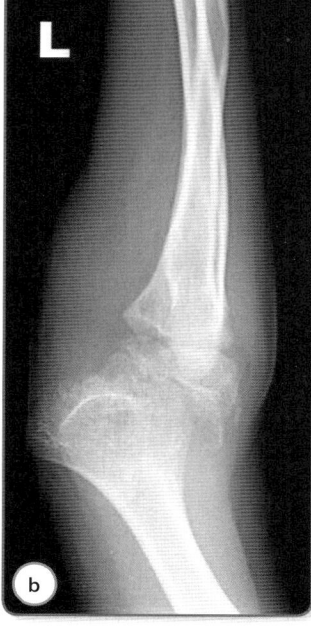

Figure 78.2 Flexion type supracondylar fracture. (a) AP radiograph and (b) lateral radiograph.

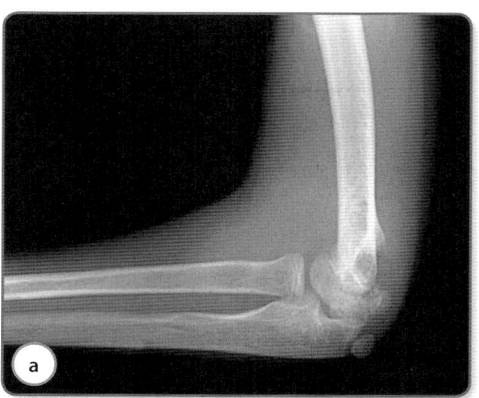

- 3 – displaced fracture with no meaningful cortical contact (**Figure 78.3**)

Around 2% of supracondylar humeral fractures are flexion-type injuries (**Figure 78.2**) and hence not classifiable by this system.

Treatment

Nonoperative management

Gartland 1 and 2a fractures can usually be managed in an above-elbow cast with the elbow flexed to <90° for 3–4 weeks. Check

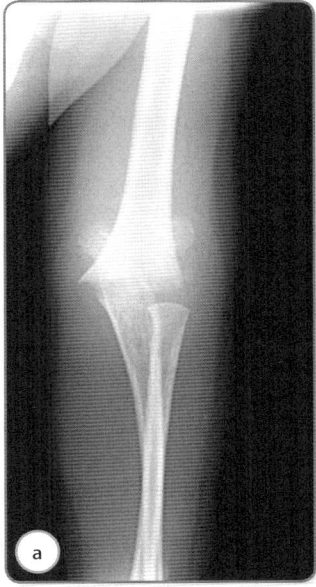
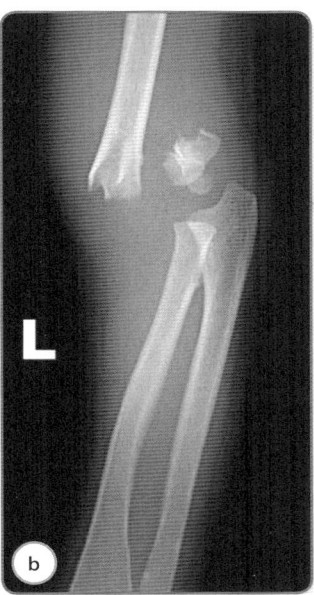

Figure 78.3 (a) AP and (b) lateral radiographs showing a Gartland 3 supracondylar humeral fracture.

radiographs are necessary at 5–7 days to verify there has been no further displacement.

Operative management

Gartland 2b and 3 fractures are usually managed operatively. Surgery should ideally be on the day of admission but overnight operating is mandated only by neurovascular deficit.

Surgical technique consists of use of a tourniquet, arm table and image intensifier. Initial reduction is attempted closed with flexion and pronation of the forearm. Once reduction has been achieved, stabilisation of the fracture with 2 mm K-wires is performed. This may be achieved using a lateral divergent or a bi-cortical crossed-wire technique (**Figure 78.4**). If using crossed wires, care must be taken to avoid ulnar nerve injury and dissection to bone is advisable to ensure this is avoided. Exploration of the brachial artery is not necessary if the hand is well perfused, whether or not a radial pulse is palpable. After fixation, the limb should be placed in

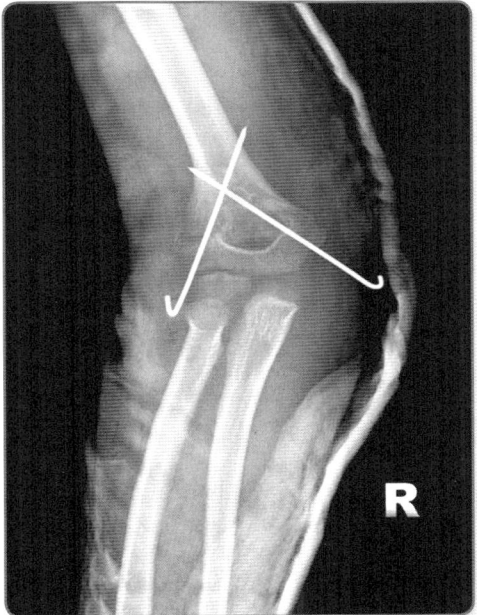

Figure 78.4 Bicortical crossed K-wire fixation of a supracondylar fracture.

a bivalved above elbow plaster. Immediate postoperative review and documentation of neurovascular status should be performed in the recovery room and hourly neurovascular observations made thereafter.

Follow-up

Check radiographs should be performed between days 4–10 postoperatively to ensure that there is no further displacement. Wires should be removed at 3–4 weeks and routine long-term follow-up is not necessary.

Complications
Immediate

- Neurovascular injury – any perfusion problem should be discussed with the regional vascular team. Nerve palsies tend to resolve spontaneously If a nerve injury is identified on open reduction, the nerve ends should be tagged intraoperatively and the patient referred to a nerve injury unit
- Compartment syndrome – any suspicion should prompt urgent fasciotomies of the forearm. Patients should be monitored for up to 24 hours postoperatively for development of compartment syndrome

Early

- Pin migration – this occurs in around 2% of cases and may require closer radiological surveillance
- Infection – pin site infections can occur and usually resolve with a course of oral antibiotics

Late

- Stiffness – this is relatively rare and usually settles after 3–6 months
- Malunion – 30% of supracondylar fractures have been associated with a delayed cubitus varus 'gunstock' deformity. This results from medial angulation, posteromedial rotation, medial communition and osteonecrosis or delayed growth of the medial condyle. These deformities tend to be cosmetic and without functional impact. Cubitus valgus is a rare, associated more with lateral condylar fractures. Both of these deformities are associated with failure of the initial attempt at anatomical reduction

Further reading

Abzug JM, Herman MJ. Management of supracondylar humerus fractures in children: current concepts. J Am Acad Orthop Surg 2012; 20:69–77.

Babal JC, Mehlman CT, Klein G. Nerve injuries associated with pediatric supracondylar humeral fractures: A meta-analysis. J Pediatr Orthop 2010; 30:253–263.

Choi PD, Melikian R, Skaggs DL. Risk factors for vascular repair and compartment syndrome in the pulseless supracondylar humerus fracture in children. J Pediatr Orthop 2010 30:50–56.

Omid R, Choi PD, Skaggs DL. Supracondylar humeral fractures in children. J Bone Joint Surg 2008; 90:1121–1132.

Related topics of interest

- *Topic 73* Paediatric forearm fractures
- *Topic 75* Paediatric humeral condylar fractures
- *Topic 76* Paediatric humeral fractures

79 Paediatric tibial fractures

Key points
- Tibial fractures are a very common injury in children, with a wide range of severity
- Most can be treated by immobilisation alone
- Associated swelling can be severe and a high index of suspicion of compartment syndrome is required

Epidemiology
Tibial fractures are the third most commonly occurring paediatric fracture, with a median age of 8 years at time of injury. 70% are isolated injuries, with 50–70% overall occurring in the distal third of the tibia.

Pathophysiology
Tibial injuries have different pathophysiologies, based on which anatomical region is affected:
- Tibial eminence fractures are rare and a consequence of avulsion of the bony attachment of the anterior cruciate ligament (ACL). As with adult ACL injuries, they usually occur in hyperextension and may be associated with meniscal, collateral ligament or osteochondral injuries
- Avulsion fractures of the tibial tubercle are associated with a Salter–Harris type III proximal tibial physeal fracture and should be distinguished from Osgood–Schlatter disease, where there is no physeal involvement. These fractures are more common in boys than girls and have peak incidence between 12–15 years of age. The mechanism of injury is typically forced passive flexion of the knee during active extension
- Tibial epiphyseal injuries are a rare but significant injury with risk of associated vascular injury. They usually occur as a result of a high-energy hyperextension of the knee in combination with a varus or valgus force. The tibial metaphysis usually displaces posteriorly, hence the risk to the popliteal artery. Salter–Harris type II injuries predominate (>40%), usually occurring in the adolescent age group
- Proximal tibial metaphyseal injuries tend to occur with a low-energy valgus force in patients between 3–6 years of age and are associated with a valgus deformity, termed a Cozen fracture
- Diaphyseal tibial fractures are the most common fractures seen in children:
  - A toddler's fracture is an undisplaced spiral or oblique fracture in a child <3 years of age, usually resulting from a rotational mechanism
  - Higher energy mechanisms can cause concomitant fibula fractures as well as tibial shaft fractures. Despite the inherent bony instability, angulation is reduced by the tough periosteum
  - Nonaccidental injury must be considered in children who are not yet walking and any concerns should be discussed with the appropriate safeguarding team

Clinical features
Pain, limp, deformity, swelling, bruising and a reluctance to bear weight are all associated with tibial fractures. More proximal injuries may cause knee swelling and in a tibial tubercle avulsion there may be an associated extensor lag or inability to straighten the leg. Disproportionate pain and more severe swelling suggest an associated vascular injury.

Investigations
Orthogonal views of the tibia, including knee and ankle, should be performed. CT can help diagnose or classify more complex fractures and plan their management, especially if intra-articular extension is suspected. Its angiographic variant may be required if vascular injury is suspected, but the case should be discussed with vascular surgeons

prior to this. MRI is indicated if suspicious of associated soft tissue injuries.

Classification

- Tibial eminence – Meyers and McKeever
  - I – Undisplaced
  - II – Minimally displaced, intact posterior hinge
  - III – Completely displaced
- Tibial tubercle – Ogden
  - I – Fracture of secondary ossification centre, near patella tendon insertion
  - II – Fracture which extends from proximal to the junction of the primary ossification centre
  - III – Fracture extending posteriorly to cross the primary ossification centre
- Tibial epiphysis and metaphysis – Salter–Harris

Treatment

Tibial eminence

- Nonoperative – suitable for type I and reducible type II fractures, immobilisation in extension is advocated by some surgeons. It has been argued, however, that immobilising the leg in extension, may put high stresses on the ACL and therefore encourage displacement
- Operative – for irreducible type II and type III fractures, arthroscopic or open reduction and internal fixation (ORIF) is performed, usually via a sub-meniscal approach

Tibial tubercle

- Nonoperative – for types I and II injuries, long leg immobilisation in extension for 4–6 weeks can be followed with targeted rehabilitation
- Operative management – reduction and fixation can be performed minimally invasively or by conventional open techniques, via either an anterior or lateral parapatellar approach

Tibial epiphysis and metaphysis

- Nonoperative – Salter–Harris I and II fractures can be managed in long leg immobilisation with slight flexion for 4–6 weeks, with progressive weight-bearing via Sarmiento cast if necessary
- Operative – in displaced fractures, anatomical reduction and fixation should be followed with a period of 4–6 weeks of immobilisation

Tibial diaphysis

- Nonoperative – suitable for the majority of diaphyseal fractures, a long-leg cast is applied in slight flexion with the foot plantar-flexed. An acceptable position offers at least 50% apposition, <1 cm of shortening and up to 10° angulation in the sagittal and 5° in the coronal plane. Concomitant fibular fracture carries a higher risk of valgus deformity due to the action of the long flexors of the leg. Close radiological surveillance is necessary to ensure reduction is maintained
- Operative – fixation is rare in these fractures but may be indicated in open or grossly unstable fractures or those with associated neurovascular injury. The indication will usually determine whether fixation is by ORIF or external fixation.

Complications

Immediate

- Neurovascular injury and compartment syndrome
- Soft tissue compromise

Early

- Infection in open fractures

Late

- Malunion
- Nonunion
- Leg length discrepancy due to physeal disruption and growth arrest

Further reading

Egol K, Koval KJ, Zuckerman J. Pediatric tibia and fibula. Handbook of fractures, 5th edn Netherlands: Wolters Kluwer; 2014.

Flynn JM, Sarwark JF, Waters PM, et al. The operative management of pediatric fractures of the lower extremity. J Bone Joint Surg Am 2002; 84:2288–2300.

Related topics of interest

- *Topic 84* Principles of nonoperative management of fractures
- *Topic 85* Principles of operative management of fractures

80 Pathological fractures

Key points

- Pathological fractures arise from disordered architecture or homeostasis of bone, and may result from significantly lower energy injuries
- After fragility fractures, the most common pathological fractures are those through metastatic deposits from primary malignancies of other organs
- Recognition of impending fracture, tumour type and staging, prognosis and performance status are all considerations in the management of pathological fractures
- The ideal fixation strategy permits weight-bearing, mobilization and optimal care and nursing
- A multidisciplinary approach is vital

Epidemiology

Breast, prostate, lung, thyroid, and kidney cancers account for 80% of all skeletal metastases. Age-adjusted incidence of fracture is 31.6 per 1000 person-years in patients with prostate cancer, versus 22.1 per 1000 person-years in those without cancer. A large UK study of skeletal complications of breast cancer revealed an incidence of pathological fractures as high as 34%.

Pathophysiology

In normal physiological conditions, bone resorption and bone formation are balanced by the actions of osteoclasts, osteoblasts and haematopoietic cells, mediated through immunomodulators, hormones and local bone-derived growth factors. In metastatic disease, this process is disrupted and results in osteolytic or osteoblastic activity at the site of the metastasis.

Breast cancers tend to exhibit osteoclastic, resorptive properties, as opposed to the osteoblastic characteristics of prostatic metastases. Several osteolytic factors have been implicated in breast cancer metastasis, including receptor activator of nuclear factor kappa-B ligand (RANKL). Understanding of the role of RANKL in the pathogenesis of breast cancer resulted in the development of denosumab, an anti-RANKL monoclonal antibody which inhibits osteoclast activity thereby suppressing bone resorption.

Clinical assessment

History

Typically, patients present with history of bone pain, usually at night and on bearing weight. Manifestations of the primary tumour may help with diagnosis – changes in bowel habit, appetite, constitution or new lumps may suggest an origin. In established cancers, it is important to know if the patient has had radiotherapy and chemotherapy treatments.

Physical examination

A conventional orthopaedic assessment should be made of the relevant limb, noting any skin changes which may be associated with radiotherapy or slow-healing wounds subsequent to chemotherapy. If spinal metastases are suspected, neurological assessment should be performed and recorded. Finally, systematic examination should be performed for problems such as lymphadenopathy and ascites.

Investigations

Laboratory tests

All patients should have full blood count, urea and electrolytes, liver function test and bone profile tests performed as a minimum. Coagulation testing should also be performed. Abnormalities in differential cell counts may suggest haematological malignancy. Protein and urine electrophoresis is vital in multiple myeloma. The level of serum alkaline phosphatase reflects the degree of bony turnover in the process. In cases of unknown primary disease, measurement of tumour markers may be helpful.

Imaging

Plain radiographs provide information on the extent of the tumour, whether it exhibits malignant features and the degree of involvement of surrounding soft tissue. In multiple myeloma, skeletal surveys can be useful, with hallmarks of multiple well-circumscribed 'punched out' lytic lesions (pepperpot skull) and endosteal scalloping. CT of chest, abdomen and pelvis can be used to stage disease and help identify carcinomas of unknown origin. Bone scintography or, more recently, PET-CT may help detect further skeletal deposits. MRI should be used to evaluate potential spinal metastases.

Biopsy

The potential exists to provide histological diagnosis, but this should be discussed with the oncology team before surgery. Ideally, reamings obtained during intramedullary nailing should not be used to diagnose the primary carcinoma.

Treatment

Management of metastatic bone disease can be broadly grouped into two strategies – prophylactic fixation of bones with metastatic lesions which are at risk of impending fracture, and stabilisation or reconstruction of such bones where fracture has already occurred. In majority of the cases, this is without curative intent and should be aimed at relieving pain, restoring functional activity and improving quality of life. Renal metastases are usually highly vascular and should be embolized prior to surgery where possible. Fixation should allow the patient unrestricted weight-bearing and adjuncts such as polymethylmethacrylate (PMMA) cement should be considered to increase the stability of the construct and help ensure its time to failure will exceed the life expectancy of the patient.

In cases of impending pathological fractures, Mirel's criteria can inform the decision whether to stabilise the fracture (Table 80.1). The risk of pathological fracture at 6 months is high as the Mirels' score rises above 7. In the original description, lesions with a score <6 were thought to be safe to be treated by radiation and lesions scoring >8 required skeletal stabilisation. Harrington described four indications for fixation of the proximal femur: cortical bone destruction >50%; metastatic deposit >2.5 cm; pathological fracture involving the lesser trochanter; pain on bearing weight.

Fixation options

- Endoprosthetic replacement should be considered for intra-articular, uncontained metastatic deposit of the proximal humerus
- Proximal humeral plating or nailing augmented by PMMA should be considered for well-contained metastatic deposits in the proximal humerus
- Total elbow arthroplasty should be considered for intra-articular, uncontained lesion of the distal humerus
- Single- or double-plating with PMMA should be considered for extra-articular, well-contained metastatic lesions of the distal humerus
- Humeral and femoral diaphyseal fractures are generally treated by intramedullary nailing
- Consider endoprosthetic reconstruction for solitary metastatic deposits around the subtrochanteric region
- Distal femoral endoprosthetic reconstruction should be considered for

Table 80.1 Mirel's criteria for prediction of pathological fracture risk at 6 months

Score	Site	Nature of metastatic deposit	Size of metastatic deposit relative to width of the bone	Pain
1	Upper limb	Blastic	<1/3	Mild
2	Lower limb	Mixed	1/3 to 2/3	Moderate
3	Pertrochanteric	Lytic	>2/3	Functional

intra-articular, unconfined metastatic lesions of the distal femur
- When dual-modality fixation is used, there should be sufficient overlap of the two constructs to prevent any subsequent fractures at the stress riser
- Intercalary prosthesis following segmental resection of the diaphysis of the tibia should be considered for solitary diaphyseal metastases

Complications

Immediate
Fat embolism syndrome is seen after reaming of the medullary canal of the long bones. Emboli occlude pulmonary and cerebral vasculature, causing fatal cardiopulmonary complications. Venting the femur may reduce the risk of this.

Early
In addition to the generally immunocompromised state of many of these patients, the use of radiation in the perioperative period is associated with higher risk of wound-healing complications.

Late
Complications are usually implant-related – dislocation of endoprostheses and failure of internal fixation (usually due to disease progression) are usually associated with high morbidity. Radiotherapy use can result in the development of avascular necrosis of the articular surfaces of the long bones.

Further reading

Ahlborg HG, Nguyen ND, Center JR, Eisman JA, Nguyen TV. Incidence and risk factors for low trauma fractures in men with prostate cancer. Bone 2008; 43:556–560.

Cheung FH. The practicing orthopaedic surgeon's guide to managing long bone metastases. Orthop Clin North Am 2014; 45:109–119.

Eastley N, Newey M, Ashford RU. Skeletal metastases – the role of the orthopaedic and spinal surgeon. Surg Oncol 2012; 21:216–22.

Melton LJ, Hartmann LC, Achenbach SJ, et al. Fracture risk in women with breast cancer: a population based study. J Bone Miner Res 2012; 27:1196–1205.

Plunkett TA, Smith P, Rubens RD. Risk of complications from bone metastases in breast cancer. Eur J Cancer 2000; 36:476–482.

Scolaro JA, Lackman RD. Surgical management of metastatic long bone fractures: Principles and Techniques. J Am Acad Orthop Surg 2014; 22:90–100.

Steeg PS, Theodorescu D. Metastasis: a therapeutic target for cancer. Nat Clin Pract Oncol 2008; 5:206–219.

Related topics of interest

- Topic 9 Bone structure and physiology
- Topic 35 Fracture healing

Pelvis – acetabular fractures

Key points

- Acetabular fractures represent an injury distinct from pelvic ring fractures
- They have a bimodal distribution, with high-energy fractures occurring in young patients and lower energy fractures in older patients with poor bone density
- The key prognostic factor is the degree of displacement of the intra-articular fragments
- Management strategies range from reduced weight-bearing in the elderly to extensive reconstruction combined with total hip arthroplasty (THA) in younger patients

Epidemiology

Fractures of the acetabulum account for a low percentage of all fractures but consume a disproportionate amount of healthcare resources. They occur predominantly in the fourth or fifth decade of life, overwhelmingly in association with road traffic collisions. In this young, high-energy population, more men than women are injured.

A second peak of injury is seen in the elderly, where mechanisms are more innocuous and varied.

Pathophysiology

In high-energy injuries, the fracture is sustained by directional loading, with the fracture personality often indicating the origin of the force. Posterior wall fractures, for example, may be associated with vehicular collision and force transmission up the femora in a seated position, sometimes also dislocating the hip posteriorly. By contrast, if sustained in a fall onto the feet from height, a dome fracture is more likely.

Clinical assessment

The patient may complain of hip pain and, in the higher-energy group, may well have other distracting injuries or a reduced level of consciousness. Abnormal hip posture may suggest an associated dislocation, reported in up to 39% of acetabular fractures. Although acetabular fractures are distinct from pelvic ring fractures, they can and do co-exist and so a thorough approach to the polytraumatised patient must be followed. Close attention to haemodynamic stability and genitourinary or rectal injury is essential. Neurological status must be assessed and documented – sciatic nerve palsy is common but femoral nerve palsy is rarely seen. Soft tissues are commonly injured, with a relatively high rate of de-gloving injuries reported. Associated injuries are reported in more than half of acetabular fractures with rates of chest injury up to 18% and spinal injury 4%. It is therefore vital that the management of these patients anticipates secondary problems, identifies associated injuries early and facilitates secondary transfer within the trauma network if required.

Investigations

Traditionally, Judet radiographs were obtained to clearly demonstrate the anterior and posterior walls of the acetabulum using iliac and obturator oblique beams. In modern practice, many patients will undergo CT 'traumagram' as part of their initial assessment and so reformats of these images can be used, with three-dimensional reconstructions, to give a detailed picture of the often complex fracture patterns. Be sure to check for femoral head and neck fracture.

Classification

A number of classifications exist but that in most common usage probably remains the Letournel–Judet system (**Table 81.1**), which describes five elementary and five associated fracture patterns. While this is a useful system, it bears observation that many fractures are more complex than the

Table 81.1 The Letournel–Judet classification of acetabular fractures

Elementary fracture patterns				
Posterior wall	Posterior column	Anterior wall	Anterior column	Transverse
Associated fracture patterns				
T-shaped	Posterior wall and column	Transverse with posterior wall	Anterior wall or column with posterior hemitransverse	Both columns

elementary types and, once cross-sectional imaging is available, classification is often by the closest approximation to the pattern rather than an exact match.

Treatment

The ultimate goal is to achieve a stable, congruent hip with pain-free function. Nonoperative or operative methods may be preferable depending on the fracture pattern and patient factors. Displacement >2 mm is likely to lead to post-traumatic arthritis necessitating early arthroplasty.

Nonoperative

The fundamental tenet of nonoperative management is that there must be a stable hip, with an intact femoral head articulating with and contained by a congruent acetabulum. Patients with such fractures may be managed by reduced weight-bearing for 6–12 weeks with appropriate venous thromboembolism (VTE) prophylaxis. In older patients, the acceptance of displacement is likely to be higher due to the high morbidity of surgery. This strategy requires intensive follow-up and the team must be alert to further displacement on serial radiographs.

Operative

Surgery is necessary when congruence is lost or when the fracture pattern is inherently unstable. This stability can be assessed by considering where loading will occur during weight-bearing – a posterior wall and posterior column pattern, e.g. offers little buttress to the femoral head during loading and so is unlikely to be stable. Surgery is also mandated by an irreducible hip dislocation or by a new-onset nerve palsy after closed reduction.

Definitive fixation is complex surgery with difficult and high-morbidity approaches. In a patient where surgery may be delayed by physiological compromise, skeletal traction offers an easy temporizing measure to incorporate into damage control surgical resuscitation. For definitive fixation, the Kocher–Langenbeck and ilioinguinal approaches offer single-column access to posterior and anterior columns, respectively. Extensile approaches such as the extended iliofemoral and triradiate are associated with very high morbidity and more rarely used. Modern surgical tactics often hinge on a single-column approach to address the more displaced fracture, relying on indirect reduction of the less displaced one.

Early rehabilitation is a key to success, but must be balanced with appropriate protection of the fixation construct. A knee brace can prevent hip flexion and hence loading of posterior fixation.

Predictors of successful outcome are the quality of reduction, surgeon experience and a delay of <3 weeks between injury and surgery. A failure rate of 10% at 2 years has been reported, and these patients will derive less satisfaction from their subsequent THA than matched controls undergoing THA for osteoarthritis.

Complications

Immediate

- Hip dislocation
- Nerve injury
- Vascular injury

Early

- Tissue necrosis from de-gloving injuries
- Venous thromboembolism

- Vascular injury from surgery
- Nerve injury from surgery
- Infection
- Failure of fixation and loss of reduction

Late
- Malunion and post-traumatic arthritis
- Nonunion
- Heterotopic ossification

Further reading

Letournel E, Judet R. Fractures of the Acetabulum, 2nd edn. Berlin: Springer, 1993.

McMaster J, Powell J. Acetabular fractures. Current Orthop 2005; 19:140–154.

Related topics of interest

- *Topic 17* Damage control orthopaedics and trauma physiology
- *Topic 82* Pelvis – pelvic ring fractures

82 Pelvis – pelvic ring fractures

Key points

- Pelvic injuries can be severe and rapidly life-threatening
- It is critical to distinguish between stable and unstable injuries
- Management is aimed firstly at gaining or maintaining haemodynamic control, then reconstruction of the pelvis
- Early involvement of colorectal and urological surgeons is mandatory, especially in patients with open fractures of the pelvis
- Patients should be counselled about chronic pain and sexual dysfunction, even after successful reconstruction of the pelvic ring

Epidemiology

Estimates from the United States show an incidence of 0.82 per 100,000 of unstable pelvic fracture between 2000–2009. The data also demonstrated in-hospital mortality of 8.3% for closed fractures and 21.3% for open fractures. It is estimated that between 5–15% of injuries will have genitourinary involvement. In the UK, the incidence of pelvic ring injuries was reported as 8% in those patients recorded in Trauma Audit Research Network database between 1989–2001 with a 3-month cumulative mortality rate of 14.2% for the same period. A similar epidemiological study from Asia reports an incidence of pelvic fractures 17.17 to 19.42 per 100,000 for the period 2000–2011. German Trauma Registry figures quote an incidence of 37/100,000 for this group of fractures.

Pathophysiology

Disruption of the pelvic ring tends to occur in two places, as it is hard to disrupt an annular structure without two points of deformation. The visceral contents of the pelvis and the plexus of relatively friable veins closely associated with the bony structures renders these patients susceptible to catastrophic vascular injury. The pattern of pelvic injury is relatively predictable from the deforming force.

Clinical assessment

History

The key points from the history pertain to mechanism, associated injuries and any subjective neurological deficits the patient may have noted. Ensure the environment in which the injury was sustained is documented, noting risks of contamination, prolonged periods of entrapment and similar.

Physical examination

Note the position and symmetry of the lower extremities, with any associated shortening and rotation of the leg. This may indicate concomitant femoral neck fractures or dislocation of the hip. A thorough examination of the skin is vital to look for open wounds, contusion, or degloving with particular attention to the perineum. Urethral, scrotal, vaginal, rectal, and prostatic examinations are required. A thorough neurological examination should be performed.

'Springing' the pelvis offers little clinical utility and may disrupt the valuable 'first clot', in many cases the result of nearly fully expended clotting products. Missed injury rates of up to 20% have been reported in pelvic injury, and with the widespread availability of CT scanning there should be an extremely low threshold for this investigation.

Investigations

Plain radiograph

The role of plain radiograph of the pelvis is diminishing with the advent of management of these injuries in major trauma centres, where the majority of the patients are investigated by trauma CT. Plain anteroposterior radiographs of the pelvis can demonstrate disruption of the pelvic ring, with fractures seen typically at two points in the ring; fractures in the elderly being an exception. This population can sustain isolated rami or sacral fractures due to minor trauma and osteoporosis.

Computed tomography

This is the gold standard in the evaluation of pelvic ring fractures. It helps identify associated acetabular injuries, retroperitoneal haemorrhage and the source of bleeding (if using contrast). It also offers the opportunity for interventional radiology in certain centres.

Classification

The most commonly used classification is that of Young and Burgess (**Table 82.1**). The direction of force vector to the pelvic ring is believed to cause a specific injury pattern – anteroposterior compression (APC), lateral compression (LC) and vertical shear (VS). The fourth type, complex injury pattern, is a combination of any of the three primary patterns.

The higher-grade LC and APC injuries are associated with haemorrhage, bladder, urethral and rectal injuries. Depending on the magnitude of force, VS injuries can cause damage to the small and large intestine in the pelvic brim.

Treatment

Initial management

Haemodynamic instability should be managed by use of a massive transfusion protocol, as the volume of blood loss can be anticipated to be large. Early administration of intravenous tranexamic acid has shown to reduce the risk of death in bleeding trauma patients and its routine use is now advocated in all the major trauma centres.

Closing the pelvic ring with a binder, which may be as simple as a folded sheet, reduces the volume of the pelvis. Packing offers a rapid means of haemorrhage control. External fixation has a place in temporising management, but as pelvic surgery services become more available and more safety data emerges suggesting binders can remain in place for longer, more units are choosing to keep patients in binders until fixation.

BOAST 3 guidelines advocate a low index of suspicion of urethral injury and hence to perform a cystourethrogram. All visceral injuries mandate involvement of the appropriate surgical teams.

Table 82.1 Young and Burgess classification

	Direction of vector of force	Grade 1	Grade 2	Grade 3
APC	AP-directed force	<2.5 cm widening of pubic symphysis. No clinical/radiological signs of posterior instability	>2.5 cm widening of pubic symphysis. STL, SSL and ASIL disrupted, PSIL intact	Complete hemipelvis separation. Anterior and posterior sacral ligaments disrupted
LC	Laterally based and directed medially	Transverse fracture of the rami. Ipsilateral sacral compression fracture	LC1 + Crescent (Iliac wing, ipsilateral) fracture	LC2 + contralateral APC3 type injury of the hemipelvis
VS	Axially loaded force over one or both hemipelvis lateral to the midline	Vertical displacement of the hemiplevis, sacrum is driven caudally relative to the iliac wing		

Abbreviations: APS, anteroposterior compression; lateral compression, LC; vertical shear, STL, sacrotuberous ligament; SPL, sacrospinous ligament; ASIL, anterior sacroiliac ligament; PSIL, posterior sacroiliac ligament; STL and SPL, pelvic floor ligaments.

Definitive management

Anteroposterior compression injuries

Anteroposterior compression type 1 injuries are generally managed nonoperatively, with examination under anaesthesia (EUA) used to demonstrate stability if required. APC2 injuries usually require anterior stabilisation of the pelvic ring. Routine stabilisation of the posterior ring is not mandatory – following anterior stabilisation, if dynamic stress views demonstrate sagittal plane instability then posterior fixation with an ilio-sacral screw is indicated. In case of APC3 injuries, both anterior and posterior fixation is recommended.

Lateral compression injuries

Lateral compression type 1 injuries are treated nonoperatively in majority of the cases. In patients with LC1 injury who experience serve pain on protected weight bearing, EUA is required. If EUA demonstrates sagittal plane instability (>1 cm displacement), both anterior and posterior fixation is recommended. LC2 and LC3 injuries are generally managed surgically.

Vertical shear injuries

Surgical fixation is indicated in all VS injuries, with anatomic reduction and fixation of the posterior pelvic ring being the primary goal. In order to neutralise the anterior forces of displacement, it is mandatory to use concomitant anterior fixation. Stabilisation of the posterior pelvic ring is achieved by ilio-sacral screws, sacral plating and/or spinopelvic fixation.

Complications

Immediate
- Haemorrhage

Early
- VTE
- Infection
- Neurological injury (especially L5 and S1 roots)

Late
- Pain
- Depression
- Dyspareunia and erectile dysfunction

Further reading

Alton TB, Gee AO. Young and Burgess classification of pelvic ring injuries. Clin Orthop Relat Res 2014; 472:2338–2342.

Langford JR, Burgess AR, Liporace FA, Haidukewych GJ. Pelvic fractures: part 2. Contemporary indications and techniques for definitive surgical managment. J Am Acad Orthop Surg 2013; 21:458–468.

Langford JR, Burgess AR, Liporace FA, Haidukewych GJ. Pelvic Fractures: Part 1. Evaluation, classification and resuscitation. J Am Acad Orthop Surg 2013; 21:448–457.

Mauffrey C, Cuellar DO 3rd, Pieracci F, et al. Strategies for the management of haemorrhage following pelvic fractures and associated trauma-induced coagulopathy. Bone Joint J 2014; 96B:1143–1154.

Stahel PF, Mauffrey C, Smith WR, McKean J, et al. External fixation for acute pelvic ring injuries: Decision making and technical options. J Trauma Acute Care Surg 2013; 75:882–887.

Yoshihara H. Demographic epidemiology of unstable pelvic fracture in the United States from 2000 to 2009: Trends and in-hospital mortality. J Trauma Acute Care Surg 2014; 76:380–385.

Related topics of interest

- *Topic 17* Damage control orthopaedics and trauma physiology
- *Topic 37* Guidelines in trauma
- *Topic 86* Resuscitation and massive transfusion

83 Peripheral nerve injury

Key points
- Thorough history-taking and assessment and documentation of sensory and motor function is paramount in managing peripheral nerve injury
- Epineural repair is appropriate in most situations
- Sensory recovery is often better than motor

Pathophysiology

Injury to peripheral nerves can occur through a variety of traumatic mechanisms, whether a laceration to the overlying limb, traction, compression, or contusion. It can be life-changing due to the variable and incomplete nature of nerve healing and possibility of permanent impairment. A peripheral nerve injury is characterised by specific changes at the site of injury, both proximally and distally. After a nerve transection following a laceration, degeneration occurs proximally to the nearest node of Ranvier, the gap junction between Schwann cells. The distal portion undergoes Wallerian degeneration, the anterograde degeneration of first the axon then the myelin sheath. This begins approximately 24 hours postinjury and is followed by macrophage infiltration to deal with the debris.

After this breakdown, there remain columns of Schwann cell nuclei and their basement membranes. These basement membranes form endoneural tubes, bands of Bunger, which guide regenerating axons to their targets. This regeneration occurs at a rate of 1 mm per day and can be monitored crudely by assessing for an advancing Tinel's sign.

Axonal regrowth occurs in response to neurotrophins such as nerve growth factor, epidermal growth factor and insulin-like growth factor, with axonal sprouts from the proximal cut end forming a growth cone. These must then enter the distal tract to regrow – only half the fibres produced will be pointing in the right direction.

Muscles innervated by the injured nerve will atrophy, with up to 70% of their substance lost by 2 months and death of fibres beginning to occur after 6 months. The optimal outcomes from surgical re-innervation will be gained if it occurs within 3 months of injury, but a viable re-innervation can usually be achieved at 1 year postinjury. Sharp transections, those closer to the motor end plate (i.e. more distal) and those occurring in younger patients have the best outcomes.

Classification

Classification is important in peripheral nerve injury, as the level and degree of injury determine treatment.

Seddon
- **Neuropraxia:** Anatomy of nerve is preserved and no Wallerian degeneration occurs. Full recovery is possible, but takes from weeks to months
- **Axonotmesis:** Axon damage within the nerve. Wallerian degeneration occurs. Recovery rate is 1 mm per day once healing begins. Fibrillations are present on electromotor testing. Complete recovery is possible without surgery if axonal regeneration is able to progress across the zone of injury
- **Neurotmesis:** Nerve is transected, with destruction of surrounding structures. Wallerian degeneration occurs. Surgical intervention is required to achieve best possible outcome.

Sunderland (modified by Mackinnon)
- **First-degree injury (neuropraxia):** Axons are in continuity but local conduction is impaired, amenable to nonoperative management
- **Second-degree injury (axonotmesis):** Some nerve fibres are disrupted but Schwann cell basal lamina intact. Can be managed nonoperatively, recovery usually within months. Progress can be monitored by advancing Tinel sign

- **Third-degree injury:** Perineurium and epineurium remains intact, but axon and endoneurium are damaged, with some areas of Schwann cell basal lamina disrupted. Treatment is usually nonoperative and recovery reasonable
- **Fourth-degree injury:** Loss of continuity of intraneural structures but epineurium remains intact. Scar blocks all regrowth, with little or no recovery. Operative treatment is required
- **Fifth-degree injury (neurotmesis):** The nerve is completely transected and no recovery is likely without operative management
- **Sixth-degree injury:** mixed pattern nerve injury with segmental damage

Recovery can be graded by the Medical Research Council (MRC) scale for both sensory and motor function.
- S0 (No recovery) insensate
- S1 Pain (deep)
- S1+ Pain (superficial)
- S2 Light touch
- S2+ Hyperaesthesia to light touch
- S3 2 point discrimination >15 mm
- S3+ 2 point discrimination 7–15 mm
- S4 (Complete recovery) 2 point discrimination 3–6 mm
- M0 No contraction
- M1 Perceptible contraction (e.g. twitch)
- M2 Contraction with gravity eliminated
- M3 Contraction against gravity
- M4 Contraction against resistance
- M5 Full contraction

Surgical management

Epineural repair represents the gold standard, and is commonly used for digital nerves. Advantages include a shorter operative duration, an atraumatic approach with no violation of intraneural contents and ease of surgery. The main disadvantage is the risk of mal-alignment of the fascicles.

Nerve grafting is the procedure of choice when a gap is present, using autograft where possible. It offers a biologic scaffold containing neutrophic factors and viable Schwann cells supporting axonal regeneration. Commonly used donor nerves include the sural nerve, lateral antebrachial cutaneous nerve, medial antebrachial cutaneous nerve and terminal sensory branch of the posterior interosseous nerve. Nerve conduits may also be used for short (<3 cm) gaps in noncritical, small diameter sensory nerves. Vein graft is commonly used for this.

Rehabilitation

Any primary repair must be protected by splintage in the first instance. Early mobilisation, sensory and motor re-education are usually led by occupational therapy or physiotherapy teams and are key drivers of favourable outcome. In nonoperative management of closed injuries, baseline nerve conduction studies should be sought. If no clinical or neurophysiological signs of recovery are seen at 12 weeks postinjury, surgical exploration may be indicated.

Further reading

Jabaley ME. Current concepts of nerve repair. Clin Plast Surg 1981; 8:33–44.

Maggi SP, Lowe JB III, Mackinnon SE. Pathophysiology of nerve injury. Clin Plast Surg 2003; 30:109–126.

Sunderland S. A classification of peripheral nerve injuries producing loss of function. Brain 1951; 74:491–516.

Related topics of interest

- *Topic 10* Brachial plexus injury
- *Topic 15* Complex regional pain syndrome

84 Principles of nonoperative management of fractures

Key points

- The aim of fracture management is the restoration of pain-free function
- Many fractures are managed nonoperatively with excellent results
- Both patient and fracture characteristics influence suitability for nonoperative management
- There is growing evidence comparing the outcome of nonoperative versus operative management of fractures

Pathophysiology

Bone is a specialised type of connective tissue whose material properties result from its composition. It can be classified anatomically (long or flat) or structurally (lamellar or woven). Woven bone is seen in early callus formation as well as immature and pathological bone. Composition of long bones is further subdivided into cortical and cancellous bone, which have differing properties. The overall material properties of bone also change throughout life; in childhood there is a higher proportion of cartilage explaining why it is more deformable than adult bone. It also has a relatively thicker periosteum, which plays a greater structural role. By comparison, adult bone is more rigid and hence liable to fracture than undergo plastic deformation. In disease states and old age, weaker bone may result in insufficiency fractures. An understanding of bone characteristics is essential for the nonoperative management of fractures.

A fracture is associated with a failure in the structural integrity of bone. Bone may fail under compression, tension or a rotational force. Several such forces may contribute to more complex fracture patterns. The material property of bone influences the type and location of fractures sustained from an injury. Fracture healing involves a complex set of events to restore injured bone to its pre-fracture condition.

A fracture, which is managed nonoperatively, will typically heal indirectly by callus formation. The theory linking the local environment of the fracture to the resultant outcome of the healing, in terms of the type of new tissue formed, was proposed by Stephan Perren in 1980. This theory helps differentiate direct and indirect healing (which is also termed primary and secondary healing). If the strain (or change in length as a proportion of original length) is very low (in a very stiff construct) then primary bone healing can occur. This needs <2% strain (absolute stability). If there is 2–10% strain (relative stability), then indirect, or secondary healing can occur. If there is a lot of movement at a fracture (>100%) then granulation tissue results and this is seen as a 'nonunion'. Absolute stability is achieved by rigid internal fixation. Having healed by callus formation, a fracture will then gradually remodel over months to years.

Both the mechanism of injury and patient specific variables, such as age, gender, co-morbidity and medication use influence fracture location and configuration.

Clinical features

A fracture is typically associated with pain and impairment of function immediately after injury. There may be a visible deformity, such as limb angulation, shortening or rotation along with swelling and bruising. An assessment of skin integrity, the state of the surrounding soft tissues and neurovascular status should be undertaken. The management of an open fracture, or fracture with associated neurovascular injury should follow national guidelines.

Investigations

Plain radiographs will demonstrate most fractures. Radiographs are two-dimensional representations of often complex three-dimensional structures and multiple views are necessary. A seemingly innocuous fracture in one plane may appear significant in another. Anteroposterior, lateral and oblique views are routine. Special views, such as scaphoid views, can reveals fractures not seen on standard views. 'Stress' views, such as weight-bearing, can add useful information about stability when deciding if a fracture is to be managed operatively or nonoperatively. CT scan or MRI can be used to further delineate a fracture and to investigate for a suspected fracture not visible on radiographs.

Radiographs may be repeated to check fracture position and for evidence of fracture healing at regular intervals.

Diagnosis

Fracture diagnosis is often straightforward. A clear mechanism of injury, such as a fall onto an outstretched hand, resulting in a painful, swollen and visibly deformed wrist guides the clinician to the likely diagnosis of a distal radius fracture. Radiographs confirm the clinical suspicion and should be assessed for:
- Intra-articular involvement
- Comminution
- Displacement (in length, translation or rotation)
- Evidence of additional injuries

Treatment

To successfully treat fractures nonoperatively requires: understanding of fracture mechanism and healing process, techniques of closed reduction and being skilled in the methods of stabilisation (typically, the use of plaster of Paris). Typically it will encompass:
- Reduction to regain satisfactory fracture position
- Immobilisation to allow healing by callus formation
- Rehabilitation to regain function

An undisplaced extra-articular distal radius fracture is often ideal for nonoperative management and could be placed straight into a splint or cast. A displaced extra-articular distal radius fracture requires further thought. Questions should include:
- Will the radiographic displacement result in a functional limitation left untreated?
- Is the fracture configuration stable or is it liable to further displacement?

Displaced adult wrist fractures are often manipulated into an improved position and immobilised with a plaster of Paris backslab in the emergency department. Post-manipulation radiographs are essential. Follow-up in an orthopaedic fracture clinic is usually at around 1 week and repeat radiographs are performed to ensure the fracture position has been maintained.

In instances where the fracture position is felt to be suboptimal, a further manipulation can be performed in the fracture clinic. A period of time handing the affected wrist from finger traps may be helpful prior to manipulation. Three-point fixation can be achieved with a well moulded cast afterwards.

In general, there is approximately a 2-week period after injury where a change from nonoperative management to operative fixation can be undertaken without additional difficulty arising from fracture healing.

Complications

Complications may relate to the healing of the fracture, such as nonunion, malunion or delayed union. This may result in a limitation of function or pain and stiffness. A surgical procedure, such as an osteotomy to improve the position of the bone may then be required.

Complications may also arise as a result of the nonoperative treatment of fractures. Immobilisation in cast may result in a deep vein thrombosis, which may be complicated by a pulmonary embolism. An improperly applied cast can cause pressure ulcers and muscle contracture.

Long periods of immobilisation will also result in joint stiffness may also increase an individuals' risk of developing a complicating chronic regional pain syndrome.

Further reading

Charnley J. The Closed Treatment of Common Fractures. Cambridge: Cambridge University Press, 1999.

Perren SM, Cordey J. The concept of interfragmentary strain. In: Uhthoff HK (Ed). Current Concepts of Internal Fixation of Fractures. Berlin: Springer, 1980:63–77.

Willett K, Keene DJ, Mistry D, et al. Close contact casting vs surgery for initial treatment of unstable ankle fractures in older adults: A randomized clinical trial. JAMA 2016; 316:1455–1463.

Related topics of interest

- Topic 9 Bone structure and physiology
- Topic 35 Fracture healing
- Topic 85 Principles of operative management of fractures

85 Principles of operative management of fractures

Key points
- Surgery should be considered if it will help restore function, and relieve pain better than available nonoperative treatments for fractures
- The nature of fixation dictates whether primary or secondary bone healing will occur
- Outcome is influenced by patient factors, fracture characteristics, the surgery performed and postoperative rehabilitation
- There is growing evidence examining the outcome of operative versus nonoperative management of fractures

Introduction
When considering surgical treatment, understanding the natural history of a fracture and the intention of an operative intervention is essential. Surgery should improve fracture alignment and stability whilst respecting soft tissues. Where both operative and nonoperative options exist, patients should be involved in the decision-making process. Patients with modifiable risk factors for complications, such as impaired wound and bone healing as a result of smoking, should be counselled accordingly.

Soft tissues
Soft tissues should be carefully assessed prior to surgery. Common assessment methods involve the use of the Tscherne or Gustillo and Anderson classification systems (for closed and open fractures respectively). Surgical fixation in the presence of swollen and bruised soft tissues may result in an over-tensioned closure, wound breakdown, metalwork exposure and infection. Delaying immediate fixation with a period of immobilisation and elevation prior to surgery gives the soft tissues a chance to settle and can reduce the risk of wound complications. When surgery is performed, the approach should, as far as possible, avoid the zone of soft tissue injury.

Surgical planning
Preoperative planning is essential to both execute successful surgery and pre-empt potential intraoperative difficulties. Broadly, fracture fixation can be internal or external, the former being intramedullary or extramedullary.

Concepts highlighted by the AO Foundation are centred around the way in which fractures heal; either by primary or secondary healing. A comprehension of how any metalwork involved in fracture healing will respond to the loads put through it is an essential part of the planning process. Consideration should be given to equipment positioning in the operating theatre. Image intensifier screens should be within easy view. Having imaging investigations visible on a large monitor in theatre can also be helpful. In fracture dislocations, review of prereduction films, if taken, may provide useful information about which structures may require fixation or stabilisation. Good knowledge of the operating equipment prior to surgery is essential and simulation training can form a key role in this.

Patient positioning
The patient should be placed in the centre of the operating room, especially when using clean air systems such as laminar flow. The intended surgical field should be easily exposed and positioned to allow easy use of image intensifier, if required, and access to instrument trays. Limb tourniquets should be positioned high enough that they will not interfere with the sterile field. Adjuncts such as wedges, sand bags and appendages such as arm tables can help with optimal positioning. Radiolucent operating tables can also help when image intensifier use is required.

Manipulation under anaesthetic

A manipulation under anaesthetic is often sufficient in the management of a clinically deformed but stable injury. Consideration of the mechanism of injury is helpful in fracture reduction as replicating the deformity may be required, such as with a 'bayonet' deformity of the distal radius. Often a sustained period of longitudinal traction with the aid of an assistant providing counter-traction is the basis for a provisional reduction. To maintain fracture reduction often requires skilled plastering techniques; involving awareness of such concepts as three-point fixation, casting index and total contact casts.

Principles of fixation and fracture healing

Fixation may achieve absolute or relative stability. Absolute stability results in direct bone healing by remodelling, whereas relative stability results in indirect healing by callus formation, followed by eventual remodelling. Direct healing requires anatomical reduction and fixation with absolute stability and is preferable in intra-articular fractures. In extra-articular and diaphyseal bone, relative stability and indirect healing is acceptable. Relative stability is achieved in the presence of fracture comminution. These concepts are guiding principles when planning fracture fixation. Fixation devices may be load-bearing, such as plates, or load-sharing, such as intramedullary nails. There may be several fixation options appropriate for a fracture.

Open reduction, internal fixation

The surgical approach to the fracture should be performed with an awareness of the nearby neurovascular structures, a good understanding of the fracture configuration and consideration of soft tissue injury (as mentioned). Fracture exposure should be as minimal as possible to preserve soft tissue attachments. Removal of any interposed soft tissue should be performed before reduction of the fracture. This reduction can be performed directly, using equipment such as with clamps, or indirectly for example by the use of carefully placed plates and screws.

A screw may provide absolute stability, when used in compression mode or relative stability, or in combination with a bridging plate. With certain fractures, and often with osteoporotic bone, locking plates may help with maintaining reduction. Other techniques involve using plates to compress fractures, the use of anatomical plates, and the use of tension band wiring (which converts a distracting force into a compressive force). Kirschner wires are useful both to hold a fracture reduced prior to fixation with screws and also as fixation in their own right.

Awareness of material properties of the fixation is also important. Combining different metals in one fracture fixation may cause such complications as galvanic corrosion and early failure.

Intramedullary nails

Intramedullary nails act as an internal splint and are load-sharing devices. They achieve relative stability and thus indirect bone healing. Intramedullary nailing often allows immediate full weight-bearing. Removal of locking screws can encourage fracture healing by dynamisation. This may also occur when locking screws fatigue and break. Intramedullary nails depend upon bone healing and in the context of a nonunion will eventually fail.

External fixation

External fixators may act as either temporary or definitive fixation. In open fractures with significant soft tissue injury or loss, application of an external fixator allows time for the soft tissues to recover and orthoplastic input with a view to coverage by graft or flap. External fixator pins should ideally be placed where there will be minimal impact on subsequent procedures, such as soft tissue coverage and definitive fixation. In complex intra-articular injuries, such as tibial plateau fractures, a combination of internal fixation plus the application of a circular frame may be utilised.

Complications

The consenting process should cover serious and frequently occurring complications. There are risks generic to most orthopaedic procedures and some specific to certain procedures (**Table 85.1**).

Follow-up

The metalwork implanted should be recorded, in case it requires removal in the future.

A clear postoperative plan should be documented on the operation note. This should cover:
- Requirements for elevation
- Weight-bearing status (where appropriate)
- Instructions for venous thromboembolism prophylaxis and duration
- Timing of follow-up and purpose, e.g. wound check, cast change, check X-ray

Table 85.1 Potential complications of fracture fixation

Time frame	Examples of potential complications
Immediate	Iatrogenic injury to nerves, blood vessels and tendons Tourniquet injury
Early	Infection Venous thromboembolism Compartment syndrome
Late	Nonunion, malunion, delayed-union Metalwork failure Painful arthritis

Further reading

Achten J, Parsons NR, McGuinness KR, et al. UK Fixation of Distal Tibia Fractures (UK FixDT): protocol for a randomised controlled trial of 'locking' plate fixation versus intramedullary nail fixation in the treatment of adult patients with a displaced fracture of the distal tibia. BMJ Open 2015; 5:e009162.

Costa ML, Achten J, Parsons NR, et al. Percutaneous fixation with Kirschner wires versus volar locking plate fixation in adults with dorsally displaced fracture of distal radius: randomised controlled trial. BMJ 2014; 349:g4807.

Gustilo RB, Anderson JT. Prevention of infection in the treatment of one thousand and twenty-five open fractures of long bones: Retrospective and prospective analyses. J Bone Joint Surg Am 1976; 58:453–458.

Related topics of interest

- *Topic 68* Open fractures
- *Topic 84* Principles of nonoperative management of fractures
- *Topic 91* Soft tissue coverage in trauma

86 Resuscitation and massive transfusion

Key points
- Traumatic injuries are often associated with significant blood loss and massive haemorrhage, which can either be evident or concealed
- Resuscitation is a process which aims to correct the physiological derangement induced by trauma across all organ systems in order to preserve life, prevent further deterioration and minimise morbidity

Principles of damage control resuscitation

Damage control resuscitation represents a philosophy of resuscitation which runs concurrently with damage control surgery. It aims to prevent and treat the lethal triad of hypothermia, coagulopathy and acidosis. The guiding principles are:
- Restoring normal tissue perfusion in order to minimise anaerobic respiration
- Prevention of coagulopathy
- Maintenance or restoration of normal temperature
- Facilitation of damage control surgery

Damage control resuscitation should start as close to the time of injury as possible, ideally prehospital. It should not delay rapid surgical management of any haemorrhage or contamination and should be continued until normal physiology has been restored.

Resuscitation fluids

The circulating volume can be restored using either fluid or blood products. Fluids can be either crystalloid or colloid and are often used either for initial resuscitation or for correction of nonblood losses. No artificial resuscitation fluid currently offers oxygen carrying capacity or coagulation factors.

Crystalloid fluids are solutions of salts and/or sugars in a concentration relatively isotonic to blood. They are generally cheap, readily available and innocuous. Balanced solutions such as Hartmann's are available which more closely approximate the chemical composition of plasma than simple solutions such as 0.9% sodium chloride, resulting in less acidosis and physiological derangement.

The main disadvantage to crystalloids is their wide volume of distribution. Glucose is rapidly metabolised, which results in the infusion being distributed throughout the fluid compartments of the body with little remaining in the circulation. Salt suspensions are theoretically slightly more restricted by their sodium content to the intravascular and extracellular spaces, but will still leak rapidly from the intravascular space. When given in large volumes all of these fluids are sequestered into tissue, causing oedema.

Colloids offer a theoretical solution to this problem; a suspension of large molecules which are too large to cross membranes exert an oncotic pull to bring fluid into the intravascular space. In practice, however, there is no evidence of benefit over crystalloids. The glycocalyx layer appears to be important in maintaining integrity of the border between the intravascular and extracellular space and is readily broken down during the stress response to injury, illness or major surgery. This allows the colloid molecules to leak into the extracellular space, removing the oncotic gradient and causing side effects such as itching.

Common colloids include gelatins, starches and albumin. Gelatins are large, naturally derived molecules suspended in a starch solution which confer a small but significant risk of anaphylaxis.

Starches are large chain sugar molecules that are not readily metabolized. Some older starch solutions have been demonstrated to impair coagulation. Two large multicentre randomized controlled trials demonstrated an increased risk of death and renal failure when they are used to resuscitate patients with septic shock and their use has fallen out of favour.

Human albumin solution may have a role in the resuscitation of patients with septic shock, but there is conflicting evidence of its efficacy and it may be more harmful than crystalloid when used to resuscitate burns victims.

Blood products

Blood products offer oxygen carriage, coagulation factors and platelets, as well as circulating volume. For this reason, whole blood is the ideal resuscitation fluid following massive haemorrhage. It has, however, a very short useful life and is rarely practical for routine use in civilian healthcare systems. Donated blood is, therefore, separated into components in order to derive the most utility from each donation and maximise useable life.

Packed red blood cells

Red blood corpuscles are stored in a solution containing saline, adenine, glucose and mannitol. With a haematocrit of approximately 70%, this solution is dense and viscous. It contains effectively no clotting factors and can be stored at 4°C for up to 28 days. Oxygen carrying capacity is reduced compared to native blood due to the effects of storage, and haemolysis resulting in hyperkalaemia is possible when older units are transfused.

Fresh frozen plasma

The major component of whole blood after removal of the red blood cells is plasma, which contains the majority of clotting factors and albumin. It has a very short useful life when chilled to 4°C, but can last for 3 years when frozen. Fresh frozen plasma (FFP) is relatively low in fibrinogen. It is suspended in citrate which chelates calcium and prevents coagulation. The time taken to defrost the FFP must be factored into any resuscitation strategy.

Platelets

Platelets are vital to effective clotting but are fragile and have a short life of 5 days. They are kept at room temperature and constantly agitated to prevent aggregation. The number of platelets in an individual donation is low and therefore platelets are either pooled from four donations or donated by a single donor using apheresis. Platelets are stored in citrate.

Cryoprecipitate

When plasma is frozen, a white layer separates out on top which is rich in fibrinogen. This is then pooled and frozen separately as cryoprecipitate which is stored in citrate. It is used to treat fibrinogen deficiency.

Other components

Fibrinogen concentrates are occasionally used instead of cryoprecipitate, and require reconstitution from powder. Prothrombin complex concentrates offer some of the clotting factors in FFP without the volume and risk of transfusion-associated lung injury. Recombinant activated factor VII is now rarely used after data demonstrated an increased risk of death when it was administered in unselected major haemorrhage patients.

The early administration of tranexamic acid following major multisystem trauma has been shown to improve mortality, and the benefit is greater the earlier it is given. Tranexamic acid is an antifibrinolytic which prevents the breakdown of clots.

Hypotensive resuscitation

Prior to definitive control of haemorrhage, full resuscitation to a normal blood pressure may be harmful, as there is evidence that it may disrupt fragile clot formation, worsen hypothermia and haemodilute the patient. Partial resuscitation to maintain flow, titrated to the presence of a radial pulse may reduce this. A lower target is often set in cases of major thoracic trauma, such as a carotid pulse.

There are some patients where a hypotensive strategy may carry risk:
- Patients with head injuries. There may be a reduction in cerebral perfusion pressure in the injured brain that is no longer able to autoregulate blood flow effectively

- Pregnant patients, where reduced placental flow may threaten fetal viability
- Children, where hypotension manifests very late in shock

In animal models, a worse outcome is seen if a hypotensive strategy is continued for longer than 1 hour after injury.

Complications of massive transfusion

Massive transfusion refers to the transfusion of more than the patient's entire circulating volume of blood products within a single 24-hour period. Resuscitation with a large volume of blood products carries a number of issues:

- The same risks associated with the transfusion of any single unit of a blood product: infection, incompatibility reactions, transfusion associated acute lung injury. These risks rise proportionately with the number of units transfused
- Hypothermia: most blood products are kept chilled and transfusion of a large volume of cold fluid can induce hypothermia. Use of a blood warmer is essential to avoid this
- Hyperkalaemia: stored packed red blood cells will degrade in storage and undergo cell lysis. This will release the potassium inside the cells and when large volumes are transfused, this can cause life-threatening hyperkalaemia
- Hypocalcaemia: most blood products except packed red cells are suspended in citrate which has an anticoagulant effect by chelating calcium. Hypocalcaemia occurs after transfusion of a large volume of these products. This will result in coagulopathy, negative inotropy and arrhythmias

Further reading

Association of Anaesthetists of Great Britain and Ireland. Blood transfusion and the anaesthetist: management of massive haemorrhage. Anaesthesia 2010; 65:1153–1161.

Mercer SJ, Tarmey NT, Woolley T, Wood P, Mahoney PF. Haemorrhage and coagulopathy in the Defence Medical Services. Anaesthesia. 2013; 68:49–60.

Related topics of interest

- *Topic 17* Damage control orthopaedics and trauma physiology
- *Topic 62* Major trauma – Advanced Trauma and Life Support principles

87 Septic arthritis – paediatric

Key points

- Septic arthritis is an infective, critical condition which rapidly threatens the articular surfaces of the affected joint
- The signs and symptoms of septic arthritis can be subtle and younger children will not be able to give a history or co-operate with examination, so a meticulous approach which takes this into account is required
- The hip is the most commonly affected joint in children, but any joint may be affected
- An early diagnosis usually offers a better prognosis, so early detection is key
- Transient synovitis mimics septic arthritis in children

Epidemiology

The incidence is 4 per 100,000 in the developed world and higher in low income areas. Half of all cases of paediatric septic arthritis occur in children under the age of 2 years. The hip is the joint most commonly affected.

Neonates, haemophiliacs and immunocompromised children are at increased risk of developing septic arthritis.

Pathophysiology

The routes of transmission are multifold. Direct transmission can be from penetrating trauma or surgery. Innoculation can also occur from haematogenous spread or from adjacent bones. Osteomyelitis can spread contiguously to adjacent joints. This usually occurs from infection in the metaphysis of bone in the hip, shoulder, elbow and the ankle.

Proteolytic enzymes (metalloproteinases) are responsible for the destructive process on cartilage and bone. These enzymes are released by inflammatory cells in the synovium and the cartilage. Together with inflammatory cytokines, macrophages and bacteria, the increase in pressure within the joint causes compromise to the intra-articular blood vessels leading to ischaemia and destruction of cartilage and osteonecrosis of bone. In the hip, this can cause ligament damage, destruction of the femoral head, dislocation and osteomyelitis.

Organisms

- Neonates to 12 months: *Staphylococcus*, group B *Streptococcus*, Gram-negative bacteria, e.g. *Escherichia coli*
- 6 months to 5 years: *Staphylococcus aureus*, *Streptococcus pneumonia*, group A *Streptococcus*, *Haemophilus influenzae*
- 5–12 years: *Staphylococcus aureus*
- 12–18 years: *Neisseria gonorrhoea* – monoarticular or polyarthopathy presentation with associated red papular rash, *Staphylococcus aureus*
- Others: *Salmonella* should be suspected in children with sickle cell anaemia. *Mycobacterium tuberculosis* should be considered in children where the risk factors are prevalent. HACEK (*Haemophilus*, *Actinobacillus*, *Cardiobacterium*, *Eikenella* and *Kingella*) are a group of bacterium prevalent in the toddler age group

Clinical features

The history is a very important part of establishing a diagnosis. The child may present with a history of a preceding illness, rash, lymphadenopathy or general malaise. The child may be febrile and refuse to walk or move their hip. It is important to ask about onset of illness or pain, mono- or polyarthropathy, previous episodes of joint pain or septic arthritis, past medical history, drug history and any recent travel.

The signs and symptoms of septic arthritis can be subtle and so it is important to have a low threshold to exclude it as a diagnosis and treat it accordingly. On examination, it is important to look for erythema, effusions, swelling and feel for a hot joint. If there is an effusion in the hip joint, the child will tend to lie with their hip flexed, externally rotated and abducted as this is the position in which the hip lies comfortably with maximised capsular volume. It is important to examine the contralateral hip and the adjacent joints – specifically the knee and ankle.

Investigations

Radiographs should be taken of the relevant joints. If septic arthritis of the hip is suspected, then anteroposterior, lateral and frog leg views of the pelvis should be taken. In the majority of cases, the radiographs may appear completely normal. Sometimes it may be possible to see widening of the joint space indicative of an effusion, subluxation or even dislocation of the femoral head. If there is evidence of osteomyelitis, then progressive bony changes may be seen.

An ultrasound is sensitive for effusions and in some situations can guide an aspiration for a diagnosis.

Diagnosis

It is important to establish between a septic arthritis and a transient synovitis in a child as both have very different paths of management. Kocher's criteria includes four independent predictors which were found to have excellent diagnostic powers in differentiating between a transient synovitis and a septic arthritis. These are: (1) an inability to weight bear, (2) white blood cell count >12000 cells/μL, (3) temperature >38.5ºC and (4) erythrocyte sedimentation rate >40 mm/h.

When:
- 4/4 criteria are met – 99% chance of septic arthritis
- 3/4 criteria are met – 93% chance of septic arthritis
- 2/4 criteria are met – 40% chance of septic arthritis
- 1/4 criteria are met – 3% chance of septic arthritis

A hip aspiration can be used to confirm a diagnosis. This fluid should be sent off urgently for a differential cell count, gram staining, culture and sensitivities, glucose and protein levels. A high white blood cell count (>50000 cells/mm^3) and glucose 0.5 mg/mL than serum levels indicates a septic joint. Blood cultures should be taken if the child is febrile and joint fluid can also be inoculated into blood culture bottles for growth.

Treatment

A nonsurgical approach with intravenous antibiotics alone can be used. This is not the standard approach used for treating septic arthritis.

An urgent surgical incision and drainage is the standard for nearly all septic joints, with samples sent for the above mentioned test. It is common to use the anterior approach to the hip joint for this using the superficial intervous plane of sartorius (femoral nerve) and tensor fascia lata (superior gluteal nerve) and the deep plane of rectus femoris (femoral nerve) and gluteus medius (superior gluteal nerve). The capsule of the hip is stretched by adducting and externally rotating the hip and a mini-capsulotomy will gain access to the joint. The joint should be irrigated with copious amounts of saline. Antibiotics should be started promptly after the samples are taken and this should then be discussed with microbiology when sensitivities of cultures are back.

The following antibiotics are recommended in the treatment of septic arthritis in the child:
- *Staphylococcus aureus*, group B streptococci, gram-negative bacilli – 1st generation cephalosporin, e.g. cephalexin
- *Streptococcus pneumonia*, group A streptococci, H. influenzae – second or third generation cephalosporin, e.g. cefuroxime or cefotaxime
- *Neisseria gonorrhoea* – oxacillin

There are many schools of thought on how long intravenous antibiotics should continue for. This should be guided by the clinical picture before a switch to oral antibiotics is made. It is important to start early mobilisation once the incision and drainage has been performed to avoid stiffness and swelling of the joint. Once the child is mobilising, appears clinically well and the biochemical parameters have reached near normal limits, then it would be sensible to convert to oral antibiotics. Liaising with the microbiology department is important for this. However, antibiotic therapy should continue for a minimum of 4–6 weeks. Clinical assessment should continue during this time as an outpatient.

Complications

Recurrence of infection can occur if an incomplete debridement has been performed. In this situation, a further surgical debridement and washout of the joint may be necessary. If the infection was so severe that there was bony involvement, this can lead to femoral head destruction of the hip which subsequently can lead to varus/valgus deformity, biomechanical instability, pain, dislocation and joint contractures. If the physeal growth plate has been affected, this could lead to growth disturbance and growth arrest which in turn can lead to limb length discrepancy.

Further reading

Howard A, Wilson M. Septic arthritis in children. BMJ 2010; 341:c4407.

Kocher MS, Zurakowski D, Kasser JR. Differentiating between septic arthritis and transient synovitis of the hip in children: an evidence-based clinical prediction algorithm. J Bone Joint Surg Am 1999; 81:1662–1670.

Related topics of interest

- *Topic 55* Infection
- *Topic 88* Septic arthritis and crystal arthropathy – adult

88 Septic arthritis and crystal arthropathy – adult

Key points
- Septic arthritis can be difficult to differentiate from crystal arthropathy
- Septic arthritis can rapidly cause destruction of articular cartilage
- Treatment of septic arthritis can vary, but early diagnosis and appropriate treatment is imperative

Epidemiology
The incidence of septic arthritis in the UK is approximately 8/100,000, and four times higher in the those over 75 years. *Staphylococcus* and *Streptococcus* are the most commonly implicated pathogens, with variation between age groups. Commonly affected joints include the knee, hip, shoulder, wrist and ankle. Co-morbidity and immunosuppression are risk factors.

Crystal arthropathy is arthritis caused by crystal deposition within the joint. Gout and pseudogout are the two most common crystal arthropathies. The UK incidence of gout is around 186/100,000, with a prevalence of 1.4%. Male sex and increasing age are both risk factors. Pseudogout affects both sexes equally and incidence increases with age.

Pathophysiology
Septic arthritis
Seeding of the pathogen into the joint may be via haematogenous spread, by spread from locally infected soft tissue and bone or by a penetrating injury into the joint. Once present, the pathogen multiplies and the immune system responds, releasing pro-inflammatory mediators. The inflammatory response results in a rise in intra-articular pressure and the joint cartilage is starved of its supply of oxygen and nutrients. Further, the release of proteolytic enzymes by the inflammatory cells induce irreversible cartilage damage within 8 hours, which is why this is deemed an orthopaedic emergency.

Crystal arthropathy
Gout is caused by an accumulation of monosodium urate crystals within the joint, whilst pseudogout is caused by calcium pyrophosphate crystals. The crystals trigger an inflammatory response, resulting in cartilage damage.

Clinical features
A septic joint or crystal arthropathy causes warmth, joint pain, swelling, erythema, restriction in range of movement and difficulty weight-bearing. The joint may be held in a flexed position to relieve pain from capsular stretch. Clinical examination is often limited, with pain on palpation and passive movement of the joint. With septic arthritis, the virulence of the organism will determine how quickly and how aggressive the symptoms present.

Investigations
Observations, including temperature, are useful in assessing for evidence of systemic sepsis. Blood cultures should be taken in the emergency department along with a full blood count, renal profile and C-reactive protein. Erythrocyte sedimentation rate and a serum urate may also be helpful. Alternative sources of sepsis should be investigated with a chest radiograph and urine dip. Radiographs of the affected joint are often performed, and may reveal evidence of a joint effusion. Certain radiographic findings, such as 'punched out' periarticular erosions or soft tissue crystal deposition may help lead to the diagnosis of a crystal arthropathy. A native joint aspirate can routinely be taken in the emergency department and sent for an urgent gram stain plus culture and sensitivity. A hip joint aspirate is usually performed

under ultrasound or image intensifier guidance by radiology or in theatre. Where there is suspicion of a septic arthritis in a joint prosthesis, an aspirate should be performed in theatre to minimise the risk of introducing infection.

Routine blood tests, radiographs and a joint fluid aspirate sent for microscopy are routine in the diagnosis of a crystal arthropathy.

Diagnosis

Initial diagnosis of a septic arthritis is made with a Gram stain and confirmed on culture of an organism. A negative Gram stain is reassuring, but does not exclude a diagnosis of septic arthritis. An organism may only be grown with enrichment cultures. Where antibiotics treatment was initiated prior to joint fluid aspirate or tissue sampling, a causative organism may never be identified.

Gout or pseudo-gout is diagnosed at microscopy by assessment of their crystals. Gout is characterised by thin, needle shaped, strongly negatively birefringent crystals, whereas pseudogout has rhomboid-shaped crystals which are weakly positively birefringent.

Treatment

Septic arthritis

Once a joint aspirate or joint tissue samples have been obtained, empirical broad-spectrum intravenous antibiotic treatment should be initiated based on local trust antibiotic prescribing guidelines. Where a patient is systemically unwell and a joint aspirate cannot be obtained in a reasonable time, the risks and benefits of initiating empirical treatment without a sample should be judged on a case-by-case basis. Source control of a septic arthritis may require joint wash-out in theatre in combination with antibiotic treatment. Fully aspirating pus from a joint combined with intravenous antibiotic treatment can provide equivalent results to joint washout in some joint infections.

Crystal arthropathy

Analgesia and anti-inflammatory medication is useful in an acute episode. Long-term prophylaxis may be initiated once the acute episode has resolved. In more severe cases, disease modifying antirheumatoid medications, such as methotrexate may be required.

Complications

Without swift diagnosis and treatment, a septic arthritis can cause significant cartilage damage, resulting in long-term joint pain, stiffness and loss of function. Early complete joint aspiration and intravenous antibiotics can be a recognised treatment for some joint infections. Arthroscopic washouts minimise soft tissue injury. In deeper joints, such as the hip, open washout may be favoured; it is deemed mandatory in septic arthritis of the paediatric hip.

Crystal arthropathies may lead to degenerative change in the long-term.

Further reading

Smith S, Thyoka M, Lavy C, Pitani A. Septic arthritis of the shoulder in children in Malawi, a randomised, prospective study of aspiration versus arthrotomy and washout. J Bone Joint Surg Br 2002; 84B:1167–1172.

Related topics of interest

- *Topic 55* Infection
- *Topic 87* Septic arthritis – paediatric

89 Shoulder dislocations

Key points
- Shoulder dislocations are common and recur frequently
- Shoulder instability can be due to structural or nonstructural factors

Epidemiology

Shoulder dislocations are amongst the most common shoulder injuries with a reported incidence of 24 per 100,000 person-years. The incidence is higher in young men and the majority of injuries are sustained in falls or participating in sports.

Pathophysiology

Dislocation of the shoulder occurs more commonly in an anterior direction than posterior. Anterior dislocation occurs with supramaximal external rotation and abduction of the shoulder and is typically associated with trauma. Posterior dislocation occurs with internal rotation and adduction and is associated with involuntary muscular contraction, such as those seen in electrocution or seizure, and occurs due to the difference in strength between the pectoral muscles and the external rotators. Inferior dislocation of the shoulder, luxatio erecta, is the least common form of shoulder dislocation and occurs due to hyperadduction. It is the most likely form of shoulder dislocation to be associated with neurovascular complications, due to the proximity of the dislocated humeral head to the brachial plexus.

Recurrent instability of the shoulder can occur due to a combination of factors.

Associated injuries are outlined in Table 89.1.

Table 89.1 Injuries commonly associated with shoulder dislocations

Injury	Description
Bankart	Classic pathological lesion associated with anterior dislocation of the shoulder. It is a tear of the antero/inferior labrum with a variable amount of bone. Represents a loss of the labrum and a glenoid detachment of the glenohumeral ligaments
HAGL lesion	Represents failure of the glenohumeral ligament at its humeral rather that glenoid insertion
Hill–Sachs lesion	Compression fracture of humeral head by edge of glenoid during anterior dislocation. An engaging Hill–Sachs can contribute to shoulder instability; a reverse Hill–Sachs is associated with posterior dislocation
Greater tuberosity fracture	Most commonly occurs with anterior dislocations in patients >50 years. Represents an avulsion of the posterosuperior cuff
Lesser tuberosity fracture	May occur with posterior dislocations; represents avulsion of anterior cuff
Neurological injury	Injury to brachial plexus is more common and more severe with higher energy injury but may occur with any dislocation. Axillary nerve most commonly injured
Proximal humeral fracture	Fracture-dislocations of the proximal humerus are a separate entity and mandate reduction in operating theatre with a plan for fixation
Rotator cuff	More common than recurrent instability in the older patient and should be suspected if rehabilitation is not progressing
ALPSA	Occurs when labrum comes away with associated periosteum and medialises down the glenoid neck, becoming stuck in this position.
GLAD	Bankart lesion with associated articular cartilage defect

ALPSA, anterior labral periosteal sleeve avulsion; GLAD, glenoid labral articular defect; HAGL, humeral avulsion of the glenohumeral ligament

Clinical assessment

Patients with unstable shoulders may present acutely in the emergency department or in the outpatient setting.

In the emergency setting, first-time dislocation of the shoulder typically presents with pain and deformity following an injury. Patients with recurrent dislocations may have little pain. Posterior dislocations may be more subtle – if it is not possible to externally rotate the shoulder a posterior dislocation must be presumed until proven otherwise. A careful, documented neurovascular assessment of the limb before and after any attempts at reduction is mandatory.

In the outpatient setting a careful history including age, occupation, sports, mode of first dislocation, age at first dislocation, number and direction of dislocations and any previous treatment should be taken. Examination should include a Beighton score, examining for periscapular muscle bulk, scapular dyskinaesia, a sulcus sign, anterior and posterior apprehension, examination of the cuff and a neurovascular examination.

Investigations

In the first instance, anteroposterior, scapular Y view and axillary view radiographs should be obtained. It is not possible to exclude a posterior dislocation radiologically without an axillary view. In the event of diagnostic uncertainty, CT scanning both confirms the diagnosis and permits assessment of the bony injury.

In the outpatient setting, if surgery is being considered for shoulder instability, MR arthrography offers good visualisation of labral (Bankart) and associated soft tissue injuries injuries. CT offers better assessment of bone loss. Ultrasonography is useful for identifying rotator cuff injuries, and may be more readily available, but does not allow for assessment of the degree of fatty infiltration of the muscles of the cuff.

Classification

Shoulder instability can be described according to the direction of the dislocation; anterior, posterior, inferior or multidirectional. The concept of direction of dislocation and associated trauma as discrete pathologies has now largely been superseded by the 'Stanmore triangle' (**Figure 89.1**), describing three polar types of instability but based on the interplay between multiple poles in nearly all patients.

Treatment

Initial management

The majority of shoulder dislocations should be reduced urgently with the use of analgesia or anaesthesia. The exception to this may be patients who experience recurrent dislocations. Reduction with a traction-countertraction technique is preferable, as leverage techniques such as Kocher's are associated with higher rates of fracture. Posterior dislocations are frequently irreducible and associated with a significant impaction of the humeral head. These should usually be reduced in the operating theatre after CT scanning to help plan definitive management. A surgeon who is capable of open reduction and definitive management should be present.

Nonoperative management

A period of sling immobilisation followed by a controlled therapy programme is the treatment of choice for the majority of first time dislocations. There is some evidence that immobilisation in external rotation may be beneficial, but it is not unequivocal and compliance is difficult.

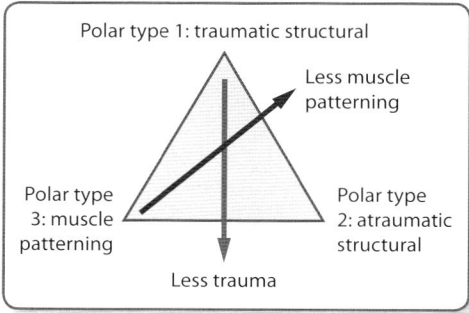

Figure 89.1 The Stanmore triangle of shoulder instability.

Table 89.2 Common surgical procedures for shoulder instability	
Surgical procedure	Description
Bankart repair	May be carried out open or arthroscopically. Arthroscopic is the 1st line surgical procedure of choice in the majority of units. It is as effective as open stabilisation with potentially faster rehabilitation. It is indicated for soft tissue Bankart lesion with <20% bone loss and may be combined with a capsular shift
Bristow-Latarjet	Transfer of coracoid to inferior glenoid bone defect. Provides both a bony block to dislocation and a dynamic sling. Indicated for bone defects, revision surgery. May be considered as primary procedure for patients keen to return to contact sport
Remplissage	Using the posterior rotator cuff to fill the defect in the humeral head caused by a Hill–Sachs lesion

Patients with a muscle patterning type of dislocation should be managed in an appropriate, specialised unit.

Surgical management

Some of the options for surgical management are described in **Table 89.2**.

Complications

Immediate

- Neurological injury – most frequently occurs at the time of injury. All pre- and postintervention neurological assessments must be documented
- Fracture – excessive force in manipulation of a dislocated humeral head

Early

- Recurrent instability – incidence is inversely proportional to patient age at index dislocation
- Stiffness

Late

- Post-traumatic osteoarthritis

Further reading

Hill AM, et al. The clinical assessment and classification of shoulder instability. Curr Orthop 2008; 22:208–225.

Lewis A, Kitamura T, Bayley JIL. (ii) The classification of shoulder instability: new light through old windows! Curr Orthop 2004; 18:97–108.

Youm T, Takemoto R, Park BK. Acute management of shoulder dislocations. J Am Acad Orthop Surg 2014; 12:761–771.

Related topics of interest

- *Topic 10* Brachial plexus injury
- *Topic 49* Imaging modalities

90 Shoulder – scapula and glenoid fractures

Key points
- Fractures of the scapula are often high-energy injuries and so may co-exist with significant chest injury
- Scapula body and neck fractures are most frequently managed nonoperatively
- Glenoid rim fractures are associated with instability of the shoulder

Epidemiology

Significant fractures of the scapula and glenoid are uncommon, representing <1% of all fractures seen. They should be differentiated from the small glenoid rim fractures which represent bony Bankart lesions and are much more common. Fractures of the scapula and glenoid tend to affect either younger men and be higher energy injuries or older women and result from a simple fall.

Higher energy scapula fractures tend to be associated with significant chest injuries, as the scapula itself is well protected by surrounding muscle and so a large amount of energy needs to be imparted to the thorax to be sufficient to fracture the relatively deep scapula.

Pathophysiology

Scapular body, neck and glenoid body fractures occur as a result of a direct blow, whereas glenoid rim fractures occur as a result of an episode of shoulder instability. Scapular neck fractures represent disruption of one of the 'struts' of the superior shoulder suspensory complex, a bone and soft tissue arch which suspends the whole arm. The other strut of this complex is the clavicle and disruption of both of these represents a floating shoulder.

Clinical assessment

In the context of the potentially high energy of injury, initial assessment of the patient should take place according to Advanced Trauma Life Support protocols. The clavicle, acromioclavicular joint and acromion should be examined and a careful neurovascular examination of the limb performed. An assessment of the shoulder joint should be made looking for an obvious dislocation without moving the arm in order to avoid unnecessary pain. Examination of the chest is mandatory, looking for associated injuries including rib fractures, flail segments, lung injury and haemopneumothorax.

Investigations

Plain radiographs including an anteroposterior, lateral and axial views of the shoulder should be obtained to look for marked displacement of the fracture or an associated dislocation. Given the three-dimensional (3D) anatomy of the scapula, and the difficulties in interpreting plain radiographs due to overlying ribs, CT scanning, preferably with 3D reconstruction should be considered for all fractures as both the pre- and potentially postoperative investigation of choice. Appropriate imaging of the chest should be undertaken as the patient's clinical condition dictates.

Classification

Several classification systems exist for scapular fracture, but in terms of guiding management it is most important to know the location of the fracture and the degree of displacement. The location of the fracture can be grouped into the body of the scapula, the neck of the scapula, the glenoid fossa and the glenoid rim.

The glenopolar angle can be used to assess the degree of displacement of scapular neck fractures and is the angle between the face of the glenoid and a line drawn from the most cranial portion of the glenoid to the inferior angle of the scapula.

Treatment

The vast majority of scapular fractures can be satisfactorily treated nonoperatively with rest in a sling until the pain settles then mobilisation. Operative management is indicated in:
- Scapular neck fractures with over 1 cm of medialisation of the glenoid or angulation of >40°
- Displaced glenoid fossa fractures
- Glenoid rim fractures associated with instability (bony Bankart lesions)

For the majority of scapula fracture fixation a modification of the Judet approach is used.

Complications

Immediate
- Those associated injuries reflecting high-energy thoracic trauma, such as pulmonary contusions

Early
- Rotator cuff dysfunction
- Shoulder instability

Late
- Osteoarthritis of the shoulder

Further reading

Cole PA, Gauger EM, Schroder LK. Management of scapular fractures. J Am Acad Orthop Surg 2012; 20:130–141.

Obremskey WT, Lyman JR. A modified Judet approach to the scapula. J Orthop Trauma 2004; 18:696–699.

Van Oostveen DP, Temmerman OP, Burger BJ, van Noort A, Robinson M. Glenoid fractures: a review of pathology, classification, treatment and results. Acta Orthop Belg 2014; 18:88–98.

Related topics of interest

- *Topic 89* Shoulder dislocations
- *Topic 99* Trauma scoring systems

91 Soft tissue coverage in trauma

Key points
- A joint, consultant-led orthoplastic approach from the outset is key
- Debridement must be adequate from the outset
- Understanding the zone of injury guides management
- Skeletal stability is essential prior to coverage
- Amputation exists on a continuum with debridement and may be the most pragmatic option for severe limb injuries

Epidemiology

The annual incidence of open lower limb fractures is approximately 5 per 100,000 population. The most common mechanisms of injury are fall from height, road traffic collision and interpersonal violence.

Assessment

Initial evaluation and treatment of the traumatised patient should be in accordance with Advanced Trauma Life Support principles. The British Orthopaedic Association Standard for Trauma 4 (BOAST 4) guidelines should also be adhered to, which in practical terms dictate that many patients may be transferred to trauma centres for treatment. Initial assessment must be made of the vascular and neurological status of the limb, clearly recorded, and reassessed if any manipulation or splintage takes place. Photographs prior to application of dressings are also helpful. Thereafter, the next opportunity for assessment is at debridement – once the wound has been excised, extended and explored, the bone ends delivered and all nonviable fragments removed, a plan can be made for both stabilisation and coverage. The severity of soft tissue damage as assessed at this point is a predictor of the clinical course and eventual outcome. The most common classification of open fractures is that of Gustilo and Anderson.

Gustilo and Anderson classification

Type 1
Open fracture with a puncture wound <1 cm long, clean.

Type 2
Open fracture with a laceration >1 cm long without extensive soft tissue damage, flaps or avulsions

Type 3
High-energy – open fracture with extensive damage to soft tissue. Subdivided into:
- 3A: Adequate soft tissue coverage of a fractured bone when closed primarily
- 3B: Extensive soft tissue injury with periosteal stripping, bony exposure and contamination, requires local flap or free tissue transfer for closure
- 3C: Open fracture associated with arterial injury requiring repair

Reconstructive goals
- Adequate debridement of traumatised and devitalised tissue
- Achieve stability, structure, vascularity and function
- Provide suitable coverage
- Cosmesis
- Minimal donor site morbidity

Surgical management

The order and timing of surgery generally starts with initial debridement followed by skeletal stabilisation, if necessary, and finally soft tissue reconstruction. The advantages of early cover are less infection, earlier mobilisation and fewer operations. Various factors may prevent emergency or early soft tissue cover, such as plastic surgical service availability and complex or contaminated wounds. At primary surgery, the full zone of trauma may not be fully appreciated and the patient may require further debridements and temporary vacuum therapy. The patient may have multiple injuries and not be fit for a lengthy procedure.

On occasion, it is possible to achieve definitive fixation and soft tissue cover at the initial operation in a 'fix and flap' operation. This is often achieved with an intramedullary nail combined with a local fasciocutaneous flap. If more complex, staged reconstruction is required, then a temporary external fixator can be applied in tandem with vacuum therapy. In this case, meticulous attention to the vacuum device and dressing is necessary. If the limb is not salvageable, amputation at first surgery is uncommon unless the patient is at severe physiological risk. It should be discussed with the patient who in turn should be given sufficient time and access to multidisciplinary advice to consider it. Any amputation, urgent or planned, should be documented to be in the patient's best interests by two surgeons, unless to delay risks harm.

The reconstructive ladder

- Secondary intention (with or without vacuum therapy)
- Direct closure
- Skin graft
- Local flap
- Regional flap
- Free tissue transfer (complex)

A flap is a composite block of tissue with its own blood supply. A free flap is created when this is moved from one area of the body to another, vascularised by microvascular anastomoses to recipient vessels, while in a pedicled flap the tissue is moved whilst retaining attachment to its original blood supply.

Preparation for definitive soft tissue reconstruction

A skin graft requires a suitable recipient bed such as periosteum, paratenon, fascia, or muscle. If none of these beds are available free tissue transfer may be indicated, offering a versatile range of techniques and donors. Composite defects involving multiple structures such as skin, nerve, tendon and bone require complex reconstruction and this may be achieved with a composite free flap incorporating these structures into one unit for transfer. Planning of such complex surgery requires multiple considerations and balancing of reconstructive needs with donor site morbidity.

Definitive cover of open fractures requires vascularised soft tissue. Current standards mandate that this should be performed within 7 days as there is evidence that this prevents infection and offers an opportunity to perform microsurgery before vessels become fibrosed and friable secondary to the physiological changes of trauma.

A CT angiogram may be required to understand both donor and host vascular supplies. A transfusion strategy maximising preoperative perfusion is key to the preservation and optimisation of tissue. Further debridements may be necessary prior to definitive reconstruction. Antimicrobial therapy should be targeted at organisms cultured from any intraoperative samples.

Free tissue transfer is the mainstay of covering high-energy open tibial fractures and needs to be performed at a specialist, joint orthoplastic centre.

There exists some debate over fasciocutaneous and muscle flaps: while they are useful for local cover, they are better suited to lower-energy injuries with a smaller zone of injury.

When considering soft tissue coverage of the lower limb, it can be useful to divide it into thirds:

Upper third

- Local fasciocutaneous flaps
- Gastronemius muscle flap, based on sural artery. Medial head is larger and suitable for local reconstruction of the upper third of tibial defects. This leaves no functional deficit and one is using the larger, broader belly of the muscle
- Free flap

Middle third
- Local fasciocutaneous flaps
- Soleus muscle flap, based on blood supply from posterior tibial and peroneal arteries. Leaves no functional deficit
- Free flap

Lower third
- Free flap:
  - Large defect: latissimus dorsi or anterolateral thigh
  - Medium defect: anterolateral thigh
  - Small defect: gracillis and split skin graft

Postoperative care

Overnight stay in a high-dependency unit for vigilant flap observations and optimal physiological control is common, followed by transfer to a plastic surgery ward. Thereafter, warming, venous thromboembolism prophylaxis and limb elevation are all key. Discharge will largely depend on weight-bearing status, mobility and progress with rehabilitation. These patients are usually followed up in a joint orthoplastic clinic.

Further reading

Godina M. Early microsurgical reconstruction of complex trauma of the extremities. Plast Reconstr Surg 1986; 78:285–292.

Gustilo RB, Mendzoa RM, Williams DN. Problems in the management of type III open fractures: a new classification of type III open fractures. J Trauma 1984; 24:742–746.

Nanchahal J, Nayagam S, Khan U, et al. Standards for the management of open fractures of the lower limb. London: Royal Society of Medicine Press Ltd, 2009.

Related topics of interest

- *Topic 68* Open fractures
- *Topic 85* Principles of operative management of fractures
- *Topic 98* Tibial shaft fractures

Spine – atlas and axis cervical fractures and dislocations

Key points
- Cervical spine injuries can be rapidly fatal
- Meticulous examination, imaging, investigation and documentation is mandatory
- Management is guided by the stability of the spine and the patient's suitability for surgery

Epidemiology
Injuries to the cervical spine account for over 30% of all spinal injuries, with C2 the most commonly involved vertebra. The odontoid process of C2 is specific part of the vertebra involved in majority of these injuries. The majority of immediate fatalities from cervical spine trauma result from injuries occurring at the C1 or C2 level. Younger patients are more likely to have C1 fractures, while odontoid process fractures of C2 are seen more in the elderly.

Pathophysiology
The upper cervical spine is susceptible to trauma due to both the large range of motion it experiences (50% of cervical spine rotation occurs at the C1/C2 junction and 20% of flexion and extension at the occiput/C1 junction) and the pendulum effect of the skull vault and its contents. Such a range of motion requires extensive ligamentous complexes to help stabilise the joints, all of which may also be injured.

Common mechanisms of injury include axial load, distraction, flexion, extension, horizontal shear and combinations of the above. Burst fractures of C1 (Jefferson fractures) tend to be associated with an axial load in extension (e.g. diving into shallow water) whilst odontoid process fractures are associated with shear forces and an element of axial compression (e.g. an unbroken fall from standing height onto the forehead).

Clinical assessment
Cervical spine injury should be suspected in all high-energy injuries and in the polytraumatised patient. Prehospital triple immobilisation is now the norm if any mechanism is remotely suggestive of spinal injury, or reduced consciousness levels preclude checking for back or neck pain.

A comprehensive assessment should be made of the central and peripheral nervous system, with completion of an American Spinal Injuries Association chart. Injury to the occipito-atlanto-axial complex can results in injury to cranial nerves as well as the spinal cord. In the unconscious, confused or agitated patient this is complicated and meticulous documentation is key. When the patient has significant neurological injury, secondary survey is difficult and must be undertaken with great care to ensure significant injuries are not missed.

In high cervical spine injuries with neurological injury, thorough assessment of the patient's respiratory function is also vital due to the potential for phrenic nerve paralysis (C3–C5).

Due to the proximity of the vertebral arteries to the upper cervical spine, an element of vascular injury may complicate fractures and dislocations, with resultant neurological sequaelae.

Investigations
Plain radiography should comprise three views – anteroposterior (AP), lateral and odontoid process or 'open mouth'. To be considered adequate the AP and lateral must include the C7–T1 junction. When this is not possible, a 'swimmer's view'

should be considered, whereby the arm position is altered to avoid the humeral head obscuring the distal cervical spine. This view has inherent difficulties, especially in injured patients in some degree of pain, and the ready availability of CT scanning in many centres offers a rapid and easy alternative. The atlantodens interval can be used to assess the integrity of the transverse cervical ligament (<3 mm in adults, <5 mm in children). Particular care should be taken in assessing radiographs of the paediatric cervical spine due to the potential for physiological pseudosubluxation in children up to 8 years old. The Canadian C-spine rules were developed in 2001 as an algorithm to decide which cervical spine injuries should be imaged and variations on this are in use in emergency departments throughout the UK. The Powers' ratio is used to identify occipitocervical subluxation/dislocation (**Figure 92.1**):

$$\text{Powers' ratio} = \frac{\text{Distance from basion to C1 arch}}{\text{Distance from tip of the dens to the opisthion}}$$

If there is no injury, the ratio is 1.0.

Computed tomography is the most commonly performed investigation for traumatic upper cervical spine injuries. It allows reconstructions in the sagittal and coronal planes, giving very good visualisation of complex fracture patterns, but does not provide information on ligamentous structures or the cord itself.

Magnetic resonance imaging is mandatory for the patient with neurological dysfunction but a normal CT scan, and should be considered in all but the most minor upper cervical spine injuries. Magnetic resonance angiography should be performed if there is suspicion of a vertebral artery injury.

Classification

- Dislocations/dissociations – all are rare and commonly fatal
  - Cranio-cervical dislocation
    - Atlantooccipital joint
    - Occipitocervical joint
    - Craniocervical joint
    - Atlantoaxial joint (rotatory fixation)
- Fractures
  - C0
  - Occipital condyle fracture
    - Andersen and Montesano – describes the injuring force
    - I – Compression
    - II – Direct blow
    - III – Rotation/lateral bending
  - C1 (**Figure 92.2**)
  - C2
  - Levine and Edwards – describes bony and associated injuries
    - I – <3 mm horizontal displacement
    - Intact C2/C3 disc
    - No angulation
    - II – >3 mm horizontal displacement
    - Posterior longitudinal ligament and C2/C3 disc injury
    - Significant angulation
    - III – Type I with associated bi-facet (C2/C3) dislocation
  - Odontoid process:
    - D'Alonzo and Andersen – describes fracture location:
    - I – Tip of the process
    - II – Junction of the base of the process and body of the axis
    - III – Fracture line extends into lateral mass of the axis

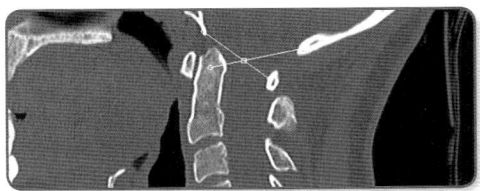

Figure 92.1 How to calculate the Powers' ratio.

Treatment

The basis of treatment in upper cervical spine injuries is based on the stability of the spine. Until the spine can be assessed, it should be regarded as unstable. The patient's prognosis and concurrent injuries, age and co-morbidities should be taken into account when suggesting any treatment.

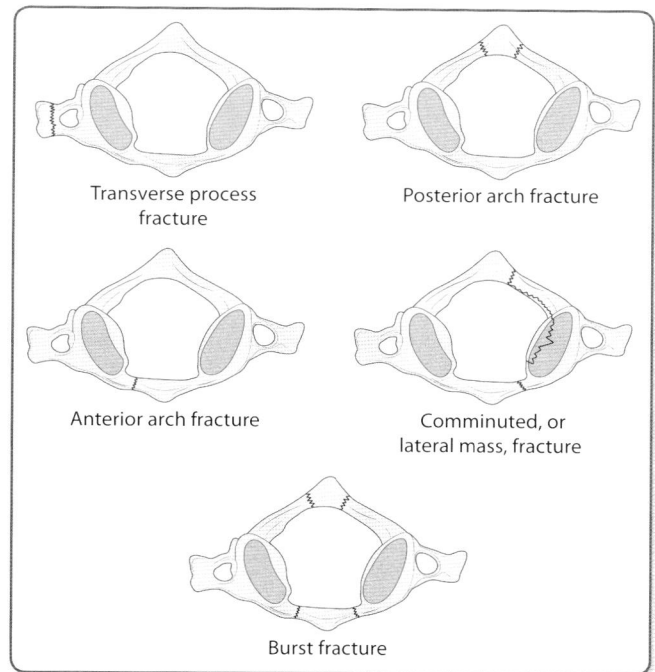

Figure 92.2 Classification of fractures to the C1/'Atlas' vertebra.

Occipital condyle fracture

This may be managed in a semi-rigid cervical orthosis for 6 weeks if stable, requiring occipitocervical fusion if not. This fusion is also the mainstay of treatment of occipitocervical and atlanto-occipital dissociations.

A C1 fracture with an uninjured transverse cervical ligament

This may be managed in a semi-rigid cervical orthosis for 6 weeks, but ligamentous injury mandates either occipitocervical or C1–C2 fusion.

C2 fractures

The management of C2 fractures depends on the risk of nonunion and the age and physiological reserve of the patient, as well as the degree of displacement.
- Odontoid peg:
  - Types 1 and 3 can be managed in a semi-rigid cervical orthosis
  - Type 2 fractures in young patients should be managed in a halo-vest or with internal fixation due to the high risk of nonunion
  - Elderly patients with type 2 fractures are managed very differently. The halo-vest and even semi-rigid cervical orthoses can create significant soft tissue problems and are often poorly tolerated. In this case, a soft cervical collar can be considered if the patient is not a surgical candidate.
- Levine and Edwards I
  - Semi-rigid cervical orthosis for 6 weeks
- Levine and Edwards II
  - Halo-vest immobilisation for 6–12 weeks, may require reduction with traction (contraindicated if the primary fracture line is horizontal)
  - Consider fusion if >5 mm displacement
    - Anterior C2/C3 interbody fusion
    - Posterior C1–C3 instrumented fusion
    - Bilateral C2 trans-pars interarticularis screws

Complications

Neurological injury remains the most significant complication of these injuries. Most dissociations or dislocations are fatal and hence rarely diagnosed in the injured patient who reaches hospital.

Late displacement of the fracture can occur, so vigilance is required. Specific complications include:
- With halo-vest: Pressure sores, skull vault injuries, pin site infection
- With semi-rigid cervical orthosis: Pressure sores, difficulty with feeding in elderly patients

Nonunion can occur with any fracture but is particularly common in type II odontoid peg fractures due to the poor blood supply of the fracture site. Risk factors for nonunion include >5 mm displacement, comminution, patient age over 50 years, angulation of the fracture fragment of more than >10° and delayed presentation.

Further reading

Fisher CG, Dvorak MF, Leith J. Wing PC. Comparison of outcomes for unstable lower cervical flexion teardrop fractures managed with halo thoracic vest versus anterior corpectomy and plating. Spine 2002; 27:160–166.

Koivikko MP, Kiuru MJ, Koskinen SK, et al. Factors associated with nonunion in conservatively-treated type-II fractures of the odontoid process. J Bone Joint Surg Br 2004; 86B:1146–1151.

Saltzherr TP, Fung Kon Jin PHP, Beenen LFM, Vandertop WP, Goslings JC. Diagnostic imaging of cervical spine injuries following blunt trauma: A review of the literature and practical guideline. Injury 2009; 40:795–800.

Related topics of interest

- *Topic 93* Spine – cord injury
- *Topic 94* Spine – subaxial cervical fractures and dislocations
- *Topic 95* Spine – thoracic and lumbar fractures

93 Spine – cord injury

Key points

- Spinal cord injuries (SCIs) are debilitating and life-changing
- Early recognition, documentation and management help limit disability, inform prognosis and preserve quality of life

Epidemiology

Spinal cord injury is a potential complication of any injury to the spine, whether fracture or dislocation. The incidence in the United Kingdom is estimated to be up to 16 per million. 75% of these cases are due to trauma, and of these cases up to 60% are due to injury to the cervical spine. The proportion of complete and incomplete SCIs is approximately equal. Road traffic collisions are the most common mechanism of injury with men affected significantly more than women at a mean age of 19 years old.

Pathophysiology

Acute, traumatic SCI occurs by two different mechanisms: primary injury occurs when the initial deforming force of the injury transfers energy, damaging the spinal cord; and secondary injury is mediated by complex biochemical and inflammatory cascades, which cause further cellular damage including ischaemia and free-radical production over the subsequent days and weeks.

The anatomical variation within the spinal canal makes the cervical spine particularly prone to SCI, primarily due to its high level of mobility and pendulum effect of the head. The spinal cord is relatively large compared to the canal in the cervical region, leaving little room for deformity to occur before the cord is injured. The thoracolumbar junction, in contrast, has a more capacious canal and narrower cord with much less flexibility.

The Torg ratio (of anteroposterior dimensions of the spinal canal to the vertebral body) has an inverse correlation with likelihood of SCI, with a figure of <0.8 indicating relative spinal stenosis.

Different mechanisms of injury are associated with different types of SCI.

Clinical assessment

A detailed assessment of peripheral and central nervous system function is mandatory. Documentation of this assessment has been simplified by the American Spinal Injuries Association (ASIA) chart (not shown here), which allows an accurate and reproducible assessment of the patient's level of function whilst aiding classification of the injury.

It is essential to identify the spinal level of the injury: this informs the prognosis and decisions in the intensity of care required. Tests of movement pinpoint the myotomes affected by the injury and identify the corresponding spinal level (**Table 93.1**). The degree of injury is classified on a scale of A to E, according to the ASIA classification system (**Table 93.2**).

The sensory cord injury level is defined as the most caudal level with normal neurological function whilst the motor cord injury level is defined as the most caudal level with a Medical Research Council (MRC) power grade of 3/5 or better. The motor level

Table 93.1 Myotomes and corresponding motor function

Motor function	Myotome
Diaphragm	C3-C4-C5
Shrugging shoulders	C4
Flex elbows	C5, C6
Extend elbows	C7
Abduct fingers	C8
Active chest expansion	T1-T12
Hip flexion	L2
Knee extension	L3-L4
Ankle dorsiflexion	L5-S1
Ankle plantar flexion	S1-S2
Eversion of foot	L5
Inversion of foot	L4

is thought to be more sensitive at predicting outcome than the sensory level.

Injury at or above C5 is highly likely to require some form of respiratory support, with functional outcomes improving as the level becomes more caudal.

Assessment should be alert to spinal shock, flaccid areflexia occurring after injury to the spinal cord. This usually resolves within 48 hours of injury, signified by the return of the bulbocavernosus reflex. A full assessment of the injury cannot be made until resolution, and initial assessments must be considered in this context.

Neurogenic shock is an equally important but distinct phenomenon. Mediated by loss of sympathetic tone below the level of the injury, it leads to loss of systemic vascular resistance manifesting in uncontrolled vasodilatation and venous pooling. In its truest form with a cervical lesion, a bradycardia is seen which does not respond to this peripheral vasodilatation. This requires management in the intensive care unit.

Sacral sparing (of the sacral nerve roots), indicated by voluntary external anal sphincter contraction and pin-prick sensory preservation confers a better prognosis and suggests an incomplete SCI.

Assessment of the patient should identify and manage any other, nonspinal injuries.

Investigations

Imaging of the bony and soft tissue anatomy of the spine is mandatory in the assessment of spinally injured patients. Plain film radiography for this has been superseded by CT scan for bony injury and MRI for soft tissues and the spinal cord. The British Orthopaedic Association Standard for Trauma 8 (BOAST 8) mandates that all centres managing patients with acute SCI should have 24-hour access to these modalities. High levels of suspicion of other organ system injuries, masked by the cord injury, are paramount when planning investigations.

Classification

The ASIA system (**Table 93.2**) is universal, reliable and reproducible. There are a number

Table 93.2 The ASIA classification system for spinal cord injury

Classification	Features
A	Complete cord injury No sensory or motor function below the level of injury
B	Incomplete Sensory but no motor function below the level of injury
C	Incomplete Motor and sensory function below the level of injury ≥50% of muscle groups have ≤MRC 2/5
D	Incomplete Motor and sensory function below the level of injury ≥50% of muscle groups have ≥MRC 3/5
E	Normal motor and sensory function below the level of injury

of classically described clinical pictures of SCI, including those in **Table 93.3**.

Treatment

The immediate priority is the prevention of secondary cord injury. This requires immobilisation of the injured spine, careful monitoring of perfusion and oxygenation (a mean arterial pressure >80 mmHg should be maintained) and associated fluid balance. This is best managed in the intensive care setting, where invasive monitoring and ventilatory support are available.

The role of corticosteroids and emergent spinal cord decompression remains controversial. Current evidence suggests that outcomes are similar at 1 year, regardless of corticosteroid administration, with higher early morbidity in the treatment group. Early (within 24 hours) spinal cord decompression and stabilisation seems to confer the best outcome.

Longer-term management is centred around the prevention of complications, such as those pertaining to bladder and bowel care or pressure sores. Rehabilitation at dedicated spinal injury centres is vital to optimise outcomes and can take many months.

Potential future treatments include the use of novel pharmaceutical agents and therapeutic hypothermia to prevent secondary cord injury.

Table 93.3 Patterns of spinal cord injury

Syndrome	Features	Prognosis
Central cord	Most common – 10% >50 years old Hyperextension of a stenotic cervical spine Predominantly distal, upper limb weakness Patchy sensory involvement	Fair
Anterior cord	2% Anterior spinal artery injury, flexion compression trauma or vasculitis Appearances similar to complete cord injury Dorsal column sparing (only anterior two-thirds of cord affected)	Poor
Posterior cord	<1% Dorsal columns only affected therefore motor, nociception and light touch are preserved	(No good data)
Brown–Séquard	4% Usually due to penetrating trauma Transverse hemisection of cord Ipsilateral motor and dorsal column loss Contralateral spinothalamic tract loss due to decussation levels	Good
Conus medullaris	Injury at the level of conus medullaris Unusual patterns of injury with mixed upper and lower motor neurone signs	(No good data)
SCIWORA	Distraction injury without spinal column injury Due to normal anatomical cord tethering and traction	Good

Complications

Immediate
- Death – up to 50% of patients with complete spinal cord lesions

Early
- Respiratory – pneumonia due to inability to clear secretions
- Skin – pressure sores
- Bladder – atonic bladder requires intermittent catheterisation
- Bowel – atonic rectum requires manual evacuation

Late
- Disuse osteoporosis
- Joint contractures

Further reading

Bracken MB. Steroids for acute spinal cord injury. Cochrane Database Syst Rev 2012; 1:CD001046.

Fehlings MG, Vaccaro A, Wilson JR, et al. Early versus delayed decompression for traumatic cervical spinal cord injury: results of the Surgical Timing in Acute Spinal Cord Injury Study (STASCIS). PLoS One 2012; 7:e32037.

Related topics of interest

- *Topic 92* Spine – atlas and axis cervical fractures and dislocations
- *Topic 94* Spine – subaxial cervical fractures and dislocations
- *Topic 95* Spine – thoracic and lumbar fractures

94 Spine – subaxial cervical fractures and dislocations

Key points
- Subaxial refers to vertebral levels C3–C7
- Fractures or dislocations at these levels are potentially unstable injuries with significant associated morbidity if not detected early
- Neurological examination and imaging are mandatory in all patients with a suspected cervical spine injury
- Assessment of these injuries often requires cross-sectional imaging with both CT scan and MRI

Epidemiology

Eighty per cent of all cervical spine injuries involve the subaxial cervical spine with C6 and C7 the two most commonly injured vertebrae. The mechanism of injury is almost always blunt trauma, most commonly sustained in road traffic collisions or falls from height. The energy required to cause injuries tends to be inversely proportional to the patient's age.

Pathophysiology

The type of injury depends largely upon the force vectors involved in the injury and the position of the head and cervical spine when these forces are applied.
- Vertical loading in a forward-flexed position is capable of producing a bifacet dislocation (**Figure 94.1**). If lateral flexion and/or a rotatory force vector is applied, a unifacet dislocation can occur
- Axial loading causes compression-type fractures with the position of the load dictating the type of fracture (anterior wedge, posterior with disc extrusion). When combined with slight flexion, burst fractures can occur. Axial loading can also cause intervertebral disc rupture in any position but tends to be more common in lateral flexion +/− rotation.

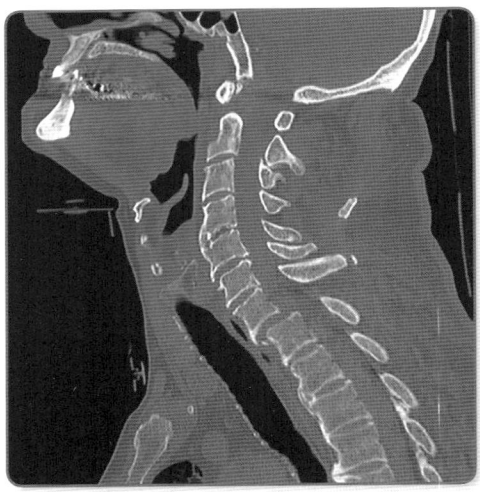

Figure 94.1 A bifacet fracture dislocation of C7 on T1.

- Axial compression in the anatomical position or with minimal forward flexion can cause a teardrop fracture.
- Extension injuries can also cause teardrop avulsion fractures and should not be confused with the more significant axial compression type (**Figure 94.2**). This often occurs at C2.

Clinical assessment

A cervical spine injury should be suspected in all high-energy injuries and in polytrauma. Prehospital triple-immobilisation is now ubiquitous and so patients are likely to arrive with cervical spine control in place.

Any assessment of the cervical spine should include a comprehensive assessment of the central and peripheral nervous system with completion of an American Spinal Injuries Association chart. In the unconscious, confused or agitated patient this is complicated and meticulous documentation is key. When the patient has

Spine – subaxial cervical fractures and dislocations

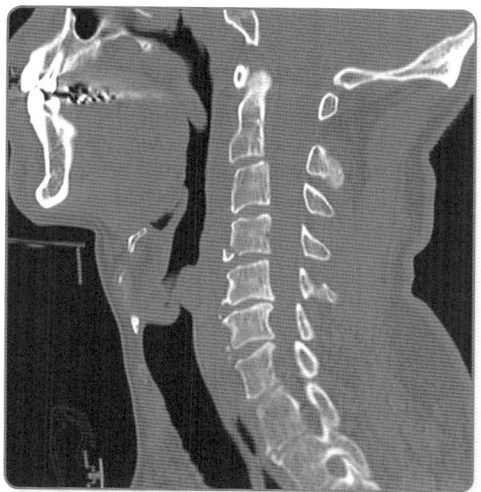

Figure 94.2 An avulsion type teardrop fracture at the anteroinferior border of C4.

significant neurological injury, secondary survey is difficult and must be undertaken with great care to ensure significant injuries are not missed.

In high cervical spine injuries with neurological injury, thorough assessment of the patient's respiratory function is also vital due to the potential for phrenic nerve (C3–C5) paralysis.

Due to the proximity of the vertebral arteries to the upper cervical spine, these can also complicate fractures and dislocations with resultant neurological sequaelae.

Investigations

Plain radiography

This comprises three views, anteroposterior (AP), lateral and odontoid process/open mouth view. To be considered adequate the AP and lateral must include the C7–T1 junction.

Flexion and extension lateral views can also be useful to assess for stability, although this must only be performed under the guidance of a spinal surgeon. They are rarely used in the acute setting as they are difficult to obtain when muscles are in spasm.

Particular care should be taken in assessing radiographs of the paediatric cervical spine due to the presence of physiological pseudosubluxation in children up to 8 years old.

Computed tomography

This is the most commonly performed investigation for traumatic subaxial cervical spine injuries and allows reconstructions in the sagittal and coronal planes. It does not provide information on the stabilising ligamentous structures. It is often used in place of plain film radiography.

Magnetic resonance imaging

This is mandatory for the patient with neurological dysfunction and a normal CT scan, and should be considered in all but the most minor cervical spine injuries. It provides vital information on the integrity of the intervertebral discs and ligamentous structures, especially in pure facet dislocations without fracture. Magnetic resonance angiography should be performed if there is suspicion of a vertebral arterial injury.

Classification

The Allen and Ferguson classification is primarily a research tool and is not routinely used in clinical practice. A radiographic descriptive classification of the pattern of injury is more commonly employed, and helps guide management. These include (often in combination):

- Compression fractures
- Burst fractures
- Hyperextension injuries (often discoligamentous)
- Flexion-distraction injuries
- Facet dislocations or fractures
- Spinous or transverse process fractures

Treatment

Management of any spinal fracture requires an understanding of its stability. Injuries which are often considered unstable, such as a unifacet dislocation, may be found to be stable if they are discovered late. The assessment of stability requires investigation of the posterior longitudinal ligament with MRI.

Injuries considered stable include teardrop avulsion fractures and mild compression fractures with no spinal cord compression or kyphosis, as well as transverse and spinous process fractures. These can be treated with a semi-rigid cervical orthosis.

Any suggestion of instability requires surgical reduction and fixation, usually with instrumented fusion and supplemental plate fixation. Indicators of instability are:
- Ligamentous injury and facet subluxation/dislocation
- Loss of initial reduction or irreducibility
- Vertebral subluxation >20%
- Discoligamentous injuries
- Anterior and posterior ligamentous injuries/fractres
- Loss of vertebral height >25%
- Kyphosis 15°

If spinal cord compression is occurring due to an anterior wedge or burst fracture then surgery requires an anterior approach for corpectomy, discectomy and fusion whilst any involvement of the posterior ligamentous structures may require posterior instrumentation also.

A pure unifacet dislocation may be managed by reduction, anterior cervical discectomy and interbody fusion. Bi-facet dislocation is a rare, absolute indication for a combined AP approach.

Complications

Immediate
- Death due to neurological injury and complete or incomplete spinal cord injury
- Nerve root injury may also occur due to disc herniation or compression from bony fragments

Early
- Worsening spinal cord injury due to haematoma or cord hypoxia
- Complications specific to the modality of management
- Radiculopathy

Late
- Degeneration of adjacent levels in the cervical spine after fusion
- Late deformity or kyphosis
- Nonunion of fusion

Further reading

Dvorak MF, Fisher CG, Fehlings MG, et al. The surgical approach to subaxial cervical spine injuries: an evidence-based algorithm based on the SLIC classification system. Spine 2007; 32:2620–2629.

Saltzherr TP, Fung Kon Jin PHP, Beenen LFM, Vandertop WP, Goslings JC. Diagnostic imaging of cervical spine injuries following blunt trauma: A review of the literature and practical guideline. Injury 2009; 40:795–800.

Related topics of interest

- Topic 92 Spine – atlas and axis cervical fractures and dislocations
- Topic 93 Spine – cord injury
- Topic 102 Whiplash

95 Spine – thoracic and lumbar fractures

Key points
- Thoracic and lumbar fractures are relatively common injuries in the polytrauma setting, but also readily missed
- Check for noncontiguous spinal fractures
- Neurological examination and documentation with an American Spinal Injuries Association (ASIA) chart is mandatory

Epidemiology

The epidemiology of thoracolumbar fractures is complex and varies widely with geography. The developing and developed worlds have differing profiles, due to a variety of socioeconomic factors. In the Western world, approximately two-thirds of young patients who sustain a traumatic fracture are male, whilst older patients tend to sustain atraumatic, osteoporotic fractures and are predominantly female.

The most commonly affected region of the thoracolumbar spine to be affected is the thoracolumbar transitional region (T11–L2) where almost two thirds of fractures occur. This is mainly due to the change between the well-supported and rigid thoracic spine to the much more mobile lumbar region, which provides little opportunity for dispersion of injuring forces.

Pathophysiology

Several mechanisms and vectors of injury exist, and often occur in combination. These include:
- Compression – axial or flexion
- Distraction or hyperextension
- Rotation
- Translation

Distraction and rotational injuries tend towards the highest severity with greatest risk of neurological compromise, whilst compression injuries have associated neurological injury far less frequently.

A complex and severe injury, the Chance fracture involves a distraction force beginning posteriorly, injuring the lamina, pedicles and exiting anteriorly through the intervertebral disc and vertebra. This is commonly associated with lap-belt injuries in road traffic collisions. The force is horizontal and is associated with significant visceral injuries as it exits anteriorly, sometimes also associated with sternal fractures. In one study, more than 60% of patients with a Chance fracture had also sustained life-threatening abdominal visceral injuries.

Clinical assessment

A full and timely neurological assessment of any patient with a suspected thoracolumbar fracture is mandatory. The ASIA has published a comprehensive assessment tool which provides a simple method of recording initial and on-going neurological function.

Any deficit must be documented and promptly investigated, remembering that this can mask other skeletal and visceral injuries.

Spinal fractures in young patients often result from high-energy mechanisms and other injuries to the axial skeleton occur in approximately one-third of patients. Femoral neck, calcaneal and pelvic fractures are easily missed and head, chest and long-bone injuries can complicate management.

Open fractures are rare but can cause significant cord damage, so must be identified early and managed appropriately.

Investigations

Prior to the widespread use of multislice CT in spinal injuries and the polytraumatised patient, thoracolumbar injuries were missed in up to 20% of patients. Care should be taken, however, in the interpretation of these studies, as they misrepresent the maximal degree of displacement which has occurred and are also performed supine and hence place no physiological axial load through the spine.

For this reason, plain radiographs may be performed in the standing position to give more information on the dynamic component of spinal instability. This is not routinely applicable to the acutely injured patient.

Full assessment of spinal stability can only be made with an MRI to demonstrate the complex osseoligamentous relationships of the thoracolumbar spine. Full spinal precautions should be undertaken until injury to the spine has been ruled-out. Any evidence of neurological injury is an absolute indication for MRI.

Classification

The two most commonly used classification systems are the Arbeitsgemeinschaft für Osteosynthesefragen (AO) thoracolumbar injury classification system (TLICS) (**Figure 95.1** and **Table 95.1**) and Denis.

The AO system has three main categories of increasing severity and multiple subgroups and specifications to classify most fractures. It has been shown to have poor inter- and intraobserver reliability.
- Type A: Compression injuries
- Type B: Distraction injuries
- Type C: Rotational injuries

The Denis classification is based on a 'three-column theory' of spinal anatomy:
- Anterior:
  - Anterior longitudinal ligament
  - Anterior annulus fibrosus
  - Anterior two thirds of vertebral body
- Middle:
  - Posterior third of vertebral body
  - Posterior annulus fibrosus
  - Posterior longitudinal ligament
- Posterior:
  - Posterior elements
    - Pedicles

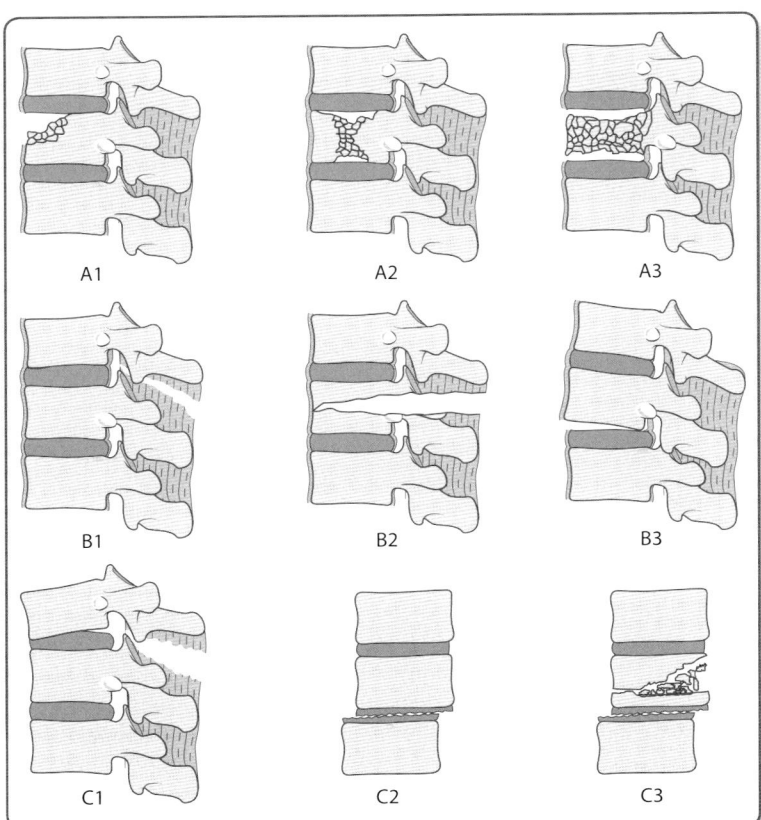

Figure 95.1 The The AOSpine Thoracolumbar Injury classification system main types and groups.

Table 95.1 The AOSpine classification system

Types	Groups	Subgroups
A: Compression	A1: Impaction	A1.1, A1.2, A1.3
	A2: Split	A2.1, A2.2, A2.3
	A3: Burst	A3.1, A3.2, A3.3
B: Distraction	B1: Posterior ligamentous	B1.1, B1.2
	B2: Posterior osseoligamentous	B2.1, B2.2, B2.3
	B3: Anterior	B3.1, B3.2, B3.3
C: Rotation	C1: 'A' with rotation	C1.1, C1.2
	C2: 'B' with rotation	C2.1, C2.2, C2.3
	C3: Shear	C3.1, C3.2

- Facet joints
- Lamina
- Spinous processes
- Posterior ligaments

Denis proposed that the middle column was key to stability and hence injury to it would render the spine unstable. Whilst this system has better inter- and intraobserver reliability than the AO system, it still has significant inherent inaccuracy.

Numerous other classification systems exist, all with advantages and disadvantages. The most important factor in planning management is the stability of the spine and consequent neurological injury. This stability can be defined as the ability of the spinal column, under normal physiological loading, to maintain anatomical alignment sufficiently to prevent compromise to the neurovascular structures contained therein and prevent disabling pain or deformity.

Treatment

There is a lack of level 1 or 2 evidence to support decision making in thoracolumbar fractures. Indications for operative intervention are subjective and vary between centres and surgeons. The aims of treatment are the:
- Restoration of alignment
- Restoration of spinal stability
- Prevention of neurological dysfunction

Studies have shown benefit in early (<12 h) stabilisation and decompression whilst others have shown no benefit in surgery earlier than 72 hours postinjury. A reasonable rationale can be summarised as below.

Nonoperative

Indications for nonoperative management include:
- Absence of neurological deficit
- Stable injury:
  - Preserved alignment
  - 'Single' column injury
  - Low energy injury
  - Preservation of trunk control

The mainstays of nonoperative management include orthotic bracing and bed-rest. Traction for thoracolumbar injuries has become much less common in the Western world.

Operative

Indications for operative management include:
- Incomplete paraplegia or early improvement in neurological status
- Worsening neurologic deficit
- Spinal cord compression
- Fracture-dislocation
- Severe ligamentous injury

Operative treatment has the benefits of allowing early mobilization in unstable injuries, easier nursing care, more rapid pain relief and helps prevent late neurological compromise. It does, however, subject the patient to the surgical risks of infection and iatrogenic neural injury.

Operative treatment of fracture dislocations is the preserve of the specialist and frequently involves posterior instrumentation with neural element decompression, often with indirect reduction techniques (**Figure 95.2**).

Around 90% of the axial compressive force in the thoracolumbar spine is borne by the anterior column, so posterior instrumentation alone may not be sufficient to stabilise the spine. Anterior instrumentation of the lumbar spine is indicated if indirect reduction cannot achieve adequate neural decompression or if posterior reduction and stabilisation does not afford sufficient reduction. If the intervertebral disc is also involved in the injury, then intervertebral fusion may be indicated.

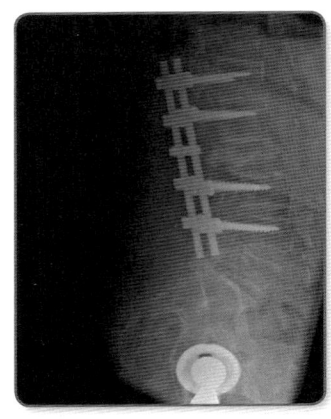

Figure 95.2 Lateral postoperative radiograph of posterior instrumentation for spinal fracture.

Complications
Immediate
- Neural injury at the time of fracture. Good prognostic indicators are:
  - Incomplete spinal cord lesions
  - Sacral sparing
  - Spinal shock <24 hours' duration
  - Early return of deep tendon reflexes

Early
- Haematoma
  - Local or central neurological deterioration
- Pressure sores
- Respiratory/urinary tract infection
- Cardiovascular compromise from neurogenic shock

Late
- Disability due to deformity
- Pseudarthrosis of fractures
- Morbidity from ongoing neural injury

Further reading

Denis F. The three column spine and its significance in the classification of acute thoraco-lumbar spinal injuries. Spine 1983; 8:817–831.

Knop C, Blauth M, Bühren V, et al. Surgical treatment of injuries of the thoracolumbar transition – 3: Follow-up examination. Results of a prospective multi-center study by the 'Spinal' Study Group of the German Society of Trauma Surgery. Unfallchirurg 2001; 104:583–600.

Vaccaro AR1, Zeiller SC, Hulbert RJ, et al. The thoracolumbar injury severity score; a proposed treatment algorithm. J Spinal Disord Tech 2005; 18:209–215.

Related topics of interest

- Topic 92 Spine – atlas and axis cervical fractures and dislocations
- Topic 93 Spine – cord injury
- Topic 94 Spine – subaxial cervical fractures and dislocations

96 Tibial pilon fractures

Key points

- Pilon fractures are high-energy injuries which usually require staged management
- The majority require operative treatment
- Patients should be warned of the high risk of secondary osteoarthritis in the ankle or other adjacent joints, even with good fixation

Epidemiology

Pilon fractures are intra-articular fractures of the distal tibia with metaphyseal extension. They usually result from high-energy trauma, in particular axial loading associated with falls from a height, or sudden torsional loading associated with motor vehicle accidents. They represent only 1% of tibial fractures and the incidence is highest amongst young men aged 15–25 years. Topliss and Atkins identified two main fracture families, a sagittal one where the primary fracture line runs from anterior to posterior, and a coronal family where the fracture runs from lateral to medial. Sagittal fractures tend to occur in the context of high-energy with varus loading whilst coronal injuries usually occur in older patients as a result of lower force and valgus loading.

Pathophysiology

There are two common mechanisms of injury, both of which relate to the relative strength of the talus in comparison with the distal tibia. With axial loading, as seen in a fall from a height, the talus is driven against the tibia and acts as a splitting wedge. In torsional injuries the distal tibia resists talar rotation by both bony congruence and the ligamentous stabilisers of the tibiotalar joint. This continues with increasing force until a sudden catastrophic failure of the distal tibia occurs, resulting in multiple fracture lines. Due to the minimal soft tissue coverage of the distal tibia, these injuries tend to result in shearing and devitalisation of the soft tissues causing significant injury.

Clinical assessment

The patient's normal level of function, employment, overall health and specific comorbidities and smoking status should be elicited in a thorough history.

On examination, inspect for the degree of soft tissue injury and exclude an open injury, compartment syndrome or neurovascular injury. Pilon fractures should be grossly aligned and immobilised in a below-knee backslab. Gross reduction is acceptable and repeated attempts should not be made to improve an adequate position; this is uncomfortable for the patient and these inherently unstable injuries require operative fixation, regardless of the quality of initial reduction.

Investigations

Plain radiographs including a lateral and mortise view of the ankle should be obtained. These complex intra-articular fractures will usually require further imaging with CT, either immediately or after the application of a temporising external fixator. This permits maximal understanding of the fracture configuration and planning of the surgical strategy and approach.

Classification

The Ruedi–Allgower classification (**Table 96.1**) is probably the most commonly used system. This may, however, lack sufficient complexity for the fracture patterns seen in these injuries. The AO-OTA classification

Table 96.1 The Ruedi–Allgower system of Pilon fracture classification	
Type	Fracture pattern
I	Undisplaced fracture
II	Displaced fracture
III	Comminution (multifragmentary high-energy fractures)

takes a different approach, classifying the injuries as 'B-type' partial articular fractures (43-B1 to 43-B3) where part of the articular surface remains attached to the metaphysis, and 'C-type' complete articular fractures (43-C1 to 43-C3) where no attachment to the metaphysis remains.

Treatment

The aims of surgery are to restore or improve articular congruity, to achieve stable and accurate alignment of the metaphysis in relation to the diaphysis to restore the mechanical axis of the limb. This should be performed in such a way that early, pain-free union is achieved without infection. The risk of secondary osteoarthritis following these injuries is significant and in high-energy injuries the surgical aims include preparing the bone stock for fusion of the ankle joint at a later date.

Nonoperative

Pilon fractures are rarely suitable for nonoperative management. In unusual circumstances where the fracture is absolutely undisplaced, where there is a minimal step in the articular surface or where the patient is not a candidate for surgery due to comorbidity, these injuries may be treated with immobilisation in a below-knee plaster cast and careful monitoring for the development of skin breakdown and loss of position.

Operative

Following the application of a temporising external fixator (**Figure 96.1**) and obtaining a CT scan, operative intervention is usually planned for around 10–14 days postinjury. When considering the CT images, it must be appreciated that bony fragments tend to be attached to specific ligamentous structures around the ankle and so there may be a functional diastasis which must be addressed (**Figure 96.2**).

Open reduction and fixation with a precontoured periarticular plate is the commonest strategy for operative

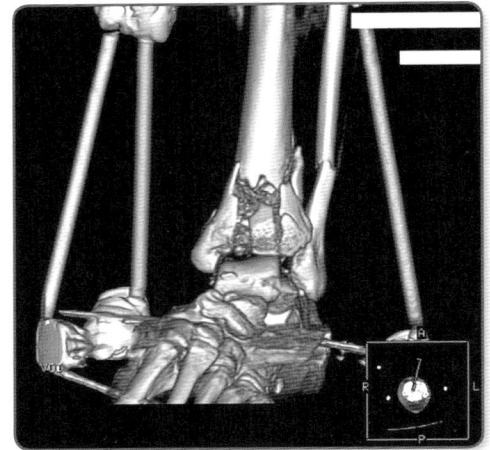

Figure 96.1 CT 3D reconstruction demonstrating a complete articular fracture with comminution along with the temporising external fixator applied before scanning.

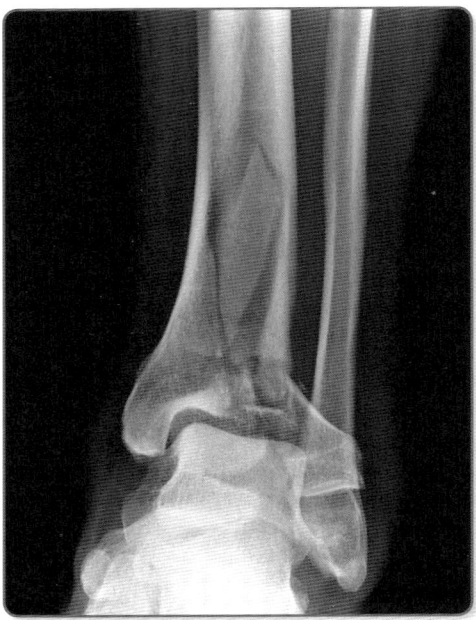

Figure 96.2 AO B-type fracture with partial articular involvement. Here the 'functional diastasis' must be recognised during fixation as the syndesmotic ligaments are attached to the anterior and posterior lateral tibial fragments.

intervention in these injuries (**Figure 96.3**). The principles of fixation are to reduce the articular surface anatomically and hold it with absolute stability whilst bridging the soft metaphyseal bone to achieve relative stability and healing with callus. The surgical approach will be dictated by the orientation of fracture fragments and some fractures may require a two-incision technique.

Historically, fixation of the fibula was performed at the same operative sitting as the application of an external fixator, but this is now discouraged as it may compromise the ability to perform an anterolateral approach for definitive fixation. The commonest approach is an anterior one which utilises the plane between the extensor digitorum longus and extensor hallucis longus. Care must be taken during superficial dissection to avoid branches of the superficial peroneal nerve, and during deep dissection to avoid the neurovascular bundle containing the deep peroneal nerve and dorsalis pedis artery.

Fractures with severe metaphyseal comminution may benefit from definitive external fixation with a circular frame. This reduces the degree of soft tissue compromise and permits early weight-bearing, whilst also offering a number of options for geometric correction and the management of bone loss by distraction or transport. In cases of severe intra-articular derangement, this may be the only reconstructive option. The technique mostly relies on the indirect reduction of fracture fragments with tensioned fine wires, although small open approaches may be used if reduction is challenging. 'Olive wires' have a metal bead formed around the wire which may be used to reduce a bony fragment and hold it in place simultaneously.

Complications

Immediate

- Vascular injury – each of the main arterial supplies in the leg (the anterior tibial, posterior tibial and peroneal arteries) may be injured at the time of fracture and, rarely, during fixation
- Neurological injury – any of the nerves supplying the foot may be injured during injury or fixation
- The deep peroneal nerve and dorsalis pedis artery are at particular risk during the anterior approach to the distal tibia

Early

- Infection – This represents a catastrophic complication of operative treatment of a pilon fracture. Treatment involves removal of the fixation, radical debridement of affected bone and soft tissue and restabilisation. This is often performed

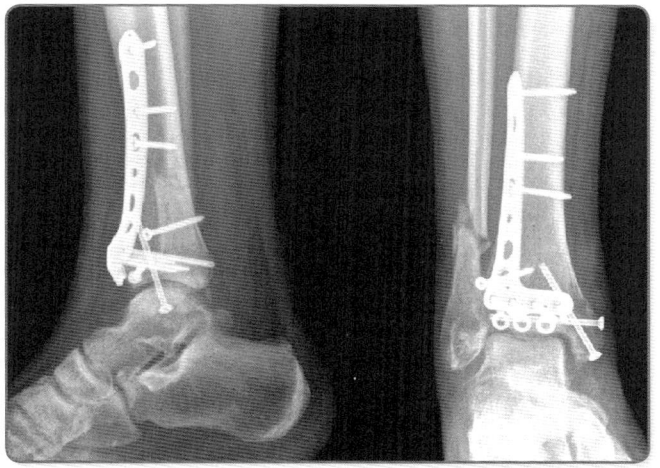

Figure 96.3 Pilon fracture after fixation.

as a staged approach with temporising external fixation. Plastic surgical coverage of the distal tibia usually requires a lengthy free tissue transfer procedure as local rotational flaps are rarely possible in this region
- Compartment syndrome – this may in fact be evident on initial presentation, or evolve during the early stages of an admission for pilon fracture

Late
- Malunion – This may be either angular or rotational and can result in inefficient gait and secondary degenerative change at adjacent joints
- Nonunion – This may complicate up to 10% of tibial fractures and can require secondary treatment with external fixation and bone grafting techniques

Further reading

Sirkin M, Sanders R, DiPasquale T, Herscovici D Jr. A staged protocol for soft tissue management in the treatment of complex pilon fractures. J Orthop Trauma 2004; 18:S32–38.

Sirkin M, Sanders R. The treatment of pilon fractures. Orthop Clin North Am 2001; 32:91–102.

Topliss CJ, Jackson M, Atkins RM. Anatomy of pilon fractures of the distal tibia. J Bone Joint Surg Br 2005; 87:692–697.

Related topics of interest

- *Topic 68* Open fractures
- *Topic 85* Principles of operative management of fractures
- *Topic 96* Tibial pilon fractures

97 Tibial plateau fractures

Key points

- Proximal tibial articular fractures have a wide spectrum of severity
- Fracture pattern and injury mechanism dictate surgical strategy
- Restoration of limb axis alignment is the most important factor influencing outcome
- High-energy fractures require staged management

Epidemiology

Fractures of the tibial plateau account for 1% of all fractures and include a wide spectrum of fracture patterns: 55–70% are isolated to the lateral plateau, 10–25% are isolated to the medial plateau and 10–30% are bicondylar. There is a range of severity, from low energy minimally displaced fractures, through to high-energy fractures with significant comminution and depression of the articular surface, and extension to the metaphysis and diaphysis.

They are often associated with major soft tissue involvement including closed degloving, open fracture, dislocation, compartment syndrome and neurovascular injury.

There is a bimodal demographic distribution, with high-energy injuries seen mainly in young men (<40 years), and lower energy injuries typically seen in older, osteoporotic women (>60 years).

Pathophysiology

The tibial plateau is fractured when subjected to either an excessive valgus or varus force, or in combination with an axial force. The fracture pattern varies according to the direction and magnitude of the injuring force, and the bone quality. In young patients, the injury mechanism is typically low energy from sports or falls, or high energy from road traffic collision. As the fracture energy increases, the comminution in the articular and metaphyseal components also increase. There is a high rate of associated ligamentous and meniscal injury (30–50%). In elderly patients with weak osteoporotic bone the mechanism may be a simple fall, associated ligamentous injury is less common.

Clinical assessment

The knee is typically swollen and may be deformed. Clinical examination of the knee itself without anaesthesia is painful and adds little to the radiographic diagnosis. Neurologic and vascular examination of the leg and foot is mandatory. Particular attention must be paid to distal pulses and perfusion (due to the proximity of the popliteal trifurcation directly posterior to the proximal tibia), and the common peroneal nerve which may be injured on its course around the fibular neck.

A careful assessment of the soft tissue envelope must be made, including prompt identification of any open injury. In closed fractures the skin should be assessed for fracture blisters and closed degloving. Tibial plateau fractures carry a substantial risk of compartment syndrome (11%). This can often occur in open fractures. A high index of suspicion and serial examinations are essential. Compartment pressure monitoring or emergent fasciotomies may also be required.

Investigations

Plain anteroposterior (AP) and lateral radiographs should be obtained. Historic classification systems are mainly based of these plain images; however, it is often felt these images alone are insufficient to adequately evaluate the fracture. Therefore, CT with multiplanar 3D reconstruction, should be obtained for all tibial plateau fractures. This allows a detailed evaluation of the fracture pattern especially the location of splits in the cortex, which assists preoperative planning including incision placement.

CT angiography may be performed where vascular injury is suspected, and MRI is useful for assessment of the soft tissues including menisci and ligaments, although rarely used in the acute setting.

Classification

The Schatzker classification system is most commonly used. This describes the location and pattern of the fracture and is important in determining likely associated injuries, treatment and prognosis (**Table 97.1**). Alternatively, the AO-OTA classification can be used and is particularly helpful in research and communication. It describes fractures according to involvement of the articular surface (extra-articular, partial articular, complete articular), fracture pattern (e.g. simple, pure split, pure depression, split-depression, multi-fragmentary) and its location (medial/lateral plateau or both). In classifying the soft tissue component of the injury, the Tscherne classification is useful in closed fractures (**Table 97.2**). Open fractures are graded in accordance with the Gustilo-Anderson system.

Treatment

The ultimate goal is to achieve a stable, well-aligned, congruent joint with an early functional return, whilst avoiding infection. Nonoperative or operative methods may be preferable depending on the fracture pattern and patient factors. However, the single most important factor in achieving a successful outcome is the preservation or restoration of the normal mechanical axis of the limb, rather than the articular surface.

Nonoperative

The minimally displaced, stable variants of Schatzker I, II, or III, or any fracture in a patient who cannot withstand surgery may be treated nonoperatively. Partial or nonweight-bearing for 6–12 weeks combined with early range of movement with or without a hinged brace is typically followed by progression to full weight-bearing.

Operative

The aim of surgery is to anatomically restore the alignment of the limb as well as the articular surface by means of a stable fixation such that early range of movement can be permitted. Surgical treatment must be timed carefully, after thorough evaluation of the fracture pattern on cross-sectional imaging and careful assessment of the soft tissues. Meticulous handing of the soft tissues is critical to success. Various surgical approaches can be utilised depending on fracture pattern and fragment location, including minimally invasive techniques.

In general, surgery is indicated in the following:

Table 97.1 Schatzker classification of tibial plateau fractures

Type	Location	Pattern	Associated injuries	Prognosis
I	Lateral	Simple split	Lateral meniscus	Good
II	Lateral	Split-depression (**Figures 97.1–97.4**)	Lateral meniscus	May develop valgus deformity
III	Lateral	Pure depression Intact rim		Usually stable to early movement
IV	Medial	Shear fracture of medial condyle – essentially a 'knee fracture-dislocation'	Ligaments, menisci, popliteal artery, common peroneal nerve	Poor
V	Medial and lateral – bicondylar	Central metaphysis still connected to the diaphysis	Anterior cruciate ligament rupture Meniscal injuries	
VI	Bicondylar with metaphysis dissociated from diaphysis	Usually comminuted	Significant soft tissue injuries 35% are open	Poor

Tibial plateau fractures

Table 97.2 Tscherne classification of soft tissue injury		
Tscherne	Soft tissue injury	Typical fracture pattern
Closed grade 0	None or minimal	Simple, e.g. spiral fracture (low energy)
Closed grade 1	Superficial abrasion or skin contusion	Simple, e.g. transverse fracture (moderate energy)
Closed grade 2	Deep contaminated abrasions and localised skin or muscle contusions	Moderate, e.g. segmental fracture (higher energy)
Closed grade 3	Extensive skin contusion, destruction of muscle or subcutaneous tissue avulsion (closed degloving)	Complex, e.g. segmental fracture, crush, bone loss (high energy)

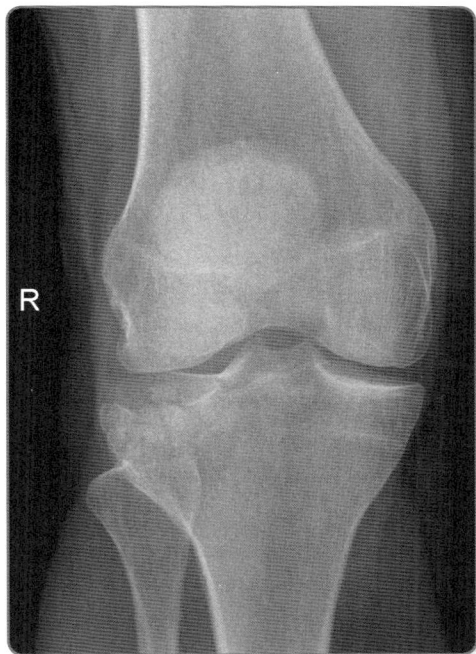

Figure 97.1 AP radiograph of split depression (type II) tibial plateau fracture.

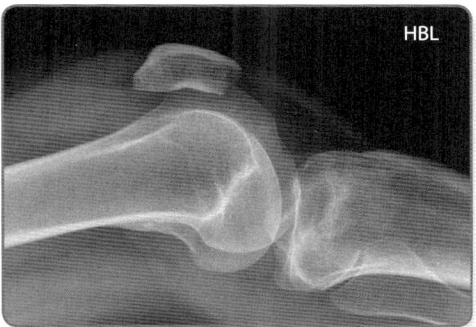

Figure 97.2 Lateral radiograph of a split depression (type II) tibial plateau fracture (same patient as in Figure 97.1).

- Articular step >2 mm
- Condylar widening >5 mm
- Instability of the knee joint
- All medial and bicondylar fractures
- Associated ligamentous or meniscal injury
- Polytrauma

Treatment can be described according to the Schatzker classification:

Type I – Undisplaced fractures can be treated nonoperatively. Displaced fractures should be anatomically reduced and stable internal fixation performed with lag screws or a buttress plate.

Type II – Minimally displaced fractures in a stable knee can be treated non-operatively, or with skeletal traction. For displaced fractures, anatomical reduction with elevation of the depressed fragment (bone graft or substitute may be used to support this) followed by stable internal fixation with raft screws should be performed.

Type III – These can be treated in a similar way to type II fractures, but they are typically more stable due to the retained integrity of the lateral rim. However, with significant displacement surgical fixation is preferred.

Type IV – Treatment is typically open reduction and internal fixation via a posteromedial approach. A lateral ligamentous injury may coexist and must be examined for after fixation of the fracture, as it may also require surgical repair to confer stability to the knee and allow early joint mobilisation.

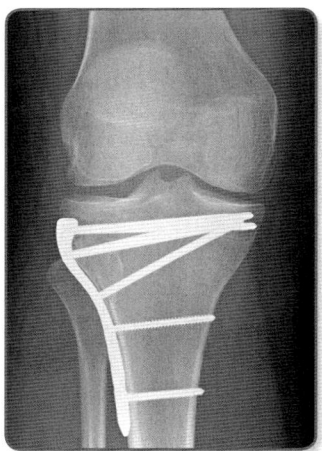

Figure 97.3 Postoperative AP radiograph of the same patient as Figure 97.1.

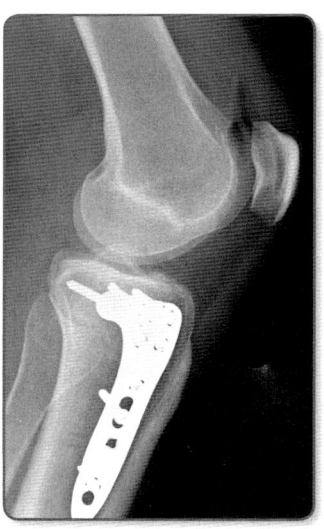

Figure 97.4 Postoperative lateral radiograph of the same patient as Figure 97.1.

Types V and VI – Early stable internal fixation and mobilisation is the ideal treatment option for these injuries, although nonoperative or traction techniques can be employed. Due to the high rate of associated compartment syndrome, wound breakdown and nonunion, a staged approach to surgical treatment is appropriate. A temporary external fixator spanning the knee is initially applied and the soft tissues (including any fasciotomies) are allowed to heal prior to definitive fixation. Definitive treatment may be with open reduction and internal fixation, or external fixation with a circular frame. Single or double approaches can be used for plating, with minimally invasive techniques often used in conjunction with fine wire circular fixation.

Complications

Immediate
- Vascular injury – popliteal artery laceration is rare but must always be assessed. It is particularly associated with type IV injuries
- Nerve injury – common peroneal nerve injury can occur with lateral plateau fractures or may be iatrogenic

Early
- Compartment syndrome – there is an 11% rate of compartment syndrome with tibial plateau fractures and a high index of suspicion is needed, along with swift treatment where it is suspected
- Infection may result from open fracture or badly timed surgery through injured soft tissue

Late
- Malunion can result from inadequate reduction, unstable fixation or implant failure and is common in Schatzker types IV and VI. This may lead to post-traumatic osteoarthritis
- Stiffness is common from scarring related to both traumatic injury and surgical treatment, as well as associated intra-articular soft tissue injury. This is a major cause of disability following tibial plateau fracture
- Post-traumatic osteoarthritis may occur in any tibial plateau fracture, but particularly where there is malalignment of the normal mechanical axis

Further reading

Koval KJ, Helfet DL. Tibial plateau fractures: evaluation and treatment. J Am Acad Orthop Surg 1995; 3:86–94.

Musahl V, Tarkin I, Kobbe P, et al. New trends and techniques in open reduction and internal fixation of fractures of the tibial plateau. J Bone Joint Surg Br 2009; 91:426–433.

Schatzker J, McBroom R, Bruce D. The tibial plateau fracture. The Toronto experience 1968–1975. Clin Orthop Relat Res 1979:94–104.

Related topics of interest

- *Topic 14* Compartment syndrome
- *Topic 61* Knee dislocations – multiligament injuries
- *Topic 68* Open fractures
- *Topic 85* Principles of operative management of fractures

98 Tibial shaft fractures

Key points
- Tibial fractures are the most common type of open fracture
- Compartment syndrome is common and must be excluded with serial clinical evaluation and double incision fasciotomy if any uncertainty exists
- Timely surgery is required
- Coverage of soft tissue defects in the tibia is challenging and early conjoint management with plastic surgeons is an audit standard in open fractures
- The aims of surgery are to restore the mechanical axis of the lower limb and achieve infection-free union

Epidemiology

Diaphyseal fractures of the tibia are both the commonest type of long bone fracture and also the commonest open fracture. The severity of injury relates to the age of the patient, the amount of energy transferred in the causative injury and the degree of soft tissue damage. There are two peaks of incidence; young patients who tend to sustain high-energy polytrauma and sports injuries, and older patients who sustain insufficiency fractures from low-energy mechanisms.

Pathophysiology

Where the tibia is subject to torsional forces, such as in sports injuries, a spiral fracture configuration tends to occur. Where a bending force has been applied, as with a leg hit by a car bumper, then there may be an oblique fracture (**Figure 98.1**). A 'bending wedge' fragment may occur if the tibia is subjected to simultaneous axial load (this may simply be the patient's own body weight). Pathological processes may result in transverse fractures, often from low-energy mechanisms.

There is very little soft tissue coverage over the tibia, in particular the anteromedial surface which is only covered by skin. This means that open injuries are common, occurring in approximately 25% of all tibial fractures.

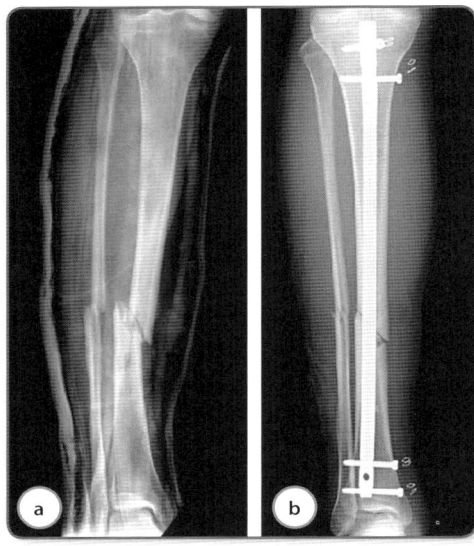

Figure 98.1 (a) An oblique tibial shaft fracture with a fibular fracture at the same level. This suggests a bending force of at least moderate energy was applied to the leg to cause this injury. Note the dressing under the plaster on the medial side which suggests that this was an open injury. (b) The same fracture after intramedullary nailing.

Clinical assessment

A careful history should be taken to elicit the circumstances of the injury, the patient's occupation, any co-morbidities and any history of smoking. Smoking increases the risk of delayed union and nonunion in tibial fractures and so smoking cessation should be discussed and support arranged if appropriate on admission.

Clinical examination should prioritise screening for compartment syndrome, detecting neurological or vascular injury and assessing open injuries. Compartment syndrome may occur in both high- and low-energy mechanisms and hence should be repeatedly screened for in each patient. The dorsalis pedis and posterior tibial pulses can be assessed in terms of both presence and nature of flow, along with capillary refill in the toes, to identify a vascular injury. Where there is any concern then further Doppler ultrasound assessment may be used or other imaging techniques such as CT angiography. Consultation with a vascular surgeon is appropriate if any uncertainty exists. Open injuries should be assessed and managed in line with the BOAST 4 standards (see Open fracture chapter).

The limb should be grossly aligned and the anterior border of the tibia gently palpated to identify any subcutaneous bone fragments which might cause skin necrosis whilst in plaster. An above knee plaster backslab should be applied for temporary pain relief.

Investigations

Plain anteroposterior (AP) and lateral radiographs should be obtained to assess the fracture pattern. Spiral fractures often extend into joint surfaces so views of both the knee and the ankle are particularly important in proximal or distal fractures respectively. Any intra-articular extension is best characterised by CT imaging.

Classification

There is no reliable prognostic classification of tibial shaft fractures guiding treatment. In practice, fractures should be described in terms of pattern and location; for example, 'There is a spiral fracture in the central third of the tibial diaphysis with an associated fibular fracture' conveys more important information than attempts at classification in this heterogeneous group of injuries.

Treatment

The aims of surgery are to achieve pain-free bony union of the tibia without infection, with normal mechanical alignment and adequate soft tissue cover, permitting a return to the patient's activities of daily living. Rotation or angular malalignment may cause secondary degeneration in adjacent joints and care must be taken intraoperatively to minimise this.

Nonoperative

Undisplaced diaphyseal fractures or those in patients who are not candidates for surgery may be treated nonoperatively. Such patients should have a well-moulded, above-knee plaster cast applied with particular attention paid to the avoidance of pressure areas. If the fracture is displaced, a general anaesthetic or sedation is generally required for reduction. The patient should remain nonweight-bearing for a minimum of 6 weeks and will require prophylaxis against deep vein thrombosis; this should be prescribed in line with trust guidelines but chemoprophylaxis will generally be required. The position of the fracture must be monitored weekly in the outpatient clinic for 4 weeks, with repeated radiographs to ensure alignment is maintained. A patellar tendon weight-bearing Sarmiento plaster cast may be applied at 6 weeks. Although the patient may bear weight in this cast, they require regular review to ensure the fit of the cast is maintained. Union takes between 3–6 months and removal of the cast is based on evidence of clinical and radiographic progression.

Operative

Many operative options exist for the treatment of diaphyseal tibial fractures, with intramedullary nailing the most commonly performed procedure. The technique is limited both proximally and distally by the level at which the nail can achieve purchase with locking bolts. Nails are inserted in an anterograde fashion using an incision over the patellar tendon, with the tibia reamed to permit a close fit between the nail and the diaphyseal isthmus. The patellar tendon itself can be either split or moved to one side in order to allow preparation of the tibia and passage of the nail. In fractures of the middle third of the tibia the mediolateral and AP alignment of the fracture tend to be well corrected by nail insertion itself. In proximal third fractures (**Figure 98.2**) there is a tendency for the fracture to angulate posteriorly (apex anterior) and to displace into valgus. The use of blocking or 'Poller' screws aids reduction in this situation (**Figure 98.3**), as can the use of suprapatellar nailing,

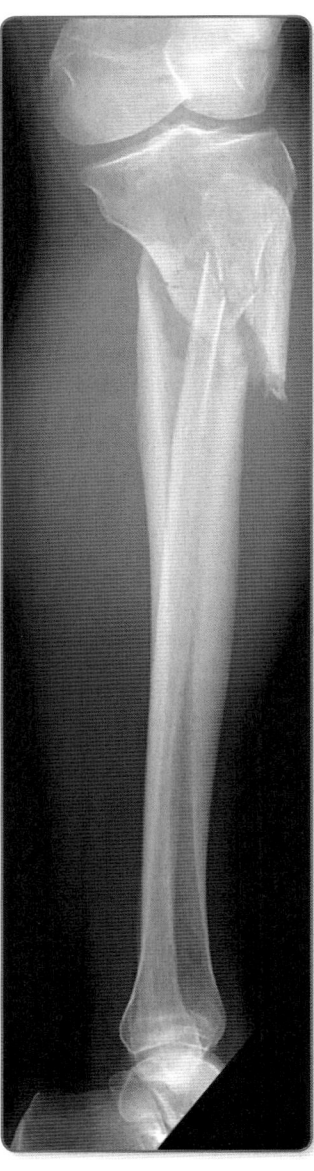

Figure 98.2 Proximal third tibial fracture. This is a high-energy injury and the fracture may exit into the tibial plateau. Note the nearly AP view of the knee and lateral of the ankle, which suggests significant rotation of the limb at the fracture site.

disruption of the zone of soft tissue injury and does not permit early weight-bearing. A bridge-plating technique is commonly used, allowing minimally invasive insertion. Plate fixation is best employed in very distal or very proximal extra-articular fractures or in those with an intra-articular component.

Diaphyseal fractures associated with extensive comminution and bone loss may be treated primarily using a definitive circular frame fixator such as an Ilizarov or Taylor spatial frame. The advantages of these techniques include the ability to perform bone regenerative techniques over time, including bone transport where a segment of bone is slowly transported down the limb over time to fill a bone defect, and the Masquelet technique where a defect is initially filled with cement then later replaced with bone graft after formation of a pseudomembrane to protect bone biology.

Complications

Immediate

- Vascular injury – each of the main (anterior tibial, posterior tibial and peroneal) arteries in the leg may be injured during tibial fracture and, rarely, during fixation
- Neurological injury – The common peroneal nerve may be injured, particularly in association with a high fibular fracture. The deep peroneal nerve may be injured where an AP locking bolt is used during distal locking of intramedullary nails. The tibial nerve may be injured in a distal fracture where it becomes tethered in the tarsal tunnel

Early

- Infection – treatment involves removal of the fixation, radical debridement of affected bone and soft tissue, restabilisation and, commonly, plastic surgical procedures to cover soft tissue defects
- Compartment syndrome – this may complicate the treatment of any tibial fracture at any early stage. Immediate management involves decompression of the four compartments of the leg via a double-incision fasciotomy, debridement

which uses specific instrumentation and a semiextended position. In distal third fractures there is a similar tendency towards malreduction and blocking screws may again be useful.

Open reduction and internal fixation is an option for fixation of diaphyseal fractures, although it involves a greater degree of

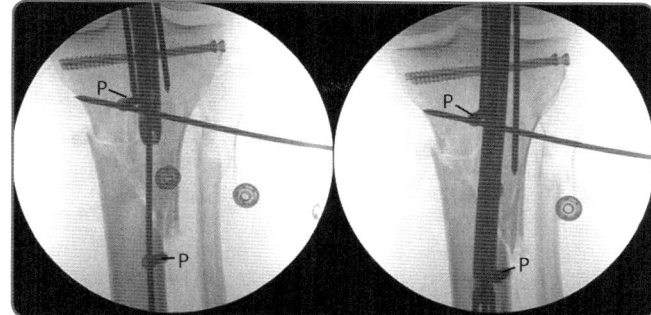

Figure 98.3 Intramedullary nailing of a proximal tibial fracture. Note the blocking screws (P) and supplementary blocking wires allowing passage of the nail whilst improving the fracture reduction and resisting deforming forces.

of any nonviable muscle and delayed closure at a further operation, sometimes in conjunction with split skin grafting

Late

- Malunion – this may be either angular or rotational, resulting in inefficient gait and secondary degenerative change at adjacent joints
- Nonunion – this may complicate up to 10% of tibial fractures and can require secondary treatment with exchange tibial nailing or conversion to an external fixator
- Anterior knee pain – this occurs in around 50% of patients treated with tibial nailing. Attempts to remove the nail do not provide reliable results in improving the pain and can, rarely, even worsen symptoms

Further reading

Bhandari M, Guyatt G, Tornetta P 3rd, et al. Randomized trial of reamed and unreamed intramedullary nailing of tibial shaft fractures. J Bone Joint Surg Am 2008; 90:2567–2578.

British Orthopaedic Association (BOA) and British Association of Plastic Reconstructive and Aesthetic Surgeons (BAPRAS) Standard for Trauma. BOAST 4: The management of severe open lower limb fractures. London: BOA and BAPRAS; 2009.

McQueen MM, Duckworth AD, Aitken SA, Sharma R, Court-Brown CM. Predictors of compartment syndrome after tibial fracture. J Orthop Trauma 2015; 29:451–455.

Related topics of interest

- *Topic 14* Compartment syndrome
- *Topic 68* Open fractures
- *Topic 85* Principles of operative management of fractures
- *Topic 96* Tibial pilon fractures
- *Topic 97* Tibial plateau fractures

99 Trauma scoring systems

Key points

- One of the most important roles of trauma scoring systems is that of predicting the clinical outcomes of trauma, such as using objective measures of injury severity
- They aid prehospital triage and resource allocation
- Trauma scoring systems have an important role in research and clinical governance, permitting the grouping of patients into populations for clinical trials and the comparison of practice between different units
- Whilst many different scoring systems have been developed in attempt to improve their predictive power and accuracy, trauma is inherently complex and affects different individuals variably

Type of scores

Generally, trauma scoring systems are based on anatomical or physiological aspects of the injury. Anatomical scores focus on the site of injury and tend to require detailed clinical assessment prior to calculation. Physiological scores focus on the systemic derangements following trauma and are particularly useful in triage situations. Anatomical and physiological scores may also be combined for superior prediction of survival, but often at the expense of ease of use. **Table 99.1** shows examples of a range of trauma and injury scores.

Physiological scoring systems

The Revised Trauma Score (RTS) is a physiological scoring system based on the initial recorded Glasgow Coma Scale (GCS), systolic blood pressure (SBP) and respiratory rate (RR). When used for prehospital triage, each parameter is coded from 0 to 4, creating a maximum score of 12. A triage-RTS (T-RTS) of 11 or less indicates that immediate life-saving intervention is required and transport to a trauma centre is advised. This system is challenging to use in paralysed, intubated or intoxicated patients. It can be calculated using the formula:

$$RTSc = (0.9368 \times GCSc) + (0.7326 \times SBPc) + (0.2908 \times RRc)$$

where c indicates coded value

In this system, greater weight is placed on the GCS to reflect the significance of head injury on trauma outcome. Its value ranges from 0 to 7.8408 and its interobserver reliability and accuracy has made it one of the most widely used triage scoring systems for trauma.

Anatomical scoring systems

The Abbreviated Injury Score (AIS) was devised in 1969 in North America by the insurance industry for quantification of the impact of automotive injuries. Since then, it has been revised to allow a greater number of organ injuries to be scored. Similar to the Organ Injury Scale (OIS) developed by the American Association for the Surgery of Trauma, each injury on the AIS is graded from 1 (minor) to 6 (unsalvageable). The limitation of the AIS is that, as it does not aggregate these scores, it cannot predict outcome. Its component scores instead contribute to the Injury Severity Score (ISS).

Each organ injury is graded using the AIS and is then assigned to one of six regions (head and neck, face, chest, abdomen, extremities or pelvic girdle, and external structures). The three highest scores, only one of which can be from each region, are squared then added to give a final score ranging from 1–75 (**Table 99.2**). If any region contains an injury with an AIS of 6 then the ISS is automatically set at 75. An example ISS calculation is showed in **Table 99.2**. A paediatric version, the Modified Injury Severity Scale, accounts for the predominance of head injuries in paediatric trauma, and introduces the GCS as a variable in the scoring model.

Table 99.1 Examples of trauma scores

Physiological

Revised Trauma Score
Glasgow Coma Scale
Acute Physiology and Chronic Health Evaluation
Emergency Trauma Score

Anatomical

Abbreviated Injury Score
Organ Injury Scale
Injury Severity Score
Modified Injury Severity Scale
New Injury Severity Score
Anatomic Profile
ICD-based Injury Severity Score
Mangled Extremity Severity Score

Combined

Trauma and Injury Severity Score
Paediatric Trauma Score
A Severity Characterisation of Trauma
TARN Ps model (Ps14)

Table 99.2 Example of an Injury Severity Scale calculation

Region	Description of injury	Abbreviated Injury Score (AIS)	Square of top three AIS scores
Head and neck	Head injury with no loss of consciousness	1	
Face	No injury	0	
Chest	Flail chest	4	16
	Pneumothorax	3	
Abdomen	Seat belt abrasion	1	
Extremity	Displaced simple long bone fractures	3	9
Skin	Large laceration	2	4
		Injury Severity Score	29

Despite widespread use, the ISS has certain limitations. Injuries from different body regions are not weighted and the inability to adjust for age, co-morbidity, multiple injuries in one particular body region or reflect injury from more than three regions leaves the tool prone to under-scoring. To address these limitations, the Anatomic Profile was designed to include all injuries in any given body region, with weighting of head and torso injuries. The introduction of significant complexity with only modest improvement in predictive performance discouraged adoption and, in 1997, the New ISS (NISS) was described. This offered a minor modification to the ISS to include the three highest AIS, regardless of body region. The NISS is easier to calculate and offers improved prediction of mortality over the original ISS.

The Mangled Extremity Severity Score (MESS) is used to guide decisions on the need for amputation, with age, mechanism of injury, ischaemia and shock as contributory variables. A MESS ≥7 has a 100% predictive value for requirement for amputation but its sensitivity is low.

Combined anatomical and physiological scoring systems

The Paediatric Trauma Score is the sum of individual scores for weight, airway, systolic blood pressure, central neurological status, presence of an open wound and skeletal injuries. It ranges from 6–12 and treatment at a trauma centre is recommended for a score ≤8.

The Trauma and Injury Severity Score (TRISS) model developed by Boyd et al. permits the probability of survival to be calculated from the ISS, RTS, and patient's age using a regression method. Separate models were devised to account for blunt versus penetrating injuries. While TRISS is well validated, it is informed by scores which themselves have some limitations and so A Severity Characterization of Trauma (ASCOT) was introduced in 1990, using the AP instead of ISS for the anatomical component. It is more complex to calculate, but has improved predictive power for mortality in trauma, especially penetrating injuries. Whilst a revised model has further improved this, the inability to account for pre-existing co-morbidities remains a limiting factor.

In 2004, the Trauma Audit and Research Network (TARN) devised a new model to calculate the Ps based on the patient's age, gender, ISS and GCS. Each component is weighted using retrospective data from the TARN database, and is re-calculated to account for population changes over time. In the TARN 2014 model (Ps14), weight is assigned to certain pre-existing medical conditions using a modified version of the Charlson Comorbidity Index. This would enable the impact of these conditions to be reflected on trauma outcome, allowing more individualised scoring and in-depth comparison between patients, groups and hospitals.

Further reading

Boyd CR, Tolson MA, Copes WS. Evaluating trauma care: the TRISS method. Trauma Score and the Injury Severity Score. J Trauma 1987; 27:370–378.

Champion HR, Copes WS, Sacco WJ, et al. Improved predictions from a severity characterization of trauma (ASCOT) over Trauma and Injury Severity Score (TRISS): results of an independent evaluation. J Trauma 1996; 40:42–48.

Champion HR, Sacco WJ, Copes WS, et al. A revision of the Trauma Score. J Trauma 1989; 29:623–629.

Osler T, Baker SP, Long W. A modification of the injury severity score that both improves accuracy and simplifies scoring. J Trauma 1997; 43:922–925.

100 Trauma outcome scores: using patient-reported outcome measures

Key point

- Patient-reported outcome measures (PROMs) is an umbrella term for tools used to assess health status from the patient's own perspective

Origin of PROMs

Historically, the performance of National Health Service (NHS) services was assessed largely by productivity, with little assessment of their impact on health as perceived by patients. To make better use of limited resources, the Office of National Statistics called in 2005 for this to be addressed. With increasing recognition of the value of patient involvement in healthcare, patient reported outcomes have become a major indicator of the quality and effectiveness of care and are components of the NHS Operating Framework, CQUIN scheme and Quality Accounts. This pattern is mirrored in healthcare systems across the world, with increasing emphasis on patient-centred care.

What are PROMs?

Patient-reported outcome measures are essentially questionnaires which assess the impact of healthcare interventions on heath, illness and quality of life from the patients' perspective. The terms 'measures', 'tools', 'instruments' or 'scales' are often used interchangeably in literature.

They must be representative of the patient's own views, and not those perceived by their family, carers or healthcare professionals. Technically, PROMs do not measure patient satisfaction.

The content of different PROMs varies greatly depending on their intended purpose. Whilst some PROMs are designed to address the impact of illness or health intervention on a single health dimension (unidimensional), others assess a combination of health dimensions (multidimensional). Such dimensions are aspects of life that interact together to determine quality of life and include physical, emotional and social aspects. The most commonly assessed health dimensions include symptoms, physical function, psychological and social well-being, cognitive function, role activity (such as employment or income), personal constructs (such as bodily appearance or spirituality), global judgment of health and satisfaction with care.

PROMs can be grouped into three broad categories: generic, specific and preference-based. Some instruments may fit into more than one category. **Table 100.1** shows different types of PROMs instruments and examples.

Generic instruments assess the general aspects of health for patients with any, or indeed no particular pathology. They cover a wide range of health dimensions and hence have a wide scope of potential uses. An example is the Short Form 36 (SF-36), which has 36 items in eight sections covering physical and mental health and elements of their impact on daily function.

Specific instruments are those designed for patients with a particular condition, such as osteoarthritis of the hip, who are members of a specific population such as the over-65s, who experience a certain symptom or who participate in a certain activity. An example of such an instrument is the Oxford Hip Score, used to evaluate the outcome of total hip arthroplasty.

The scores of the various questions in these generic and specific instruments are typically summed for each dimension, then combined

Table 100.1 Different types of patient-reported outcome measures instruments and examples

Type		Example
Generic		SF-36, Nottingham Health Profile
Specific	Condition-specific	Arthritis Impact Measurement Scales
	Dimension-specific	McGill Pain Score
	Site-specific	Oxford hip/knee/shoulder scores
Preference-based/utility		EQ-5D, Health Utilities Index

Table 100.2 Factors to consider when choosing a patient-reported outcome measure

Factor	Consideration
Appropriateness	Is the instrument's content appropriate to answer the research question?
Reliability	Can the instrument provide consistent and reproducible results free from random error? How much inter-rater variability is there?
Validity	Does the instrument actually measure what it purports to?
Responsiveness	Can the instrument detect clinically important differences?
Precision	How precise are the measurements? Is the instrument able to make specific distinction between scores?
Interpretability	Can the instrument produce statistically meaningful data?
Acceptability	How easily can the instrument be completed by patients?
Feasibility	Is it easy to collect and analyse data using the instrument? What timescale, costs, and staff are required?

into a final score. In doing so, the detail of each health domain is lost. In addition, the scoring systems assigned by the instrument's designers may not be representative of the patient's priorities. The concurrent use of both generic and condition-specific PROMs can be helpful to provide greater insight.

Preference-based or utility instruments use weighted scores (also known as values or utilities) to reflect the views of the general public on a particular health state. These social value sets are obtained through experimental techniques such as standard gamble and time trade-off, by asking participants to imagine living in a particular health state or by deriving scores from prior research. A widely-used utility-based measure is the EQ-5D, which has five dimensions assessing mobility, self-care, usual activity, pain and discomfort and anxiety and depression. These values can be used to inform quality adjusted life years and health-gained calculations for health economic analysis.

Choice of PROM

A wide range of PROMs exist and careful consideration must be given to which is the most suitable for the intended purpose. **Table 100.2** outlines the key factors that should be considered.

The acceptability of the instrument is particularly important, as this can influence the response rate. Shorter forms with relevant content, written in simple language with clear instructions have better response rates, thereby reducing responder bias. The mode of administration can also affect response rates; distribution via the internet has allowed rapid responses from large audiences but has poor penetration in those groups less likely to use the internet, such as the elderly or socially deprived. It is associated with lower administrative time and costs, but the use of social media has inherent problems with patient confidentiality, and should be carefully considered and risk-assessed before use. Patient feedback is often useful for the development of instruments.

Since PROMs report the health of a patient at a particular point in time, they should be completed before and after an intervention for meaningful comparison.

Further reading

Darzi A. High quality care for all: NHS next stage review final report. London: Department of Health, 2008.

Devlin N, Appleby J. Getting the most out of PROMs. London: The King's Fund, 2010:1–92.

Fitzpatrick R, Davey C, Buxton MJ, Jones DR. Evaluating patient-based outcome measures for use in clinical trials. Health Technol Assess 1998; 2:1–74.

Related topics of interest

- *Topic 1* Amputations – mangled extremities and decision making
- *Topic 2* Amputations – prosthetics and rehabilitation
- *Topic 15* Complex regional pain syndrome

101 Triage

Key points

- Triage is the process of prioritising patients in order to most effectively distribute limited resources
- Although commonly applied in the context of major incidents, triage occurs in all environments of care, both formally and informally. It can also be applied to a single patient – which of the multiple competing priorities is most urgent?
- Triage is a dynamic process; injuries evolve with time and those missed by crude screening tools may present problems that may confound or confuse the clinical picture and plan. By contrast, rapid, simple interventions may stabilise patients sufficiently to make their further management less clinically urgent. It is important, therefore, that patients are regularly reviewed and their urgency adjusted accordingly
- Triage may be based on physiology or anatomy

Triage categories

For the management of multiple casualties, a standard nomenclature is used across all agencies. Uninjured survivors are not categorised in this system. Some services will refer to casualties as P1, P2, etc. rather than T1, T2.

T1 (immediate) – red

T1 casualties are the most severely injured, with pathology that requires immediate intervention to save life and prevent further deterioration.

This may apply to an injury such as catastrophic external haemorrhage from traumatic above knee amputation.

T2 (urgent) – yellow

T2 casualties are those with serious injuries that are likely to require intervention or hospital admission. They are currently stable, however, and do not require immediate intervention to save life. Their treatment can usually wait until T1 patients have been initially stabilised. This may apply to pathologies such as a perforated abdominal viscus without haemorrhagic complications, which will require surgery within the next few hours to control contamination.

T3 (delayed) – green

Patients in the T3 category are usually referred to as the 'walking wounded'. They are injured, but typically with minor problems whose management can wait until more urgent casualties have been managed.

Dead (black)

The threshold for declaring that a casualty is dead will depend on the severity of an incident. Where there is a single casualty, it may be reasonable to attempt resuscitation provided that the injuries are compatible with life. When a large numbers of casualties exist, however, attempting to resuscitate the dead is likely to divert significant resources away from those who could potentially be saved. This triage code should not be confused with T4, a distinct category with medicolegal meaning and implications.

T4 (expectant) – blue; or red, with one corner of the card folded over

In truly overwhelming major incidents, where the number of casualties is far greater than the number that could be coped with despite extraordinary resources, a senior commander may authorise the use of the T4 category. This is used to refer to casualties who would otherwise be labelled as T1 – immediate, but in whom the injuries are likely to be unsurvivable, despite best possible care. T4 casualties are usually set aside until potentially salvageable casualties have been treated. Such injuries may be >90% total body surface area full-thickness burns, for example. In most major incidents, instituting the use of the T4 category is limited to the gold commander, in consultation with national government.

Physiological triage

Physiological triage systems are most commonly used to assess multiple casualties in a major incident. They have the advantage of being rapid and reproducible, they do not require significant specialist knowledge and are sensitive to casualties who are decompensating. They evaluate physiological variables such as consciousness level, heart rate and blood pressure.

The early warning score, used routinely on wards to spot signs of early deterioration, is a commonplace example of such a system.

Physiological tools risk missing certain injury patterns associated with later deterioration, however, such as airway burns and represent a snapshot of physiology, which may well worsen.

Anatomical triage

An anatomical approach to triage, by contrast, relies on specialist knowledge to delineate priorities based on a known or likely injury pattern. This is seen in patient or procedure selection by surgeons. It allows prioritisation of injuries which, although not a threat to life, may cause avoidable morbidity unless treated in a time-critical fashion, such as fracture-dislocation of the ankle with threatened skin and reduced perfusion of the foot.

A high degree of specialist knowledge and experience is required to use such systems effectively.

In many incidents, a layered combination of systems is used – initial triage by a basic physiological system (triage sieve) on initial rescue, further triage by a doctor using a more advanced physiological system (triage sort) and an anatomical triage by surgeons to decide on priorities for imaging and operating.

Triage sieve

The triage sieve is a very basic system which allows a large number of casualties to be processed rapidly by a small team with minimal training. A typical sieve is shown at **Figure 101.1**. It allows noninjured and walking wounded casualties to be rapidly separated from T1 and T2 casualties. The ability to walk is regarded as a marker of minor injury, implying that the airway is maintained and the patient is able to breathe, with sufficient circulatory reserve and cognition to stand upright.

This system has inherent limitations – an isolated ankle sprain may stop a patient walking and hence prioritise them inappropriately, while casualties with evolving injuries such as an airway burn may be able to walk into a group carrying a lower triage category.

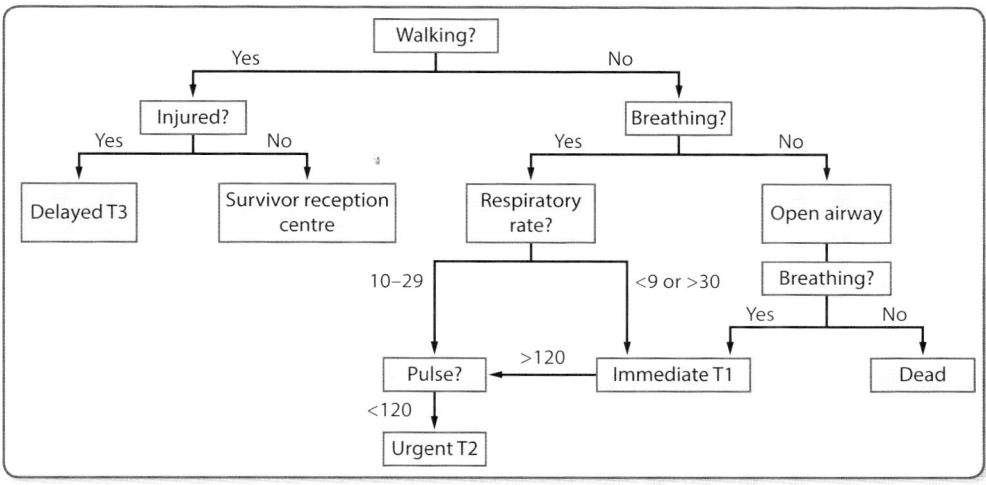

Figure 101.1 Triage sieve.

While triage is distinct from treatment, immediate interventions can be performed concurrently at this stage. These may include the application of tourniquets, turning patients on their side to clear airway obstruction and needle decompression of tension pneumothorax. The focus here is on single interventions which may reverse an avoidable, life-threatening pathology.

Triage sort

The triage sort is a more complex physiological system using three physiological parameters to give an aggregate value. It is a four-step approach, outlined in **Table 101.1**.
- The Glasgow Coma Score (GCS) is calculated
- Scores out of four are assigned to the GCS, respiratory rate and systolic blood pressure, with a lower number suggesting a worse value
- The above scores are added together to create a composite number, and a triage category assigned. 12/12 suggests grossly normal physiology and results in a T3 category. Dropping one point (minor derangement of one value only) results in a T2 category. Dropping two points (one very deranged variable, or multiple derangements) results in a T1 category
- A senior clinician can upgrade the triage category if required, based on their assessment of the pattern of injury

The triage sort is more complex and time-consuming than the sieve, and is best performed by a senior clinician with the experience to support the decision-making required in step 4.

Special circumstances

Children have different normal values for heart rate, respiratory rate and blood pressure, which will tend to over-triage them if an adult triage sieve or sort is used. Specialist paediatric triage tools are available, such as the Broselow bag system.

Casualties in a chemical, biological, radiological or nuclear incident may be up-

Table 101.1 Triage sort

1. Calculate the Glasgow Coma Scale score

Eye opening (E)		Motor score (M)		Verbal response (V)	
To voice	3	Obeys commands	6	Orientated	5
To pain	2	Localises	5	Confused	4
None	1	Withdrawal	4	Inappropriate	3
		Abnormal flexion	3	Incomprehensible	2
		Abnormal extension	2	None	1
		None	1		

GCS = E + M + V

2. Calculate the triage sort score

GCS		Respiratory rate		Systolic BP	
13 – 15	4	10 – 29	4	>90	4
9 – 12	3	>30	3	76 – 89	3
6 – 8	2	6 – 9	2	50 – 75	2
4 – 5	1	1 – 5	1	1 – 49	1
3	0	Apnoea	0	0	0

Triage sort score (out of 12) = GCS score + RR score + BP score

3. Assign a triage priority

12 = Delayed (T3)
11 = Urgent (T2)
10 or less = Immediate (T1)

4. Upgrade priority of the discretion of a senior clinician on the basis of anatomical injury/working diagnosis

triaged if they are showing signs of poisoning or irradiation. A casualty who, following a chemical attack, is dead by normal triage sieve criteria may warrant limited resuscitation if specific antidotes are immediately available.

In dangerous environments with on-going threats, the priority is to avoid increasing the scale of the incident by creating more casualties. This may mean limiting initial treatment to self- or buddy-aid, and casualties who are not breathing and to whom safe access is impossible may be considered dead until the threat is cleared.

Further reading

Advanced Life Support Group. Major Incident Medical Management and Support: The practical approach at the Scene (MIMMS), 3rd Ed. London: BMJ Books, 2011.

Joint Royal Colleges Ambulance Liason Committee/ Association of Ambulance Chief Executives. UK Ambulance services clinical practice guidelines, 2013. London: Class publishing, 2013.

Related topics of interest

- *Topic 63* Major trauma networks
- *Topic 99* Trauma scoring systems

102 Whiplash

Key points

- Whiplash represents a spectrum of disorders
- Treatment is often complex and can require a multidisciplinary approach
- It is an economically important condition with an estimated annual cost to the UK economy in excess of £3 billion

Epidemiology

The incidence of whiplash is estimated to be greater than 300 cases per 100,000 population in the United States. The cost to the UK economy exceeded £3 billion in 2012.

Ninety per cent of road traffic collisions occur at speeds <14 mph, the order of velocity which is associated with the whiplash effect. Of those patients who sustain whiplash injury, between 15 and 40% will go on to experience some form of chronic neck pain and 5–7% will become permanently disabled as a result of their injury.

Pathophysiology

The term 'whiplash' was coined by Crowe in 1928 in a presentation to the Western Orthopaedic Association. The neck sprain or strain injury classically occurs after a side-on or rear-end impact in a road traffic collision. This collision imparts acceleration to the passengers and driver with their torsos being thrown up and forwards. This in turn deforms the cervical spine, extending the lower portion and flexing the upper portion. The subsequent rebound reverses the deformity and hence the presence of a headrest leads to a reduced period and extent of deformation. The overall ranges of movement of the cervical spine as a whole are usually within the physiological range but individual motion segments may undergo nonphysiological movement, leading to injury to the joints, discs and supporting musculature. The entire process usually occurs within <500 ms.

Pain can arise from many causes, from a tear to the longus colli muscles, injuring the sympathetic trunk, to a disc herniation with associated radiculopathy. The pain is typically delayed in presentation, occurring 12–14 hours after the collision.

Clinical assessment

A detailed history should be taken, including the speed of and seating location within the vehicle, whether a seatbelt was worn and whether a headrest was present.

Inspect the skull and neck, looking especially for any bruising over the forehead (implying a flexion injury and possible impact with the steering wheel), occipital tenderness (implying rebound impact against the headrest) and temporomandibular joint tenderness.

Examine the central nervous system and look for features of sympathetic chain injury, such Horner's syndrome. Associated injuries are unusual, given, the low velocity typically seen, but must be looked for. Meticulous documentation is vital in this often-litigated injury.

Investigations

Whilst by definition whiplash is a soft tissue injury, any suspicion of bony injury should be investigated by plain film radiography in the first instance. Cross-sectional imaging may be performed if this is inconclusive or if objective clinical signs such as cervical myelopathy are noted. Radiological evidence of C5/C6 spondylosis is twice as frequent in symptomatic as asymptomatic patients.

Classification

Classification is most commonly by the Quebec Task Force grading (**Table 102.1**).

Treatment

In early whiplash, soft collars and activity modification are no longer recommended and may even worsen outcomes. A return to

Table 102.1 Quebec Task Force symptom grading

Grade	Symptoms
0	No neck pain, no physical signs
I	Neck pain, stiffness, tenderness, no physical signs
II	Neck symptoms with decreased range of movement and point tenderness
III	Neck symptoms with neurological defect
IV	Neck symptoms with fracture/dislocation

normal daily activities and physiotherapy are more effective at reducing symptoms, with use of simple analgesia and nonsteroidal anti-inflammatory drugs where necessary. Resistant pain can be treated with facet or nerve root injections and subacromial decompression for shoulder impingement has also been successful in up to 1/3 of patients.

Later stages of the injury are much more difficult to treat, with variable success. The strategy requires a multi-disciplinary approach, a key component of which is often cognitive behavioural therapy.

Complications

Immediate
- Minimal

Early
- Stiffness and ongoing pain

Late
- Chronic pain and resultant disability

Further reading

Bannister G, Amirfeyz R, Kelley S, Gargan M. Whiplash injury. J Bone Joint Surg Br 2009; 91:845–850.

Schofferman J, Bogduk N, Slosar P. Chronic whiplash and whiplash-associated disorders: an evidence-based approach. J Am Acad Orthop Surg 2007; 15:596–606.

Related topics of interest

- *Topic 10* Brachial plexus injury
- *Topic 92* Spine – atlas and axis cervical fractures and dislocations
- *Topic 94* Spine – subaxial cervical fractures and dislocations

Index

Note: Page numbers in **bold** or *italic* refer to tables or figures, respectively.

A

Abbreviated Injury Score (AIS) 356
Abductor pollicis longus (APL) 157
Acetabular fractures 299–301
    CT 'traumagram' 299
    definitive fixation 300
    Judet radiographs 299
    Letournel–Judet classification 299–300, **300**
    nonoperative management 300
Achilles tendon ruptures 8–11
    classification of 9, *9*
    gastrocnemius flaps or V-Y advancement, reconstruction with 10
    MRI for 9
    nonoperative treatment 10
    open end-to-end repair 10
    percutaneous repair 10
    tendon transfer, reconstruction with 10
    ultrasound for 9, *9*
Acromioclavicular (AC) joint 47
    dislocation 47–48
    Rockwood classification of AC joint injuries 48, **48**
Acute compartment syndrome (ACS) *see* Compartment syndrome
Acute respiratory distress syndrome (ARDS) 64, 65
    Berlin definition 65
    fat embolism and 77–79, 88, 91
    trauma and 65
Airway assessment, in trauma patients 235
Albumin 314
Allograft 25, **27**
Amputation 1, 3, 5, 30
    above-knee 4, 6
    below-knee 4, 5–6
    level of 3–4
    mangled extremity and 1–2
    and prosthetic limbs 5–6
    and rehabilitation 6–7
    scoring systems and decision for **2**, 2–3, *3*
    upper limb 4, 6
Ankle-brachial index 88
Ankle fractures 12, 17
    classification systems 12
    Lauge-Hansen classification 12, 17, **17**
    pronation–abduction (PAB) 12, 17–20
    pronation–external rotation (PER) 12–15
    supination–adduction (SAD) 12, 17–20
    supination–external rotation (SER) 12–15

Ankle fractures, in children 267–269
    and chondral injury 269
    compartment syndrome and 269
    CT scan, use of 268
    Dias–Tachdjian system 268
    radiographic views 267–268
    and reflex sympathetic dystrophy 269
    Salter–Harris classification system 268
    tillaux fractures 267
    treatment 268
    triplane fractures 267
Anterior cord syndrome **335**
Anterior cruciate ligament (ACL) injuries 217–219, 293
    in children 219
    classification 218, **219**
    meniscal injury with 217
    MRI 218, *218*
    nonoperative treatment 218
    operative treatment 218–219
    Segond fracture 218, *218*
Anterior draw test 14, 217
Antibiotic-impregnated cement beads/spacers 31
Antibiotics
    for infection prevention 209, 212
    for septic arthritis in children 317–318
Arbeitsgemeinschaft für Osteosynthesefragen (AO)/Orthopaedic Trauma Association (OTA) classification 42, 81
Arthroplasty 98–99
Autograft 25, **27**
Avascular necrosis (AVN) 103
    of proximal femur 95
    proximal humerus fractures and 189
    scaphoid fractures and 171
    subtalar dislocations and 123
    talar fractures and 22, 24
Axonotmesis 305

B

Barton's fracture 125, *125*
Basketball foot 120
Battle's sign 177
Bennett's fracture 157
Bisphosphonates
    complications of 263, *264*
    for osteoporosis 263
Blood products 314

BMP *see* Bone morphogenic proteins (BMP)
Böhler angle 107, *107,* 109
Bone densitometry 58
Bone grafts 25–26, **27**
    allogenic 25
    autogenic 25
    definition 25
    incorporation of 26
    synthetic substances 25–26
Bone healing
    factors affecting 137
    immobilisation and 137
    primary 136
    secondary 136
Bone loss 29–31
    acute shortenings of bone 30
    amputation *versus* limb salvage 30
    autologous nonvascularised bone graft 30
    bulk structural allograft 31
    causes 29
    classification of severity 29, **29**
    distraction osteogenesis 30–31
    early appropriate care (EAC) 29
    endoprosthetic replacement 31
    external ring fixators 31
    free vascularised fibula transfer 31
    initial stabilisation methods 31
    intramedullary fixation 31
    Masquelet technique of induced membrane 30
    and plating 31
    reconstruction in, options for 30–31
    traumatic, management of 29–30
Bone marrow aspirate 25, **27**
Bone mineral density (BMD) 262
Bone morphogenic proteins (BMP) 26, **27**
Bones 32, 307
    flat 32
    homeostasis 34–36, *35,* **36**
    long 32, *33,* 307
    osteoblasts 34
    osteoclasts 34
    osteocytes 34
    remodelling 34, *35*
    structure *33,* 33–34, *35*
    vascular supply 32–33, *33*
    woven 307
Bone scans 193
Bone–tendon–bone (BTB) autografts 219
Boxer's fracture 157, *158,* 162
BPIs *see* Brachial plexus injuries (BPIs)
Brace 223
Brachial plexus injuries (BPIs) 38–41
    anatomy related to 38–39, *40*
    Leffert classification 39–40, **40**
    minor 38
    moderate 38
    nonobstetric 38
    obstetric-associated 38
    Seddon and Sunderland classification 40, **41**
    severe 38
    treatment 40–41
Broselow bag system 364
Brown–Sequard syndrome **335**

C

Calcaneal fractures 105–109
    computed tomography 107, *107*
    Eastwood–Atkins classification 105–106, **106**, *106*
    Essex-Lopresti classification 105, *105, 106*
    extra-articular 105
    intra-articular *105,* 105–106, *106*
    lateral transcalcaneal approach 108, *108*
    plain radiographs 106–107, *107*
    Sanders classification 107, *107,* **108**
    tongue-type fracture 105, *105, 106*
    treatment 107–108, *108*
Calcaneocuboid (CC) joint 116
Calcium phosphate 26, **27**
Calcium sulphate 25–26, **27**
Calcium supplements, in osteoporosis 263
Calf squeeze test *see* Thompson's test
Callus formation 307
Cancellous grafts 25, **27**
Capitate fractures 153, 154 *see also* Carpal fractures
Carpal dislocations 149–151
    Gilula's lines 150, *150*
    greater arc and lesser arc 149, *149*
    radiographs *150,* 150–151
    types of 149–150
Carpal fractures 153–156
    capitate fractures 153, 154
    hamate fractures 153, 154
    lunate fractures 153, 154
    nonunion 155
    pisiform fractures 153, 154
    scaphoid fractures 153, 154
    trapezium fractures 153, 154
    trapezoid fractures 154
    triquetral fractures 153
Carpal tunnel decompression 127
Carpometacarpal (CMC) joints 154, 158
Ceftazidime 209
Cefuroxime 209, 258
Central cord syndrome **335**
Centre of rotation of angulation (CORA) 243
Cephalomedullary nails 90, *90,* 94, 98
Cephalosporin 209
Ceramics 26
Cervical spine injuries 329–332
    Canadian C-spine rules 330
    C1 fractures 331, *331*
    C2 fractures 330, 331
    classification 330, *331*
    clinical assessment 329

CT scan 330
mechanisms of injury 329
MRI for 330
and neurological injury 332
nonunion 332
occipital condyle fracture 330, 331
plain radiograph for 329–330
Powers' ratio 330, *330*
treatment 330–331
Chance fracture 339
Charlson Comorbidity Index 358
Child maltreatment 146
Chopart's joint 120
Chronic regional pain syndrome (CRPS) 216
Circular external fixator 195–198, 244
for bone transportation 195, *196–197*
construction 195
for deformity correction 197, *197–198*
history 195
indications 195
Clavicle dislocations 46–49
AC dislocations 47–48
SC dislocations 46–47
Clavicle fractures 50–52
Allman classification 51
clinical assessment 50, *50*
management **51**, 52, **52**
Neer classification 51
nonunion rates 52
plain radiographs 50
Robinson classification 51–52
Clindamycin 209, 258
Co-amoxiclav 209, 258, 259
Collagen matrices 26, **27**
Colloids 313
Compartment syndrome 53–55, 82, 91, 216
delayed union/nonunion 134
fasciotomy wound management 55
foot fasciotomy 55, **55**
forearm fasciotomy 55, **55**
with fractures 53
guidelines for 145
hand fasciotomy 55, **55**
intracompartmental pressure (ICP) increase in 53, 54
knee dislocation and 232
leg fasciotomy 54, **55**
malunion 134
and pain 53–54
radius and ulna fractures and 134
treatment 54–55, **55**
without fractures 53
Complex regional pain syndrome (CRPS) 57–60
Budapest criteria for 57, **58**
cold phase of 57, 59, *60*
multidisciplinary team (MDT), referral to 59
Orlando criteria for 57

pharmacotherapy and physiotherapy 59–60
trophic changes in 59, *59*
type 1 58
type 2 58
warm phase of 57, 59, *59*
Computed tomography (CT) scans 192
Continuous positive airway pressure (CPAP) 79
Contusions 178, *178*
Conus medullaris syndrome **335**
Coracoclavicular (CC) ligaments 47
Cortical grafts 25, **27**
CRPS *see* Complex regional pain syndrome (CRPS)
Crush injuries and crush syndrome 61–63
and compartment syndrome 61
definition 61
fasciotomy and amputation 63
hospital treatment 62–63
pre-hospital assessment and treatment 62
and rhabdomyolysis 61
Cryoprecipitate 314
Crystal arthropathy 319–320
Crystalloid fluids 313
Cubitus valgus 292
Cuboid fractures 116–117
displaced 117, *117*
open reduction internal fixation 117, *117*
Cylinder cast 223
Cytokines 64, 65

D
Deformity assessment
angular deformity 243
joint mechanics and 243
leg length discrepancy (LLD) 242–243
limb rotation 243
of lower limb 242–243
mechanical and anatomical axes and 242, *242*
symptoms 243
Delirium 140
Demineralised bone matrix 26, **27**
Denosumab 263, 296
Disseminated intravascular coagulation (DIC) 64, 65
Distal femoral fractures 80–82
AO/OTA classification 81, **81**
and compartment syndrome 82
extra-articular *81*, 81–82
intra-articular fractures 82
nonunion and malunion 82
post-traumatic osteoarthritis 82
severely comminuted fractures 82
treatment *81*, 81–82
Distal humerus fractures 182–185
AP and lateral radiographs 183, *183*
bicolumn fractures 182
closed reduction and percutaneous fixation 184
malunion 185
Mehne and Matta classification 183, *184*

Milch classification 183, *183*
and nerve injury 185
nonoperative management 183–184
open reduction and internal fixation 184, *184*
pathophysiology 182, *182*
single column fractures 182
total elbow arthroplasty 184
Distal radial fractures 124–127
Barton's fracture 125, *125*
Colles' fracture 124, *125*
and compartment syndrome 125
Frykman classification 125–126, *126*
malunion 127
rule of 11s 124, *124*
Smith's fracture 124
treatment 126–127
Distal radioulna joint (DRUJ) 128
Distraction osteogenesis 30–31, 195
Doxycycline 209
Dual-energy X-ray absorptiometry (DEXA) scan 262

E
Early appropriate care (EAC), concept of 29, 64, 65
Elastic stable intramedullary nailing (ESIN) 275
Elbow dislocation 67–70
anatomy related to 67
anterior 67
anteroposterior radiographs *68*
classification **68,** 68–69
with coronoid process fracture 68, **68,** *68*
divergent 68
lateral radiographs *68*
posterior 67
posterior Monteggia fracture-dislocation 69
with radial head fracture 68, **68,** 69
terrible triad 68
transolecranon fracture-dislocation 69
treatment **69,** 69–70
Endoprosthetic replacement 31
Erb's palsy 39
Extensor retinaculum syndrome 269
Extensor tendon ruptures, of knee 221–224
Insall–Salvati ratio 222, *222*
MRI 222, *223*
patella ligament ruptures 221, *222*
plain radiographs 222
quadriceps tendon ruptures 221
treatment 222–223, *223*
ultrasonography 222
External fixators 199–201, 244, 311
advantages of 199
bars 200
bone pin 199–200
clamps 200
constructions with differing stabilities 200, *201*

damage control 201
frame design 200–201
structure 199, *199*, *200*
Extracapsular hip fractures 96–99
AO classification 96, *97*
arthroplasty 98–99
cephalomedullary nail 98, *98*
dynamic hip screw (DHS) fixation *97,* 97–98
fixed angle plate 98
greater trochanter fracture 99
reverse oblique fractures 98
tip–apex distance (TAD) 97, *97*
Extremities, mangled 1
decision to salvage or amputate, scoring systems for **2,** 2–3, **3**
management of 1–2
mechanism of injury 1

F
Falls in the elderly 145
Fat embolism syndrome (FES) 77–79
chest radiograph 78, *78*
Gurd's and Wilson's criteria 78
Lindeque's criteria 78
prevention 78–79
Schonfield's criteria 78, **79**
Femoral fractures *see also specific type*
extracapsular fractures 96–99
intracapsular femoral neck fractures 100–103
periprosthetic 83–86
shaft fractures 88–91
subtrochanteric fractures 92–95
Femoral periprosthetic fractures 83–86
distal 83, 84, **84,** 85–86, *86*
Lewis and Rorabeck classification 84, **84**
proximal 83, **84,** 84–85, *85*
treatment 84–86, *85, 86*
Vancouver classification 84, **84**
Femoral shaft fractures (FSFs) 88–91
AO/OTA classification 89
external fixators 89
heterotopic ossification 91, *91*
intramedullary nailing 89–90, *90, 91*
malunion 91
nonunion 91
open reduction internal fixation 89
Winquist–Hansen classification 89, **89**
FES *see* Fat embolism syndrome (FES)
Fifth metatarsal fractures 117–118, *118*
diaphyseal fractures 117, *118*
Jones fractures 117, 118, *118*
tuberosity fractures 117, *118*
Figure-of-eight splint 265
Flexor digitorum profundus (FDP) 155
Flexor pollicis longus (FPL) 157
Fluoroquinolones 209

Foot
  calcaneal fractures 105–109
  Lisfranc's fracture–dislocations 110–114
  mid- and forefoot fractures 115–119
  subtalar dislocations 120–123
Forearm
  distal radial fractures 124–127
  Galeazzi's and Monteggia's fractures 128–130
  radius and ulna fractures 132–134
Fracture 307 *see also specific type*
  classification 215
  clinical assessment 214
  and complications 215–216
  definition 214, *214*
  investigations 214–215
  nonoperative management 215, 307–308
  open (*see* Open fractures)
  operative management 215
Fracture clinic services, guidelines for 145–146
Fracture healing 136–137, 307
  delayed or nonunion 137
  immobilisation and 137
  primary bone healing 136
  secondary bone healing 136
Fracture liaison services 145
Fractures, classification of 42–44
  on degree of soft tissue injury 43–44, **44**
  fracture-specific classification systems 44
  generic classification systems *42*, 42–43
  Gustilo open fracture classification system 44, **44**
  Oestern and Tscherne classification of closed fracture 44, **44**
  uses of 44
Fractures, operative treatment of 310–312
  complications of fixation 312, **312**
  external fixation 311
  fixation and fracture healing 311
  follow-up 312
  intramedullary nails 311
  manipulation under anaesthetic 311
  open reduction, internal fixation 311
  patient positioning 310
  preoperative planning 310
  soft tissues, assessment of 310
Fragility fracture of hip in adults, guidelines for 143
FRAX, for osteoporotic fracture 262
Free fatty acids (FFAs) 77
Free vascularised septocutaneous flap 31
Freeze dried grafts 25, **27**
Fresh allograft 25, **27**
Fresh frozen grafts 25, **27**
Fresh frozen plasma (FFP) 314

G
Galeazzi's fracture *128*, 128–130, *130*
Gas gangrene 211–212

GCS *see* Glasgow Coma Scale (GCS)
Gelatins 313
Gentamicin 209, 259
Glasgow Coma Scale (GCS) 177, 236, **236**, 356, 364, **364**
Glenoid fractures 324–325
Gout 319–320
Gunshot injuries 147–148
  nerve and vessel injury 147
  operative management 148
  principles of ATLS management 147
  spinal injuries 147–148
  tissue damage 147

H
Haemorrhagic shock 236
  grading of **236**
Hamate fractures 153, 154 *see also* Carpal fractures
Hamstring autografts 219
Hand and wrist
  carpal dislocations 149–151
  carpal fractures 153–156
  metacarpal fractures 157–162
  phalangeal fractures 163–166
  scaphoid fractures 168–171
  tendon ruptures 172–175
Hartmann's solution 313
Head injury 177–181
  cerebrospinal fluid (CSF) leak 177
  complications 180–181, *181*
  contusions 178, *178*
  CSF rhinorrhoea 181
  CT scan in 177–178, **178**
  extradural haematoma 179
  Glasgow Coma Score 177
  intracranial haematoma 178–179, *179*
  intracranial pressure and mass effects 180, *180*
  Monro–Kellie doctrine 180
  primary brain injury 177
  secondary brain injury 179–180
  skull fractures 178
  subdural haematoma 179, *179*
  traumatic brain injury 177
Hemiarthroplasty, for displaced femoral neck fractures 101
Hepatitis B 213
Hepatitis C 213
Hilton's law 33
Hip fracture, perioperative management of
  anaemia and 139
  best practice tariff (BPT) 139
  The Blue Book and National Hip Fracture Database (NHFD) 138–139
  delirium 140
  fluid and electrolyte balance 139–140
  nutrition 140

in older people 138–140
  pain relief 139
  postoperative care 139–140
  preoperative care 139
  pressure care 140
  venous thromboembolism and 140
Hook of hamate fractures 155
Hook (Cotton's) test 14, 19
Horner's syndrome 39
Hueter-Volkmann law 34
Human immunodeficiency virus (HIV) 212–213
Hydroxyapatite 26, **27**
Hyperkalaemia 315
Hypocalcaemia 315
Hypothermia 315
Hypoxia 235
Hypoxia inducible factor-1 (HIF-1) 8

I
Imaging 190
  and description *190,* 190–191, *191*
  fracture terminology *190,* 190–191, *191*
  fracture type 190, *191*
  interpretation of 191
  modalities 192–194
  types of fracture displacement 190, *190*
Impaction grafting 25
Implants
  circular external fixators 195–198
  monolateral external fixators 199–201
  nails 202–203
  plates 204–205
  screws 206–207
Infection 209–213, 216
  antibiotics in fractures management 209
  causative organism 209–210
  closed fractures 209
  and delay in bony healing 255, 257
  gas gangrene 211–212
  necrotising fasciitis 212
  occupational hazards 212–213
  open fractures 209
  osteomyelitis *210,* 210–211, **211**
  susceptibility to 209
  tetanus 211, **212**
Injury Severity Score (ISS) 65, 237, 239, 356–357, **357**
  New ISS (NISS) 357
Interleukins (IL) 64
Interphalangeal joints (IPJs) 163, 172
Intracapsular femoral neck fractures 100–103
  blood supply of femoral head and 100, *101*
  displaced fractures 101, 103
  Garden's classification 100–101, *102*
  in older adults 101, 103
  Pauwels' classification 101, *102*

undisplaced fractures 103
in younger adults 103
Intracompartmental pressure (ICP) 53
  in compartment syndrome 53, 54
  measurement 54
  normal resting ICP 54
Intramedullary nails 202, *202,* 244, 311
Ischial ramal containment socket 6

J
Jefferson fractures 329
Jumper's knee 221

K
Klumpke's palsy 39
Knee
  cruciate ligament injuries 217–219
  extensor mechanism injury 221–224
  meniscal injuries 225–227
  patella fractures 228–231
Knee dislocations 232–234
  anterior tibiofemoral dislocation 232
  arterial injury 234
  dimple sign 232
  initial management 233
  multiligament reconstruction 233–234
  neurological examination 232
  nonoperative management 233
  posterior tibiofemoral dislocation 232
  post-traumatic osteoarthritis 234
  Schenck classification 233, **233**
  stiffness and limited range of motion 234
  vascular examination 232

L
Lachmann's test 217
Leadbetter manoeuvre 103
Leg length discrepancy (LLD) 242–243
Limb injuries, guidelines for 144–145
Limb salvage index (LSI) 2–3, **3**, 30
Limb tourniquets 310
Limited contact dynamic compression plate (LC-DCP) 255
Lisfranc's injuries 110–114
  and compartment syndrome 114
  fleck sign 112
  Myerson classification 110–111, *111*
  open reduction internal fixation 112–113, *113*
  radiographs 111–112, *112*
  tarsometatarsal complex and 110, *110*
  treatment 112–114, *113*
Lisfranc's ligament 110
Locking screws 203, 204
Lower limb fractures, open 143
Lunate fractures 153, 154 *see also* Carpal fractures

Index

M

Macrophage colony-stimulating factors (M-CSF) 34
Magnetic resonance imaging (MRI) 193–194
Major trauma 235–237, 239
    ABCDE approach 235–236
    classifications 237
    code red alert 237
    Glasgow Coma Scale 236, **236**
    haemorrhagic shock 236, **236**
    injury severity score (ISS) 237, 239
    mangled extremity severity score (MESS) 237
    mortality rate 235
    networks 239–241
    quality of care (QoC) for trauma patients 239
    treatment 237
    UK trauma network 240–241
Major trauma centres (MTC) 235, 239
Male hormone screen 262
Mallet injury 172, 175
Malunion 242
    deformity assessment *242*, 242–243
    and deformity correction 242–244
    fixation methods 244
    mechanical and anatomical axes and 242, *242*
    osteotomy 243
    surgical indications 243
Mangled Extremity Severity Score (MESS) 2, **2**, 30, 63, 237, 357
Mangled extremity syndrome index (MESI) 3
Mass casualty incident (MCI) 245–249
    aftercare 248–249
    ambulance services, responsibilities of 246, **248**
    big bang incidents 246
    chemical, biological, radiological or nuclear (CBRN) incidents 245, 246
    Civil Contingencies Act (CCA), UK 245
    complex incidents and 245
    hospital planning and preparedness 248
    multi-disciplinary team 246
    preparations for 245
    rising tide incidents 246
    START casualty triage 247, *247*, **248**
    triage system in *247*, 247–248
    types of 246
Massive transfusion 315
    complications of 315
MCI *see* Mass casualty incident (MCI)
McMurray's test 217
Median nerve 182, *182*
Meniscal tears 225–227
    ACL injury and 225
    anatomy related to 225–226
    arthroscopic meniscectomy 226–227
    classification 226, **226**
    lateral meniscus and 225
    medial meniscus and 225
    MRI for 226

Metacapophalangeal (MCP) joints 163, 172
Metacarpal fractures 157–162
    Boxer's fracture 157, *158*
    metacarpals 2–5 157–160, *158–161*
    4th metacarpal fracture *158*
    5th metacarpal shaft fracture *160, 161*
    5th metacarpophalangeal joint, dislocation of *159*
    thumb 157
    treatment 161–162, **162**
Metalloproteinases (MMPs) 8
Minimally invasive percutaneous osteosynthesis (MIPO) 255
Monteggia's fracture 128–130, *129*
    Bado classification 129, *129*
Multiple myeloma 296, 297
Multiple organ distress syndrome (MODS) 64, 65
    trauma and 65

N

Nailbed injuries 250–253
    anatomy of nailbed and fingertip *250*, 250–251
    crush injuries and 251
    nailbed avulsion 253
    nailbed laceration 251–253
    phalangeal fracture with 251, *252*
    post-traumatic nail deformities 253, **253**
    treatment 251–253, **252**, *252*
Nail deformities, post-traumatic 253, **253**
Nails 202–203
    interlocking 203
    intramedullary nails 202, *202*
    reaming 202–203
    slotted nails 203
    working length 203
Navicular fracture dislocations *115*, 115–116, *116*
Near-infrared spectroscopy (NIRS) 54
Necrotising fasciitis (NF) 212
Negative pressure wound therapy (NPWT) 55
Neurogenic shock 334
Neuromuscular electrical stimulation (NMES) 41
Neuropraxia 305
Neurotmesis 305
NISSSA score (Nerve injury, Ischaemia, Soft-tissue injury, Skeletal injury, Shock, and Age) 3
Nonaccidental injury (NAI), in children 277–279
    bruising and fractures 278
    developmental milestones and **277**, 277–278
    long bone fractures 279
    metaphyseal fractures 278–279
    multi-disciplinary team approach for 279
    rib fractures 278
    skeletal survey in 278
    skull fractures 279
Nonunion of fractures 254–257
    atrophic/avascular 256, *256*, 257
    fixation factors 254–255
    fracture factors 254

host factors 254
hypertrophic/hypervascular 255–256, *256*, 257
infection and 255, 257
nonoperative interventions 256–257
oligotrophic nonunions 257
operative interventions 257
segmental loss 257
Nuclear medicine 192–193
Nutcracker fracture 116

O

Olecranon fractures 71–73
classification 71
management 71–72, *72*
plating of, with metaphyseal extension *72*
tension band technique *72*
Olive wires 345
Open fractures 258–259, *260*
debridement of 259, *260*
guidelines for management of 258–259
Gustilo 3A distal tibial ankle fracture *260*
Gustilo–Anderson grading system 258, **259**
open tibial fractures 258
Organ Injury Scale (OIS) 356
Osgood–Schlatter disease 293
Osteogenic proteins *see* Bone morphogenic proteins (BMP)
Osteomyelitis 210–211, 316
Cierny–Mader staging system 210–211, **211**
classification 210–211
diagnosis 210, *210*
management 211
Osteonecrosis of jaw (ONJ) 263
Osteoporosis 261–264
diagnosis 262, **262**
fracture risk assessment and osteoporosis management, guidelines on 262–263, **263**
fragility fractures in the elderly 261
nonpharmacologic treatment 263
pharmacologic treatments 263–264
risk assessment tools 262
risk factors 261–262
secondary **261**
Osteoprotegerin (OPG) 34
Osteotendinous quadriceps rupture 223
Osteotomy 243
Ottawa ankle rules (OAR) 14
Oxford Hip Score 359

P

Packed red blood cells 314
Paediatric clavicle fractures 265–266
Allman classification 265
Paediatric distal tibial and ankle fractures 267–269
Paediatric femoral fractures 270–272
femoral shaft fractures 271, 272

proximal and distal femoral fractures 271
treatment 271, *272*
Paediatric forearm fractures 274–276
acceptable angulations for 275, **275**
remodelling potential in children 275
treatment 275–276
Paediatric humeral condylar fractures 280–283
Bensahel classification of medial condyle fractures 281, **282**
displaced medial condyle fracture 281, *282*, 283
Jakob type 2 lateral condyle fracture 281, *281*, *282*
lateral condylar fractures 280, 281–282, *282*
medial condylar fractures 280, *281*, 283
Paediatric humeral fractures 284–285
acceptable angulation and displacement for **285**
classification 284
treatment 284–285, **285**
Paediatric physeal fractures 286–288
anatomy of growth plate and *286*, 286–287
Salter–Harris classification system 287, *287*, **288**
treatment 287–288
Paediatric supracondylar fractures 289–292
Baumann's humeral-capitellar angle 289, *290*
and compartment syndrome 292
flexion-type injuries 290, *290*
Gartland classification 289–290, *291*
malunion 292
and neurovascular injury 292
nonoperative management 290–291
operative management *291*, 291–292
pin site infections 292
radiographs 289, *290*
Paediatric tibial fractures 293–294
avulsion fractures of tibial tubercle 293
classification 294
diaphyseal tibial fractures 293
proximal tibial metaphyseal injuries 293
tibial eminence fractures 293
tibial epiphyseal injuries 293
treatment 294
Paediatric Trauma Score 357
Paget's disease 100
Patella fractures 228–231
classification 228–229, *229*
open reduction and internal fixation 229–230, *230*
partial patellectomy 230
post-traumatic patellofemoral osteoarthritis 231
rehabilitation 230
total patellectomy 230
Patella tendon ruptures 221–224, *222*, *223*
Pathological fractures 296–298
biopsy 297
breast cancer metastasis and 296
fixation options 297–298
history and physical examination 296
laboratory tests 296

Mirel's criteria for 297, **297**
plain radiographs 297
Patient-reported outcome measures (PROMs) 359–361
  choice of **360**, 360–361
  generic instruments 359
  preference-based 360
  specific instruments 359
  types of 359, **360**
Pelvic binder 236
Pelvic ring fractures 302–304
  anteroposterior compression injuries 304
  CT scan 303
  examination under anaesthesia (EUA) 304
  history and physical examination 302
  initial management 303
  lateral compression injuries 304
  plain radiograph 302–303
  vertical shear injuries 304
  Young and Burgess classification 303, **303**
Pelvis
  acetabular fractures 299–301
  pelvic ring fractures 302–304
Penicillin 209
Peripheral nerve injury 305–306
  guidelines for 144
  Medical Research Council (MRC) scale 306
  Seddon classification 305
  Sunderland classification 305–306
  surgical management 306
Phalangeal fractures 163–166
  displaced fractures 163
  distal phalanx fractures 164–165
  extra-articular proximal and middle phalanx fractures 165, *165*
  intra-articular fractures of proximal and middle phalanx 165–166, *166*
  malunion 166
  nonunion 166
  post-traumatic arthrosis 166
  rotational deformity, assessment for 164, *164*
  and stiffness 166
  undisplaced fractures 163
Phantom limb pain 7
Physeal injuries, in children 286–288
Pilon fractures 343–346
  AO-OTA classification 343–344
  and compartment syndrome 346
  and infection 345–346
  malunion 346
  nonoperative management 344
  nonunion 346
  operative management 344, 344–345, *345*
  Ruedi–Allgower classification 343, **343**
Pisiform fractures 153, 154 *see also* Carpal fractures

Pivot shift test 217
Platelet-derived growth factor (PDGF) 8
Platelet transfusion 142, 314
Plates 204–205
  biomechanical principles 204
  bridge plating 205
  compression plating 204–205, *205*
  design 204
  dynamic compression plate (DCP) 204
  locking compression plate (LCP) 204
  locking plates 204
  low contact dynamic compression plate (LC-DCP) 204
  precontoured anatomical plates 204
  tension band plates 205
Popliteal artery 232
Positive end expiratory pressure (PEEP) 79
Positron emission tomography 193
Posterior cord syndrome **335**
Posterior cruciate ligament (PCL) 217–219
Posterior sag sign 217
Post-traumatic osteoarthritis 216
Predictive salvage index (PSI) 3, 30
Pressure ulcers 140
PROMs *see* Patient-reported outcome measures (PROMs)
Pronation–abduction (PAB) ankle fractures 12, **17**, 17–20
  stages and injuries of 17–18, **19**
Pronation–external rotation (PER) ankle fractures 12–15, **17**
  stages and injuries of 13, **13**, *14*
  treatment 15, *15*
Prosthetic limbs 5
  above-knee amputation 6
  below-knee amputation 5–6
  pain 7
  rehabilitation 7
  upper limbs 6
Prosthetic socks 6
Proteolytic enzymes 316
Prothrombin complex 142
Proximal humeral varus 285
Proximal humerus fractures 186–189
  fracture patterns 186, *186*
  hemiarthroplasty 188
  intramedullary nail 188
  malunion 189
  Neer classification 187, *187*
  nonoperative management 188
  nonunion 189
  open reduction internal fixation (ORIF) 188, *188*
  reverse shoulder arthroplasty 188, *188*
  total shoulder arthroplasty 188
Pseudogout 319–320
Purtscher's retinopathy 78

Q
Quadriceps tendon ruptures 221–224, *223*
Quadrilateral socket 6

R
Radial head and neck fractures 74–76
    fixation of radial head 75
    Mason classification 74, *75*
    plain radiographs 74
    radial head excision 75
    radial head replacement 75
    Sail sign 74
    treatment 75, **76**
Radiographs 192
Radius and ulna fractures 132–134
    AP and lateral radiographs 132, *133*
    and compartment syndrome 134
    isolated fracture of radius 133, *134*
    neurological injury 134
    open fractures 133
    open reduction and internal fixation 133, *133*
    treatment 132–134, *133*
Raloxifene 264
Receptor activator for nuclear factor-κ B ligand (RANKL) 34, 36, 296
Recombinant human BMP (rhBMP) 26, **27**
Reflex sympathetic dystrophy 269
Resuscitation and massive transfusion 313–315
    blood products 314
    complications of 315
    damage control resuscitation 313
    hypotensive resuscitation 314–315
    resuscitation fluids 313–314
Revised Trauma Score (RTS) 356
Ring fixators 31
Rolando fracture 157
Rugger jersey finger 173

S
Sacral sparing 334
Scaphoid fractures 153–155, 168–171 *see also* Carpal fractures
    avascular necrosis in 171
    Herbert classification 169, **170**
    nonunion 170
    plain radiographs 168, *169*
    treatment 170, *170*
Scapular fractures 324–325
SCIs *see* Spinal cord injuries (SCIs)
SCIWORA **335**
Screws 206–207
    cancellous 207
    cannulated 207
    cortical 207
    functions 207
    headless 207
    locking 207
    non-locking 207
    partially threaded 207
    self-tapping 206–207
    structural characteristics 206, *206*
    structure 206–207
    types 207
Segond fracture 218, *218*
Sepsis 64
    trauma and 65
Septic arthritis, in adults 319–320
Septic arthritis, in children 316–318
    antibiotics for 317–318
    causative organisms 316
    hip aspiration 317
    history 316
    Kocher's criteria 317
    radiographs in 317
Short Form 36 (SF-36) 359
Shoulder dislocations 321–323
    anterior 321
    classification 322
    initial management 322
    injuries associated with **321**
    luxatio erecta 321
    nonoperative management 322–323
    posterior 321
    Stanmore triangle of shoulder instability 322, *322*
    surgical management **323**
Simmond's test *see* Thompson's test
Simple Triage and Rapid Treatment (START) system 247, *247*, **248**
Single-positron emission photon computerised tomography 193
Skeletal surveys 297
Skin graft 327
Skull fractures 178
Smith's fracture 124
Smoking, and fracture healing 254
Soft tissue coverage in trauma 326–328
    British Orthopaedic Association Standard for Trauma 4 (BOAST 4) guidelines 326
    fix and flap operation 327
    Gustilo and Anderson classification 326
    postoperative care 328
    reconstructive goals 326
    reconstructive ladder 327
    soft tissue reconstruction, preparation for 327
    surgical management 326–328
Spinal cord decompression 334
Spinal cord injuries (SCIs) 333–335
    ASIA classification system **334**
    clinical assessment **333**, 333–334
    myotomes and corresponding motor function **333**
    patterns of **335**
    sacral sparing 334

Torg ratio and 333
traumatic, guidelines for 143–144
treatment 334
Spine
atlas and axis cervical fractures and dislocations 329–332
subaxial cervical fractures and dislocations 336–338
thoracic and lumbar fractures 339–342
Starches 313–314
Sternoclavicular (SC) joint 46
dislocation 46–47
Stiffness, after fractures 216
Stress fractures, of femoral neck 100
Strontium ranelate 264
Subaxial cervical fractures and dislocations 336–338
avulsion type teardrop fracture 336, *337*
bifacet dislocation 336, *336*
classification 337
clinical assessment 336–337
CT scan 337
MRI 337
plain radiography 337
treatment 337–338
Subdural haematoma 179, *179*
Subtalar dislocations 120–123
avascular necrosis in 123
classification 121, **121**
CT scan 121, *121*
Hawkins sign 123
lateral dislocations 121, 122
medial dislocations 121–122
open injuries 122
subtalar joint and 120, *120*
temporary Kirschner (K) wire fixation 122, *122*
treatment 121–122, *122*
Subtrochanteric fractures 92–95
95° angle device, use of 94, *95*
and infection 95
intramedullary nailing 94, *94*
nonunion 95
Russell–Taylor classification 93, **93**
Seinsheimer classification 93, **93**
treatment 93–94, *94, 95*
Subungal haematoma 251
drainage of *252*
Suction catheters 235
Supination–adduction (SAD) ankle fractures 12, **17**, 17–20
stages and injuries of 17, **18**, *18*
Supination–external rotation (SER) ankle fractures 12–15, **17**
stages and injuries of **12**, 12–13, *13*
Supracondylar fracture of distal humerus, displaced 144
Syndrome of inappropriate antidiuretic hormone (SIADH) 181

Systemic inflammatory response syndrome (SIRS) 64
definition **64**
trauma and 64, 65

T

Talar fractures 21–24
and avascular necrosis 24
classification 22, **23**
Hawkins sign 21, 23
radiographs *21*, 21–22, *22*
Talar tilt test 14
Talonavicular articulation 115
Tendon ruptures, in wrist and hand 172–175
anatomy related to 172
extensor zones of injury 172–173, *173*, 174–175, **175**
flexor zones of injury 173–174, *174*, 175
treatment 174–175, **175**
Teriparatide 264
Tetanus 211, **212**
Thermography 58
Thomas splints 89
Thompson's test 9
Thoracic and lumbar fractures 339–342
classification systems *340*, 340–341, **341**
clinical assessment 339
mechanisms and vectors of injury 339
nonoperative management 341
operative management 341–342, *342*
Thumb metacarpal fractures 157, 161
Thyroid shields 192
Tibial plateau fractures 347–350
and compartment syndrome 347, 350
malunion 350
nonoperative treatment 348
operative treatment 348–350
post-traumatic osteoarthritis 350
Schatzker classification 348, **348**, 349
split depression 349, *350*
Tscherne classification 348, **349**
Tibial shaft fractures 352–355
classification 353
clinical assessment 352–353
and compartment syndrome 354–355
and infection 354
malunion 355
and neurological injury 354
nonoperative treatment 353
nonunion 355
oblique fracture 352, *352*
operative treatment 353–354, *354, 355*
and vascular injury 354
Tibial tubercle fractures 223
Toddler's fracture 293
Total hip replacement (THR) 98–99, 103
Trabecular bone 261
Tranexamic acid 142, 303

Transfusion in adults and children, guidelines for 142–143
Transosseous fixation 223, *223*
Trapezium fractures 153, 154 *see also* Carpal fractures
Trauma 64–66 *see also* Major trauma
  and acute respiratory distress syndrome 64, 65
  and coagulation abnormalities 65
  damage control orthopaedics (DCO) principles 64–66
  mortality following 64
  and multiple organ distress syndrome 64, 65
  post-traumatic immunosuppression and sepsis 65
  resuscitation measures 65–66
  soft tissue coverage in 326–328
  and surgery 65
  and systemic inflammatory response syndrome 64, **64**, 65
  treatment process 65–66, *66*
Trauma and Injury Severity Score (TRISS) 358
Trauma Audit and Research Network (TARN) 240, 358
Trauma, guidelines in 142–146
  British Orthopaedic Association Standards for Trauma (BOAST) guidelines 142
  fracture clinic services 145–146
  National Institute for Care and Health Excellence (NICE) guidelines 142
  surgical treatment 142–145
Trauma scoring systems 356–358
  anatomical scoring systems 356–357, **357**
  combined systems 357–358
  examples of range of **357**
  physiological scoring systems 356
Traumatic brain injury 177 *see also* Head injury
Trauma tourniquet 235

Triage 362–365
  anatomical 363
  categories 362
  physiological 363
  sieve *363*, 363–364
  sort 364, **364**
Triangular fibrocartilage complex injury 127
Tricalcium phosphate 26, **27**
Triquetral fractures 153 *see also* Carpal fractures
Turf toe 118–119

U
UK trauma network *240*, 240–241
Ulnar nerve 182, *182*
Ulna styloid fracture 129
Ultrasound 193

V
Vascular endothelial growth factor (VEGF) 8
Vascularised grafts 25, **27**
Venous blood gas (VBG) 237
Vitamin D, for osteoporosis 263
Volar fasciotomy 55
Volkmann contracture 55, 182

W
Whiplash 366–367
  Quebec Task Force symptom grading 366, **367**
  treatment 366–367
Whitesides infusion technique 54
Wick-and-slit catheters 54
Wolff's law 34, 137

X
X-rays 192